Also by America's Test Kitchen

FOR A FULL LISTING OF ALL OUR BOOKS:

CooksIllustrated.com

AmericasTestKitchen.com

Praise for America's Test Kitchen Titles

Selected as the Cookbook Award Winner of 2021 in the Health and Nutrition category

INTERNATIONAL ASSOCIATION OF CULINARY PROFESSIONALS (IACP) ON *THE COMPLETE PLANT-BASED COOKBOOK*

"An exhaustive but approachable primer for those looking for a 'flexible' diet. Chock-full of tips, you can dive into the science of plant-based cooking or just sit back and enjoy the 500 recipes."

MINNEAPOLIS STAR TRIBUNE* ON *THE COMPLETE PLANT-BASED COOKBOOK

"In this latest offering from the fertile minds at America's Test Kitchen the recipes focus on savory baked goods. Pizzas, flatbreads, crackers, and stuffed breads all shine here . . . Introductory essays for each recipe give background information and tips for making things come out perfectly."

BOOKLIST* (STARRED REVIEW) ON *THE SAVORY BAKER

"A mood board for one's food board is served up in this excellent guide . . . This has instant classic written all over it."

PUBLISHERS WEEKLY* (STARRED REVIEW) ON *BOARDS: STYLISH SPREADS FOR CASUAL GATHERINGS

"Reassuringly hefty and comprehensive, *The Complete Autumn and Winter Cookbook* by America's Test Kitchen has you covered with a seemingly endless array of seasonal fare . . . This overstuffed compendium is guaranteed to warm you from the inside out."

NPR ON *THE COMPLETE AUTUMN AND WINTER COOKBOOK*

"Here are the words just about any vegan would be happy to read: 'Why This Recipe Works.' Fans of America's Test Kitchen are used to seeing the phrase, and now it applies to the growing collection of plant-based creations in *Vegan for Everybody*."

THE WASHINGTON POST* ON *VEGAN FOR EVERYBODY

"If you're one of the 30 million Americans with diabetes, *The Complete Diabetes Cookbook* by America's Test Kitchen belongs on your kitchen shelf."

PARADE.COM ON *THE COMPLETE DIABETES COOKBOOK*

"Another flawless entry in the America's Test Kitchen canon, *Bowls* guides readers of all culinary skill levels in composing one-bowl meals from a variety of cuisines."

BUZZFEED BOOKS ON *BOWLS*

Selected as the Cookbook Award Winner of 2021 in the Single Subject category

INTERNATIONAL ASSOCIATION OF CULINARY PROFESSIONALS (IACP) ON *FOOLPROOF FISH*

"The book's depth, breadth, and practicality makes it a must-have for seafood lovers."

PUBLISHERS WEEKLY* (STARRED REVIEW) ON *FOOLPROOF FISH

"*The Perfect Cookie* . . . is, in a word, perfect. This is an important and substantial cookbook . . . If you love cookies, but have been a tad shy to bake on your own, all your fears will be dissipated. This is one book you can use for years with magnificently happy results."

HUFFPOST ON *THE PERFECT COOKIE*

"The book offers an impressive education for curious cake makers, new and experienced alike. A summation of 25 years of cake making at ATK, there are cakes for every taste."

THE WALL STREET JOURNAL* ON *THE PERFECT CAKE

"The go-to gift book for newlyweds, small families, or empty nesters."

ORLANDO SENTINEL* ON *THE COMPLETE COOKING FOR TWO COOKBOOK

Selected as the Cookbook Award Winner of 2021 in the General category

INTERNATIONAL ASSOCIATION OF CULINARY PROFESSIONALS (IACP) ON *MEAT ILLUSTRATED*

"True to its name, this smart and endlessly enlightening cookbook is about as definitive as it's possible to get in the modern vegetarian realm."

MEN'S JOURNAL* ON *THE COMPLETE VEGETARIAN COOKBOOK

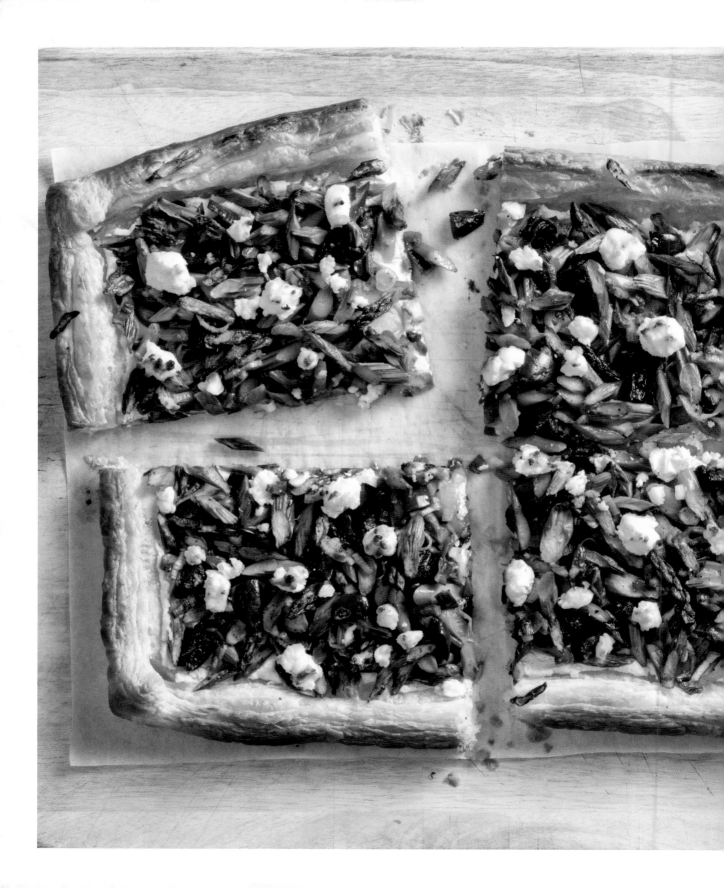

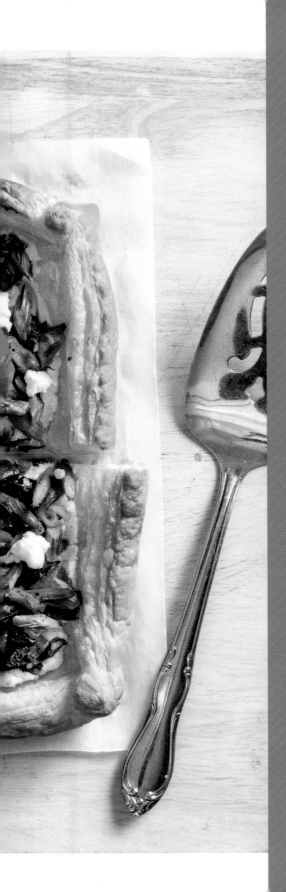

THE
Healthy
Back
Kitchen

Move Easier, Cook Simpler

How to Enjoy Great Food While Managing Back Pain

GRIFFIN R. BAUM, M.D.

AMERICA'S TEST KITCHEN

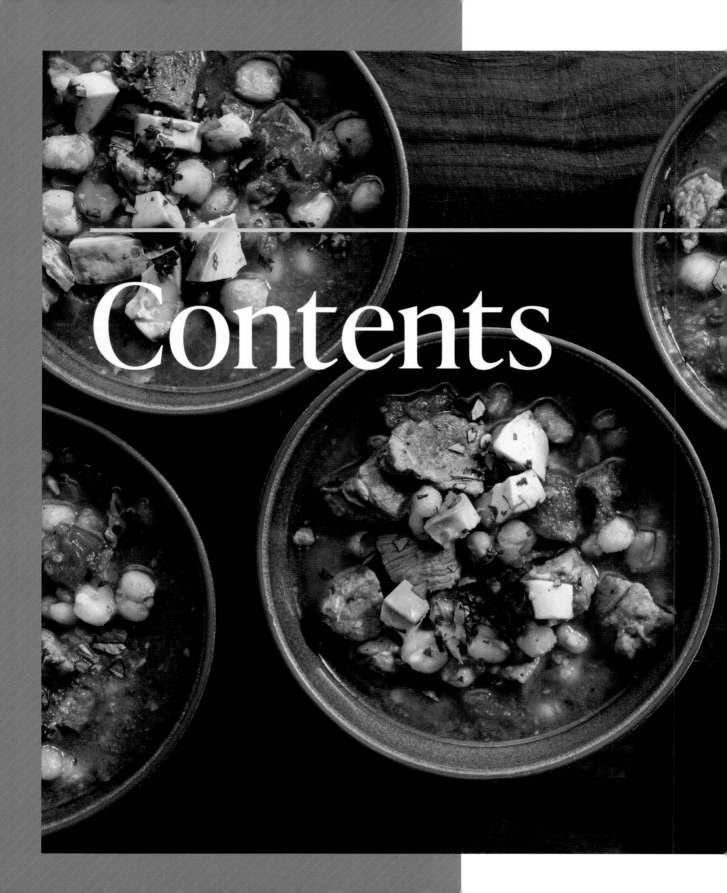

Contents

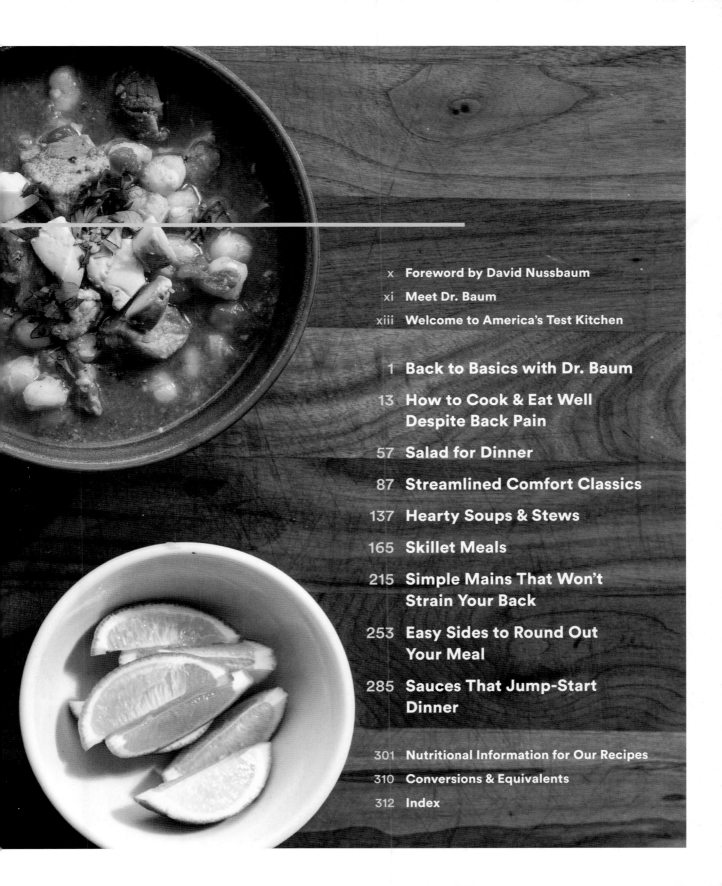

Library of Congress Cataloging-in-Publication Data

Names: Baum, Griffin R., author. | America's Test Kitchen (Firm), issuing body.
Title: The healthy back kitchen : move easier, cook simpler-how to enjoy great food while managing back pain : 120+ ergonomically designed recipes / Griffin R. Baum, M.D..
Description: Boston, MA : America's Test Kitchen, [2023] | Includes index.
Identifiers: LCCN 2023003059 (print) | LCCN 2023003060 (ebook) | ISBN 9781954210653 (paperback) | ISBN 9781954210660 (ebook)
Subjects: LCSH: Cooking. | Backache--Prevention. | LCGFT: Cookbooks.
Classification: LCC TX714 .B383 2023 (print) | LCC TX714 (ebook) | DDC 641.5--dc23/eng/20230127
LC record available at https://lccn.loc.gov/2023003059
LC ebook record available at https://lccn.loc.gov/2023003060

AMERICA'S TEST KITCHEN

AMERICA'S TEST KITCHEN
21 Drydock Avenue, Boston, MA 02210

Printed in Canada
10 9 8 7 6 5 4 3 2 1

Distributed by Penguin Random House Publisher Services
Tel: 800.733.3000

Pictured on front cover: **One-Pan Steak Fajitas (page 228)**

Pictured on back cover (from top to bottom):
Slow-Cooker Citrus-Braised Chicken Tacos (page 216), Skillet-Charred Green Beans (page 274), and Instant Pot Creamy Spring Vegetable Linguine (page 131)

FRONT COVER
Photography: **Joseph Keller**
Food Styling: **Catrine Kelty**

Author and Candid Photography: **Kevin White**

Editorial Director, Books: **Adam Kowit**

Executive Food Editor: **Dan Zuccarello**

Deputy Food Editors: **Leah Colins and Stephanie Pixley**

Executive Managing Editor: **Debra Hudak**

Project Editor: **Elizabeth Carduff**

Senior Editor: **Sara Mayer**

Test Cooks: **Olivia Counter, Hisham Hassam, and José Maldonado**

Design Director: **Lindsey Timko Chandler**

Deputy Art Director: **Katie Barranger**

Associate Art Director: **Kylie Alexander**

Photography Director: **Julie Bozzo Cote**

Senior Photography Producer: **Meredith Mulcahy**

Senior Staff Photographers: **Steve Klise and Daniel J. van Ackere**

Staff Photographer: **Kevin White**

Additional Photography: **Joseph Keller and Carl Tremblay**

Food Styling: **Joy Howard, Sheila Jarnes, Catrine Kelty, Chantal Lambeth, Gina McCreadie, Kendra McNight, Ashley Moore, Christie Morrison, Marie Piraino, Elle Simone Scott, Kendra Smith, and Sally Staub**

Illustrations: **Remie Geoffroi**

Project Manager, Publishing Operations: **Katie Kimmerer**

Senior Print Production Specialist: **Lauren Robbins**

Production and Imaging Coordinator: **Amanda Yong**

Production and Imaging Specialists: **Tricia Neumyer and Dennis Noble**

Copy Editor: **Deri Reed**

Proofreader: **Vicki Rowland**

Indexer: **Elizabeth Parson**

Chief Creative Officer: **Jack Bishop**

Executive Editorial Directors: **Julia Collin Davison and Bridget Lancaster**

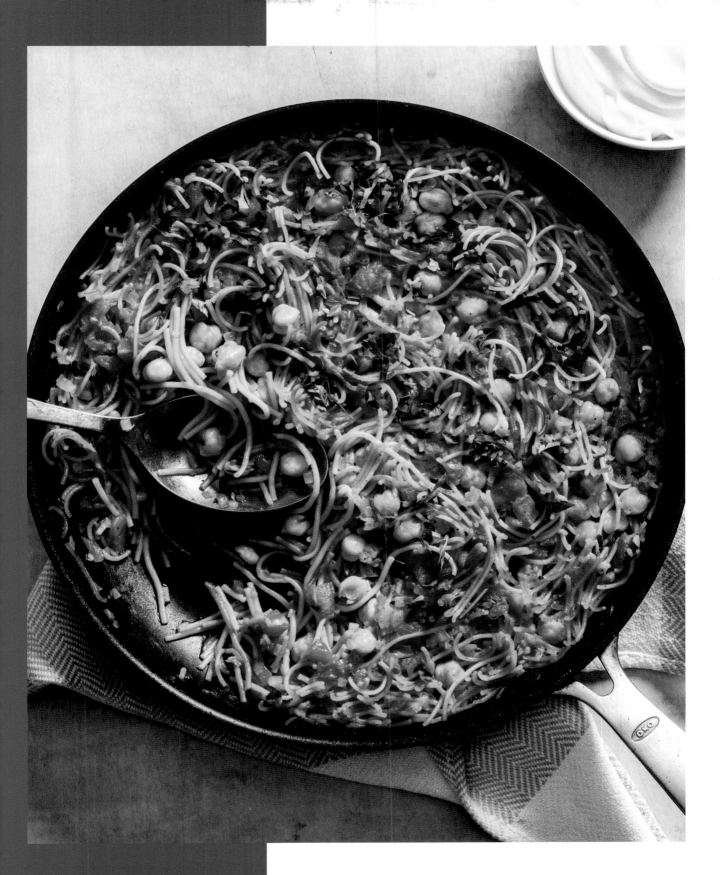

Foreword

It's rare that a book concept occurs to you when you are under pretty heavy sedation, in a fair amount of pain, recuperating from surgery. But that is exactly what happened with *The Healthy Back Kitchen*. Here's how I got to the operating table and beyond, and my final epiphany.

I have struggled with back pain for more than 20 years, and for the first 15 years of searing pain I staved off the worst of it by doing yoga, working with a private trainer, lifting weights, seeing a psychologist, and eating certain foods. However, after 20 years, there was nothing I could do to eliminate the pain. All options were exhausted.

If you have opened up this book, or downloaded a sample on your Kindle, you are someone who knows that back pain is debilitating and depressing. Every movement hurts. It is hard to travel. It's hard to carry a backpack. And it is hard to lift that backpack to the overhead compartment.

I tried back braces. I traveled with ice packs. I also traveled with heating pads. I took Advil, Tylenol, Aleve, prescription pain pills, and I drank special smoothies. I dieted. I lifted weights. Nothing helped at this stage.

So I turned to what should be the last resort. I had spine surgery. In fact, I had four spine surgeries over a period of eight years. And I used multiple surgeons at some of the best spine hospitals in NYC. But none worked until the fifth surgery, done by Dr. Baum. When I first met with Dr. Baum he impressed me because he discussed my total being: what I ate, how I moved around the kitchen when I cooked, and how I tried to compensate for the pain. He would then follow up the visit with a video restating everything we discussed so I could think about the entire journey. But we both knew that in addition to eating right and moving correctly around the apartment, I'd need surgery.

Dr. Baum specializes in revision surgery, which basically means undoing what was done by other surgeons; he starts from the beginning and focuses on the location of the pain. And within 90 days post surgery, I was pain free and moving better. As the days and weeks went by, I realized that my back felt like it did when I was 20 years old. (I wish the rest of my body felt that way, but alas, only my back does.)

It's now been two years since that surgery, and by getting the surgery done AND following Dr. Baum's strategies for cooking, moving, and standing in the kitchen, I am completely pain free. My back still feels like it did when I was 20 years old.

Dr. Baum is my spirit guide when it comes to back pain. I wish this book had existed before all of my surgeries; I would have tried everything in it first. But regardless of where you are on your back journey (those of us long-term sufferers of back pain know that it is a journey), this book should help you. Dr. Baum's exercises, which you can do during breaks in the recipes, will help you keep your back strong. And his guidelines for setting up an ergonomic kitchen, along with America's Test Kitchen's equipment recommendations, will set you up for a more manageable cooking experience. Not to mention the fantastic and back-friendly recipes that will give you the confidence to cook great meals again.

I hope you enjoy the book as much as I enjoyed working with Dr. Baum.

David Nussbaum
FORMER CEO AND CHAIRMAN OF THE BOARD, AMERICA'S TEST KITCHEN

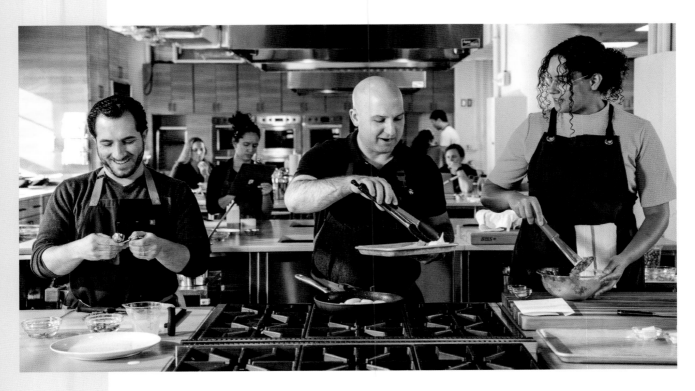

Meet Dr. Baum

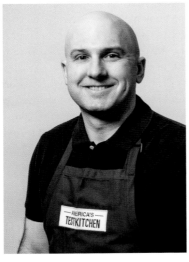

Griffin R. Baum, M.D., is a fellowship-trained, board-certified spine surgeon and Assistant Professor of Neurosurgery at the Donald and Barbara Zucker School of Medicine at Hofstra/Northwell. He treats pediatric and adult patients with scoliosis and spinal disorders at Lenox Hill Hospital located on the Upper East Side of Manhattan. Dr. Baum specializes in pediatric and adult scoliosis surgery as well as complex and revision spine surgery of the cervical, thoracic, and lumbar spine. Having trained at Columbia University Medical Center for his Orthopaedic Spine Surgery fellowship, Dr. Baum has advanced expertise in neurosurgical and orthopaedic spine surgery and has distinguished himself as a leading spine surgeon in New York City. In addition to his clinical and research efforts, Dr. Baum is a passionate teacher and educator and serves as Associate Residency Program Director for the Neurosurgery Residency Training Program at the Donald and Barbara Zucker School of Medicine at Hofstra/Northwell. In 2022, he was named Residency Teacher of the Year by the Neurosurgery Residents at the Zucker School of Medicine, the award that he is most proud of in his career. Dr. Baum lives in New York City with his wife, Sarah, and daughter, Frances, and spends all his free time cooking. He has been a passionate cook since his teens and loves to test the limits of what he can do in the kitchen.

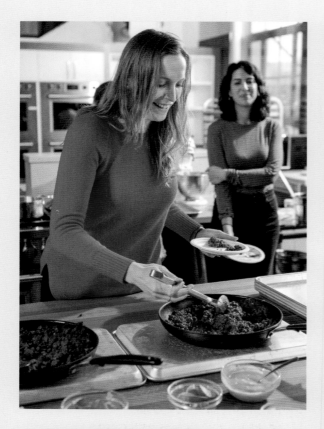

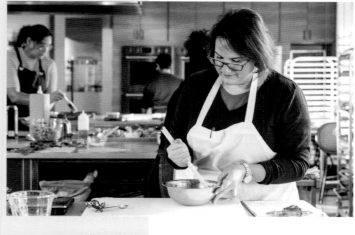

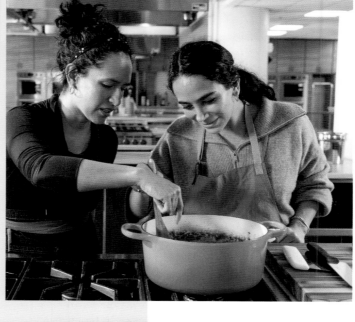

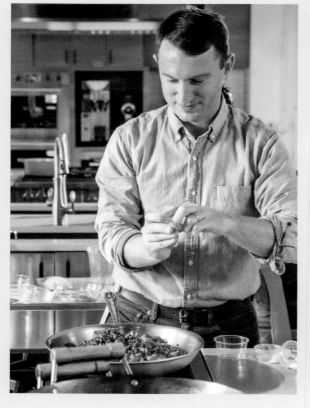

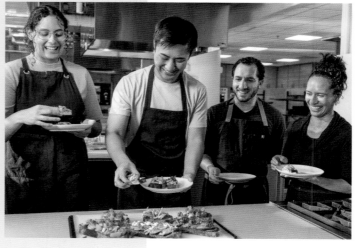

Welcome to America's Test Kitchen

This book has been tested and edited by the folks at America's Test Kitchen, where curious cooks become confident cooks. Located in Boston's Seaport District in the historic Innovation and Design Building, it features 15,000 square feet of kitchen space including multiple photography and video studios. It is the home of *Cook's Illustrated* magazine and *Cook's Country* magazine and is the workday destination for more than 60 test cooks, editors, and cookware specialists. Our mission is to empower and inspire confidence, community, and creativity in the kitchen.

We start the process of testing a recipe with a complete lack of preconceptions, which means that we accept no claim, no technique, and no recipe at face value. We simply assemble as many variations as possible, test a half-dozen of the most promising, and taste the results blind. We then construct our own recipe and continue to test it, varying ingredients, techniques, and cooking times until we reach a consensus. As we like to say in the test kitchen, "We make the mistakes so you don't have to." The result, we hope, is the best version of a particular recipe, but we realize that only you can be the final judge of our success (or failure). We use the same rigorous approach when we test equipment and taste ingredients.

All of this would not be possible without a belief that good cooking, much like good music, is based on a foundation of objective technique. Some people like spicy foods and others don't, but there is a right way to sauté, there is a best way to cook a pot roast, and there are measurable scientific principles involved in producing perfectly beaten, stable egg whites. Our ultimate goal is to investigate the fundamental principles of cooking to give you the techniques, tools, and ingredients you need to become a better cook. It is as simple as that.

To see what goes on behind the scenes at America's Test Kitchen, check out our social media channels for kitchen snapshots, exclusive content, video tips, and much more.

You can watch us work (in our actual test kitchen) by tuning in to *America's Test Kitchen* or *Cook's Country* on public television or on our websites. Listen to *Proof*, *Mystery Recipe*, and *The Walk-In* (AmericasTestKitchen.com/podcasts) to hear engaging, complex stories about people and food. Want to hone your cooking skills or finally learn how to bake—with an America's Test Kitchen test cook? Enroll in one of our online cooking classes. And you can engage the next generation of home cooks with kid-tested recipes from America's Test Kitchen Kids.

However you choose to visit us, we welcome you into our kitchen, where you can stand by our side as we test our way to the best recipes in America.

- facebook.com/AmericasTestKitchen
- instagram.com/TestKitchen
- youtube.com/AmericasTestKitchen
- tiktok.com/@TestKitchen
- twitter.com/TestKitchen
- pinterest.com/TestKitchen

AmericasTestKitchen.com
CooksIllustrated.com
CooksCountry.com
OnlineCookingSchool.com
AmericasTestKitchen.com/kids

JOIN OUR COMMUNITY OF RECIPE TESTERS
Our recipe testers provide valuable feedback on recipes under development by ensuring that they are foolproof in home kitchens. Help the America's Test Kitchen book team investigate the how and why behind successful recipes from your home kitchen.

Back to Basics

with Dr. Baum

The Anatomy of the Back

Understanding the anatomy of the back, which includes the spine (the defining and most complicated structure of the back) and the organs that surround it, will give insight into the many causes of back pain. In addition to injuries to the spine or degeneration of its parts due to aging or arthritis, it is important to note that back pain can emanate from the major blood vessels, the gastrointestinal tract, or the kidneys—places you would not expect to be the source of such pain. As a neurosurgeon, my focus is on diagnosing the cause of back pain and determining whether a surgical solution has the best chance of relieving pain and improving quality of life. Here are the anatomical structures that can contribute to back pain.

THE VERTEBRAE
The Bones of the Spine

It is fitting that we are reviewing the bones of the spine in a cookbook because in medical school doctors are taught to remember the number of bones as being the same as the typical time of day for breakfast, lunch, and dinner: There are **seven** cervical vertebrae in the neck (breakfast at 7 a.m.); **twelve** thoracic vertebrae in the mid back (lunch at noon), which all have ribs attached to them; and **five** lumbar vertebrae in the low back (dinner at 5 p.m.). Lastly, the tailbone is made up of the sacrum, which has five segments that are all fused into a single bone, and the coccyx, which is the very last segment of the spine. Each vertebra connects to the bone above and below with a pair of joints on each side of the spine. This results in a total of 52 joints in the spine, all of which have anywhere from 1 to 45 degrees of motion. When you compare this with the other joints in the body like the hip, knee, or elbow, you can see why it is so much harder to diagnose and treat back pain than other types of musculoskeletal pain.

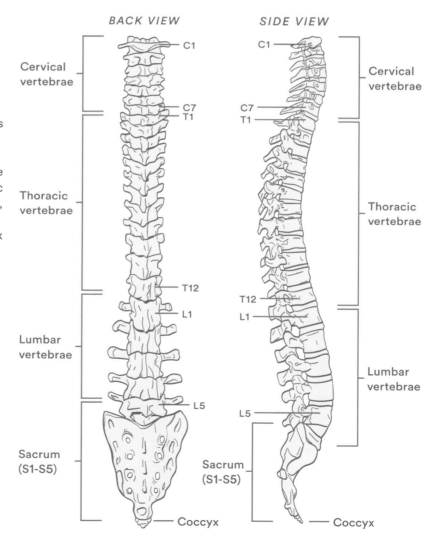

BACK VIEW   SIDE VIEW

Cervical vertebrae — C1
C7
T1

Thoracic vertebrae

T12
L1

Lumbar vertebrae

L5

Sacrum (S1-S5)

Coccyx

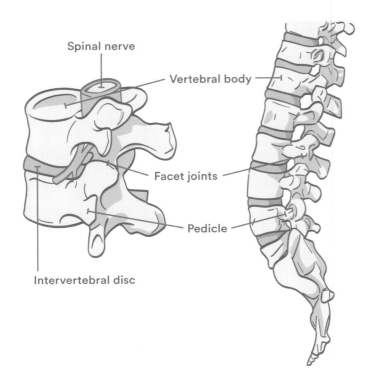

Spinal nerve

Vertebral body

Facet joints

Pedicle

Intervertebral disc

THE SPINAL NERVES
The Signal Cables of the Spine

Each spinal segment, consisting of a pair of vertebrae and a single intervertebral disc, forms a neural foramen, the opening between every two vertebrae, which allows for the passage of a single spinal nerve on each side of the spine. Without it, nerve signals could not travel to the brain and beyond, and your body could not function. This nerve is always named for the bone it passes below (i.e., the L4 nerve travels between L4 and L5). The proximity of this nerve to the intervertebral disc opens up the opportunity for a disc herniation or joint arthritis to cause mechanical compression of this spinal nerve, which can result in irritation from inflammation caused by these phenomena. This explains why medications like non-steroidal anti-inflammatories (NSAIDs) such as naproxen or ibuprofen can be so effective at treating this kind of pain.

THE INTERVERTEBRAL DISCS
The Shock Absorbers of the Spine

In between each pair of vertebrae there is a structure made up of two types of tissue, which act as shock absorbers. Spine surgeons commonly describe the intervertebral disc as a jelly donut—with an outer layer called the annulus fibrosus and a soft, spongy inner layer called the nucleus pulposus. When the intervertebral discs degenerate and begin to lose their squishiness, pieces of the nucleus pulposus can herniate through the annulus fibrosus and cause back pain, nerve pain, or inflammation. (It is no wonder that the intervertebral discs can degenerate, as they withstand up to seven times a person's body weight with every step they take every day of their life.) In cases where surgical removal is required, the fragments look and feel exactly like the imitation crabmeat in a sushi roll. It is hard to believe just how large these fragments can be and how much pain they can cause.

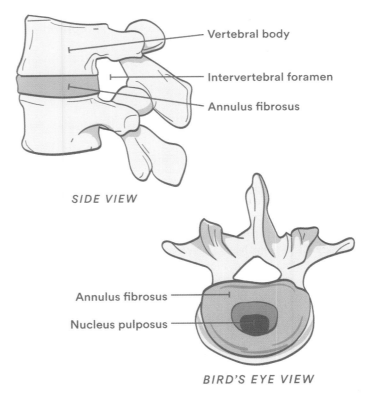

Vertebral body

Intervertebral foramen

Annulus fibrosus

SIDE VIEW

Annulus fibrosus

Nucleus pulposus

BIRD'S EYE VIEW

The Etiology of Back Pain

Back pain is real pain, as anyone who has ever suffered from even a temporary pain episode knows all too well. The most common cause of back pain is arthritis in any one of the 52 joints in the spine, which can cause inflammation and irritation of the spinal nerves. In extreme cases, this arthritis can cause compression of the nerves, which can cause numbness, tingling, or even weakness in addition to pain. This same syndrome can be caused by the degeneration and herniation of the intervertebral discs and can result in either back pain, leg symptoms, or both.

In cases where patients lose bone density due to osteoporosis or other metabolic conditions, the bones can become compressed or even fracture spontaneously. In addition to these most common causes originating from the bones and the discs, there are other causes of pain including strains or sprains in the muscles, ligaments, and tendons that wrap the spine and stabilize our bodies, which allows us to stand upright. These are especially common after accidents or traumas, such as a fall.

If you are suffering from new or different pain, be sure to talk to your doctor, as it may be time for new x-rays or an MRI to see if there has been a change that is causing your worsening symptoms. All pain has to have a cause. Remember—all pain is nerve pain. For the body to perceive pain, it has to travel to the brain where it is processed, and only then does the body become aware of it.

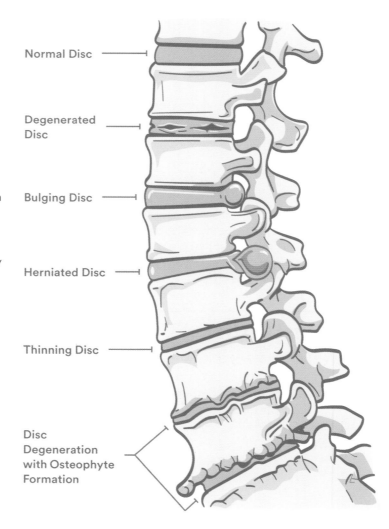

Normal Disc

Degenerated Disc

Bulging Disc

Herniated Disc

Thinning Disc

Disc Degeneration with Osteophyte Formation

When to Seek Help

Leg symptoms

Any symptoms that move from the back and down the legs into the feet can be a sign of something more serious than arthritis and should be evaluated right away.

Sensory changes

Numbness or burning-type symptoms can indicate nerve irritation and compression and if untreated can become permanent.

Weakness

Trouble standing or walking because of a weak foot (or drop foot) can be a sign of serious nerve dysfunction and can become permanent within a few months; don't delay getting this looked at ASAP.

Falls

There can be many causes of falls, from brain and inner ear problems to spinal cord or spinal nerve issues. All are disabling, and any fall is abnormal and must be addressed with your doctor.

Bowel, bladder, or sexual dysfunction

These issues are never normal and need immediate attention, as they can have a serious cause and are often irreversible if not addressed.

Symptoms persist despite treatment

If you feel as if you should be getting better but you're not, it may mean that something else is going on and you need to be re-evaluated.

Answers or a plan are needed

Pain is isolating, and suffering often happens in silence. Don't let things get out of control; sometimes just taking the first step toward relief can lead to an improvement in symptoms.

Back Pain Management Strategies

The first question when faced with pain is usually "what the heck is that?" The second question should be "is this normal, or is this dangerous?" There is a huge difference between normal pain, which can occur after exercise, a new activity, travel, or even a stressful day, and abnormal pain, which generally is accompanied by red flags. These red flags can include numbness, tingling, weakness, or persistent symptoms that last several days without relief from medication. If you are experiencing these symptoms, it is time to get help. Regardless of the source of your pain, here are some strategies to relieve pain.

MEDICATION

The first line of defense against routine back pain can be over-the-counter medications such as acetaminophen, ibuprofen, and naproxen. However, there is new data that demonstrate that patients can worsen their pain by taking medication every day. If you find yourself turning to medication as a way to get through the day, it may be time to talk to your doctor about finding the cause of the pain. Prescription medication can help as well, but only for short periods of time; medications used long-term can lose their effectiveness quickly as your body builds tolerance to them.

MINDFULNESS

The practice of mindfulness, similar to meditation, is the ability to be fully engaged in the present moment. It is all too easy to race through life, but adopting the practice of mindfulness has many benefits, and it can be a fantastic technique to help manage and control pain while building a connection with the activity at hand. I recommend mindfulness to all of my patients, and I find that I am able to use these skills myself both in the kitchen as well as in the operating room. Musicians, professional athletes, and artists describe "being in the zone," which is a state of flow facilitated by mindfulness. In the operating room, we use the "mindful moment" as a way to slow our thoughts and actions and allow for connection to the patient and our present moment.

Need to get mindful fast? Try this: Close your eyes, and take three long, slow, deep breaths. Focus on the depth of each breath, and exhale out all of your mind's racing thoughts. Open your eyes, say to yourself what you're thankful for in that moment, and proceed with the task at hand.

MOVEMENT AND EXERCISE

The pain-relieving benefits of aerobic exercise, not to mention its overall cardiovascular and pulmonary health benefits, make it a must for anyone suffering from back pain. Regardless of how, one must stay active to reduce pain. Simple things like parking farther away to boost walking or taking the stairs instead of the elevator can make a difference; in short, it is important to find small ways to recapture opportunities for movement throughout your day. For example, set an alarm to get up and stretch once an hour; or allow yourself to watch TV only if you are engaged in another activity like prep work in the kitchen; anything that gets you up and moving.

ACTIVITY MODIFICATION

If you have pain, there are things you may not be able to do anymore. Like using a step stool in the kitchen to reach a heavy pot or appliance. Or even just standing and cooking for a long period of time. Heavy lifting, reaching under things, and awkward postures are all triggers to avoid. Of course, you should do what you have to do to stay active and avoid unnecessary pain. But as we all age there will be things we simply can't do anymore. When was the last time you climbed a tree? Jumped off the high dive? Rode a roller coaster? Ran five miles? And remember that just because you don't do a certain thing anymore doesn't mean it's a bad thing—it's just because you are in a different phase in life. There are plenty of activities that won't stress your back or your body. Try chair yoga or just commit to a walk around your neighborhood every day.

"*You are not alone.*
Back pain is the #1 reason people see the doctor in the United States."

LIFESTYLE MODIFICATIONS (AND MORE)

If you have back pain, there may be things you need to reconsider. For instance, a job that requires physical labor you can't manage anymore. Or a living situation that is no longer tenable because of stairs or other hurdles. Even your kitchen may be an issue because of the arrangement of drawers or cabinets that are suddenly hard to access and reaching them triggers pain. Accept your limitations and adapt to them. Making changes isn't something to be sad about, it's an opportunity to take stock of what you need to do to make improvements. On the other hand, sometimes small lifestyle changes can have a big impact. Ask your doctor if a trial of physical therapy would be helpful. Even a few sessions focusing on core strengthening, balance, and correcting maladaptive posture can result in substantial pain relief. Engaging in a routine of simple stretches and exercises like the ones in this section can also be beneficial. Lastly, try massage therapy! Sore muscles and tight tendons can wreak havoc on your back, and many times a massage and some relaxation can be just as effective as medication.

Stretches and Exercises to Manage and Reduce Back Pain

In the Kitchen and Beyond

Avoiding all activity is not a good strategy when it comes to managing and reducing back pain. Often, correcting postural imbalances and strengthening your core muscles can help you both move better and reduce pain at the same time. These stretches and strengthening exercises can be done whenever you have an extra few minutes. And because many of the recipes in this book have designated walkaway breaks, think of the breaks as a good time to get in some high-yield stretches and exercises. If you have trouble getting down on the floor, you can do all the exercises on your bed.

KNEE TO CHEST STRETCH

This is one of my favorite stretches dating back to my days as a baseball player in college. Imagine your back being the skyscraper, and your legs are the bedrock that stabilizes the back. Tight hamstrings and hip flexors are the target of this stretch, and can be done either standing, seated, or lying on the ground. I was always taught that a stretch must last at least 30 seconds; try three to four reps for maximal effect.

CROSSED LEG GLUTEUS STRETCH

Similar to the last stretch, this one has always brought me the most relief of all of the stretches and exercises that I recommend. This one targets the gluteal and piriformis muscles, and it also provides some relief of occasional sacroiliac joint tightness. A great way to get the most out of this exercise is to do 30-second stretches paired with slow, controlled breathing. Shoot for three to four reps if possible.

SEATED ROTATION STRETCH

For minor pains and to work the low back stabilizing muscles (the multifidus and the longissimus), there is no better stretch. If you feel pain, stop and try again on another day. Severe or sharp pain is never normal, and this stretch should feel good as it releases tension in the stabilizers on either side of the spine. Positioning your opposite arm on your thigh and pressing gently will give you leverage to twist further.

CHILD'S POSE YOGA STRETCH

I recommend yoga to all of my patients, and this pose is one of my favorite recovery exercises after a long, grueling case in the OR. Known as child's pose, it is a great whole spine stretch and serves as a wonderful introduction to the basic yoga poses that every person, not just those with back pain, will enjoy. You may want to set a timer so that you don't do this for too long, as you can get a great comfy stretch and forget all about the delicious meal you're in the middle of cooking.

CAT-COW POSE YOGA STRETCH

This motion is great for strengthening not only the stabilizing muscles and the core abdominal muscles but also ensures working out any flexibility restrictions in the low back that might be contributing to pain. Start on your hands and knees, with knees under your hips and hands in line with your shoulders. Round your spine up, tuck your chin into your chest, and let your neck drop (cat pose). Arch your back and lift your head to the ceiling (cow pose). Try 12 to 15 cycles of cat and cow in each set, with two to three sets total, if possible.

SUPERMAN STRETCH

Balance is incredibly important in the musculoskeletal system, and the back is no different. By extending an opposite arm and leg at the same time while on your hands and knees, this exercise focuses on strengthening core muscles as well as the stabilizing muscles in the low back and the pelvis. Break these up in sets, with 12 reps of each pair of opposite arms and legs in each set, with four sets total.

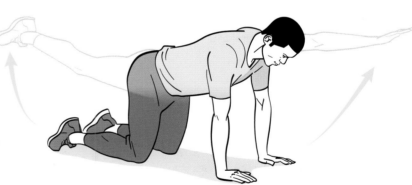

FOREARM PLANKS

Planks engage and strengthen all of the core muscles that are so crucial for back health and relief of back pain. Place elbows directly under your shoulders. Tuck your toes under; keep legs straight and your head in line with your back. Focus on your core, keep your abdominal muscles tight, and actively draw your navel into your spine. This is by far the hardest exercise in our list, but start small with 15-second sets and try to work up to a minute or more. You will work new muscles you didn't even know you had, and in turn, your back will thank you.

Ten Principles for Living Your Best Life

 1 *Acknowledge that your pain is real.*

Pain is not just in your head, and it's not your fault. Everyone has pain at some point in their life whether they admit it or not.

 2 *Control what is controllable and let go of the rest.*

There are certain things that you can control and affect, and other things that you have no power over. Don't waste time feeling badly about the things that are out of your control.

 3 *Build your medical team (and more).*

Once you know you need help overcoming back pain or simply living your best life while dealing with it, rely on your doctors, therapists, friends, and other allies. The team is there to sustain you, and it is a crucial support system. You can't be your own doctor, nurse, or therapist. Rely on the experts and follow their advice.

 4 *Establish a routine.*

Find a schedule or a rhythm that works for your daily life and stick with it. You'll be better able to handle the stresses life throws at you, especially when you have a bad day because of pain.

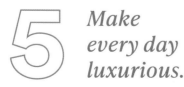 **5** *Make every day luxurious.*

Use the things you do every day as opportunities to treat yourself: A cup of good coffee. A special ingredient. A decadent dessert. Something special to mark a small achievement. These seemingly little things can boost your dopamine and serotonin levels and can literally make you happier and lessen your pain.

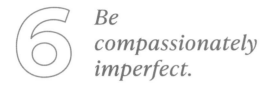 **Be compassionately imperfect.**

If you can't treat yourself with respect and compassion how can you be expected to treat others that way? Pay yourself first, whether with a compliment, a treat, love, understanding, or empathy. Imagine how you feel about your spouse or child, and find ways to show yourself the same empathy and understanding. Take care of yourself, it's the only body you have.

 Be resilient.

It's OK to bend, but you can't break. It's not an option. Keep doing the things you love, like cooking for family and friends, and make adjustments along the way to make it possible. Life isn't a sprint to the finish. Enjoy the process. Take your time, with breaks if you need them, and find ways to persevere even on your hardest days.

 Give and receive.

Gratitude and thankfulness are the keys to happiness. Love languages come in all different forms. Something as simple as making a meal for someone can show you the power of your gifts and allow you to open up to receive gifts that others are able to give you.

 Engage in things that make you happy.

Comparison is the thief of joy. Do things because they excite you or because you want to, not because someone else is doing it or it will make a great social media post.

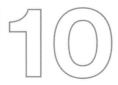 **Stay active.**

A body in motion stays in motion (one of Newton's Laws). Keep moving, and keep cooking! Your life depends on it!

How to Cook & Eat Well

Despite Back Pain

Reboot Your Cooking Life

When you suffer from back pain, cooking can be especially difficult, as it requires all sorts of movements—bending, reaching up and down, lifting, even twisting your torso—just to get prep work done and a meal in the oven, skillet, or saucepan. Perhaps the worst aspect of cooking for those with back pain is all the standing normally required. It's hard on every part of your spine, as well as other joints, such as your knees and your hips. In this book, we provide you with recipes designed to make prep work and the cooking process easier, with breaks strategically built into the recipes, prep-ahead strategies so that you can spread out the work, ideas for using pre-prepped ingredients, and even radically simplified tips for things like cutting up broccoli, chopping tomatoes, and more.

And our suggestions go beyond the cooking process to rethinking how you interact with your kitchen itself and everything in it. How is it organized? What could be better with a few small changes? We look at every important piece of cooking equipment through this lens and tell you which ones will be your allies and which ones you need to replace, and why. With the information in this section, you will learn how to set up an optimized workstation, why you need a rolling cart, why a utility knife is the one you need to buy if you don't have one, hacks for making prep easier with kitchen shears, and much more.

Embrace the Spirit of Mise en Place

Mise en place is a philosophy from the French that I find especially relevant and powerful for those with back pain who want to cook. It means "to put in its place" and refers to the process of gathering and prepping all ingredients for a recipe before starting the cooking process, and also to the philosophy of discipline and organization in the kitchen to enable the most efficient cooking process possible. The end result of this practice is that you will get more mileage out of your time in the kitchen with less standing, bending, and reaching required and fewer chances that you will hurt yourself.

In the spirit of both mise en place and my Ten Principles for Living Your Best Life (page 10), I want to encourage you to run a reboot of your kitchen and your cooking game. I want you to get shopping and embrace cooking for family and friends, because interacting with the outside world and your special people will lift your spirits immeasurably and allow you to persevere and take pleasure in every cooking achievement.

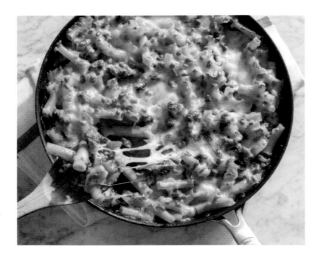

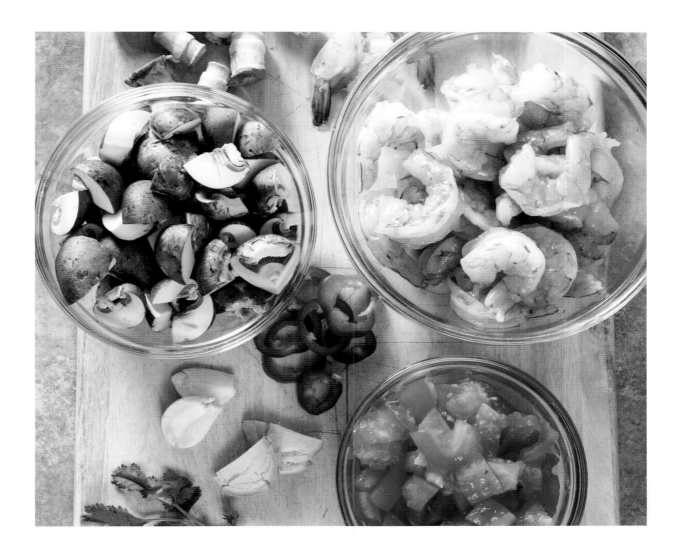

FIVE WAYS TO MISE EN PLACE YOUR COOKING LIFE

1. Gather the recipes you plan to make for the coming week and then review your pantry and make a shopping list for the store and farmers' market.

2. Store and organize ingredients, tools, and supplies in such a way that makes them easy to find when you start prepping your next meal.

3. Before cooking, collect all your knives, tools, ingredients, and spices on your rolling cart and around your workstation before starting to chop, dice, and prep.

4. Before moving from the prep to the cooking phase, use lightweight ingredient trays, cups, and bowls to store prepped ingredients prior to turning on the oven, stove, or countertop cooking appliance. If pain is slowing you down, this is a great time to take a break, do some exercises, take a mindful moment, or put your feet up on the sofa and relax for a few before regrouping.

5. As soon as you've gotten the cooking started, take advantage of any unattended cooking times to rest or take a break so that you can enjoy the meal and relax with minimal cleanup when all is said and done.

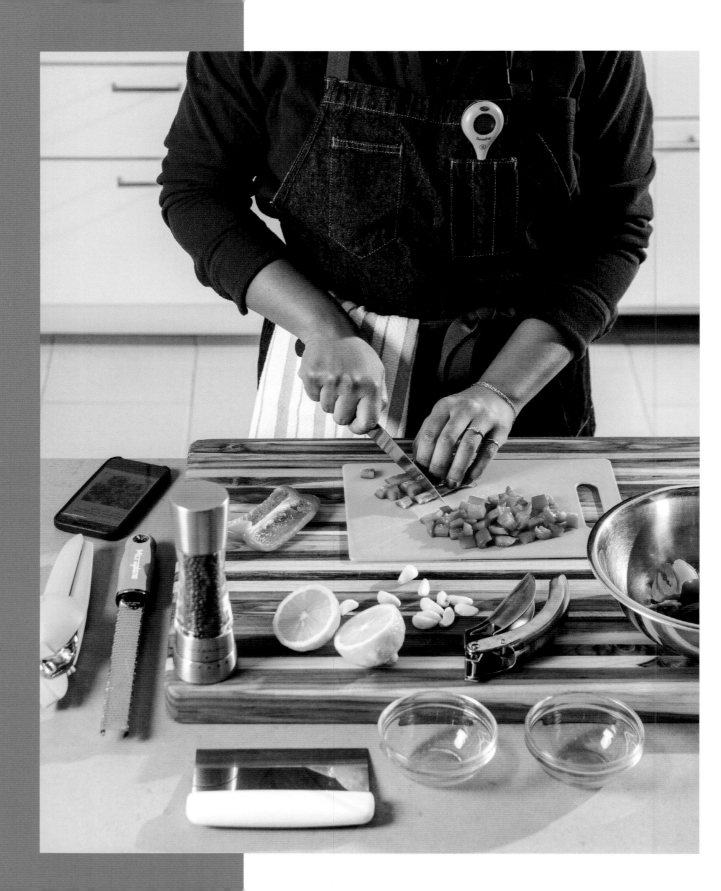

The Ergonomic Kitchen

You can have the simplest recipe in the world, but if you aren't equipped with the right tools, and your kitchen isn't well organized, cooking will be harder and will put unnecessary strain on your back and tax your energy. By contrast, creating an ergonomic kitchen, one that's set up for comfort and efficiency, will help you cook using far less time and effort—and it doesn't require a major redesign. In this section of the book, we will be asking you to think hard about your kitchen and everything in it.

As a first step, stand in your kitchen and look around. Are your counters too high or too low as they relate to your height? You cannot suddenly change your counter height, but there *are* ways to get around this if it is an issue. Small changes like the ones that follow can make a big difference and will help ensure you are more comfortable when prepping and help keep your posture in a position that won't strain your back. There are many other things to consider too. Are your pots and pans buried in cabinets and hard to reach without hurting your back? Do your cutting boards and prep bowls suddenly feel too heavy? Do you have a designated workstation set up for efficiency? We will examine all this and more and provide suggestions you can implement now, no contractor required.

The goal is to get you cooking again and cooking with pleasure—without the fear of hurting your back. An ergonomically organized kitchen is a great asset to your back health because it will help you avoid reaching and bending in ways that strain your back, minimize walking around your kitchen needlessly, and perhaps most important, help you prep faster and more efficiently with less time spent on your feet. The ergonomic kitchen starts with a workstation, but also encompasses you—your shoes, your apron, where you stand or sit, and how you prep and cook.

SET UP AN OPTIMIZED WORKSTATION

Identifying the best and most efficient place in your kitchen for prep work is the first step in making the most of your space. Much like a hospital operating room is organized to maximize efficiency and safety in the surgical field, your kitchen tools and supplies should orbit this spot as if it has a gravitational force field.

But the first thing you need to do is assess your physical relationship to the space. The relationship of your counter to your size will determine your posture when prepping. And your posture has a big effect on your back strain over time. If you have to hunch over while prepping, instead of your spine being in balance, your paraspinal muscles (the multifidius and the longissimus especially) will be working overtime, and you may have 15 minutes tops before muscle spasms and painful fatigue set in. (See page 21 for more on proper posture.) But there are simple ways around this issue. What follows are a few options to consider when setting up a workstation. While not everyone will want to invest in a big board or will even want a board that stays on the counter, the point is to have a workstation. Here you can set up the tools you need for any given recipe, a supply of dish towels, your compost bin if you use one, and more. This way you won't need to spend time while you are in the process of cooking to walk around your kitchen looking for your rasp grater or some other tool.

ESTABLISH A PERMANENT WORKSTATION

One practical (and beautiful) way to mark your workstation is to invest in a big, gorgeous cutting board. One of our favorites is the **Teakhaus Edge Grain Cutting Board (XL)**, which is 18 by 24 by 1½ inches. This thick board allows you not only to anchor your workstation, but it also raises it, which will keep you from bending over as much when prepping ingredients (if that is the case for you), or allow you to work from a padded bar stool (more to come on this). There are many boards that are even thicker, so if you are tall, one of them may be a good option. These boards are heavy (the Teakhaus board weighs 15 pounds) and should stay on your counter and serve as your main cutting board. You can simply wipe it clean after each use with a warm sponge. Make sure to position your board ergonomically.

FLEXIBLE CUTTING MATS

When you are cutting messy ingredients or meats or other items where you want to prevent cross-contamination, we recommend using a flexible cutting board on top of your large board, ensuring that the board underneath stays pristine. Made from dishwasher-safe plastic, they can be easily tucked into the dishwasher after use—a convenience that we especially appreciate when working with messy raw proteins. And these flexible cutting mats have their place elsewhere in the ergonomic kitchen even if you are not using a large board. They're generally flexible enough to roll up like a newspaper and funnel ingredients directly into a skillet or bowl. We love the **Dexas Heavy Duty Grippmats** (set of four), as they are the perfect size: large enough to fit a significant amount of food but not so big as to make cleaning and handling a pain. They also strike the right balance between strength and flexibility, and they're textured on both sides for better stability.

BUY A STANDARD BUT LIGHTWEIGHT CUTTING BOARD

Everyone needs a stable cutting board (or two) even if you also have a large stationary wooden board. Weighing just over 3 pounds, our favorite lightweight board is the **OXO Good Grips Carving and Cutting Board**, which is especially easy to lift and maneuver. Make sure you position it ergonomically on your counter: It needs to be far enough away from the edge so that you can get enough strength and leverage through your arms to your hands to power a knife properly, but not so far that it feels awkward. If it is too close, you will end up moving more of your body than is necessary.

ARRANGE YOUR CUTTING BOARD ERGONOMICALLY

This is somewhat size dependent, but in general placing your cutting board 4 to 5 inches from the counter edge should work well. You should not be reaching; try keeping your back straight and your arms at 45 to 90 degree angles to find the best distance for your body.

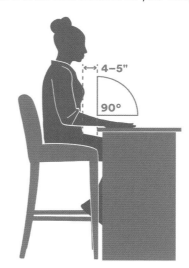

PUT A CONTAINER FOR PREP SCRAPS NEAR YOUR WORKSTATION

If you have to walk to the trash can or compost container every time you have a pile of onion skins, herb stems, bits of trimmed chicken skin, and any other prep remnants, you are just wasting time. You will be surprised how much you can gather up and put in a simple canister or plastic bowl while you are getting a recipe ready to cook. Remember, saving time saves energy.

ADD A TALL BAR STOOL FOR SEATED PREP WORK

If you have a kitchen island with an overhang, it is a great place to put a bar stool. But that said, you can put a stool in just about any kitchen next to the counter where you plan to do most of your prep work. Buy one with a back (and rungs for resting your feet) and keep it near your prep station so that you can prep sitting down at counter height when possible. There are many options when it comes to these stools, including those that swivel and those that are stationary. Some are padded and some are not. There is no one-size-fits-all solution here, but most kitchen islands (and counters) are around 36 inches high (though some are as high as 42 inches), so you want a stool where the seat fits under that (assuming an open counter or island) or aligns with your counter height, which means a floor-to-seat height of about 23 inches (or more). Seat backs come in various heights, so choose one that is comfortable. Measure carefully in order to choose a bar stool that is neither too low nor too high. Rungs that are 8 inches from the floor will be good for resting your feet and will relieve pressure on your back. For more options on the benefits of prepping while sitting, see page 29.

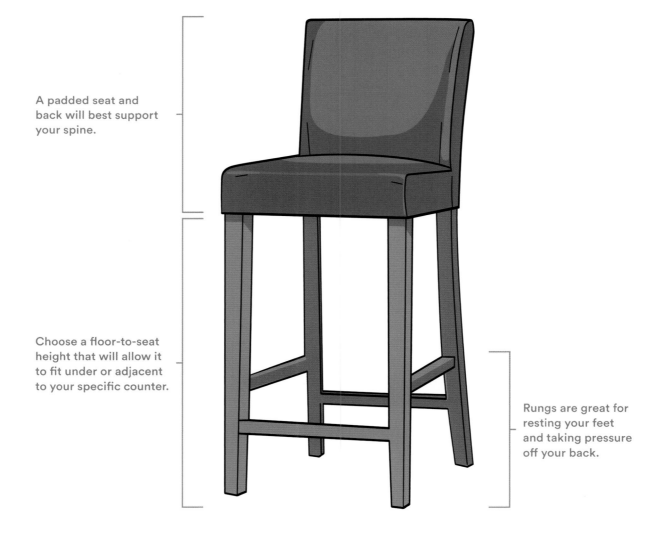

A padded seat and back will best support your spine.

Choose a floor-to-seat height that will allow it to fit under or adjacent to your specific counter.

Rungs are great for resting your feet and taking pressure off your back.

MINIMIZE WALKING WHILE COOKING WITH A SLIM ROLLING CART

You'd be surprised how much energy you can expend gathering equipment and ingredients, even in a small kitchen. The ability to bring your pantry, spice drawer, and refrigerated goods to your work space is a true game changer for cooks with back pain. Enter the rolling cart, which can help you gather everything you need and simply roll it to your workstation, eliminating the need to carry both ingredients and equipment. We recommend a cart with sides to prevent things from falling out if you are regularly moving it around. If your cart doesn't have sides, use a tray to keep items in place as you move the cart around the kitchen. As an added bonus, you can use the cart to bring serving dishes to the table.

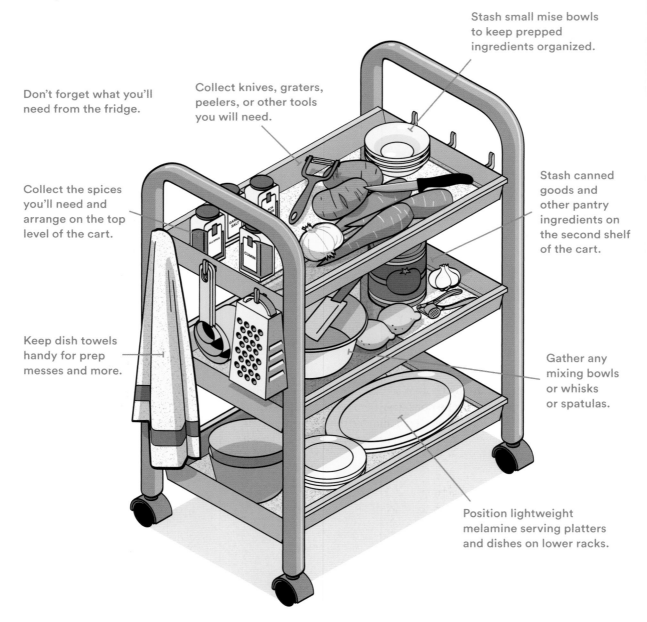

Stash small mise bowls to keep prepped ingredients organized.

Don't forget what you'll need from the fridge.

Collect knives, graters, peelers, or other tools you will need.

Collect the spices you'll need and arrange on the top level of the cart.

Stash canned goods and other pantry ingredients on the second shelf of the cart.

Keep dish towels handy for prep messes and more.

Gather any mixing bowls or whisks or spatulas.

Position lightweight melamine serving platters and dishes on lower racks.

Mind Your Posture While Prepping (or Doing the Dishes)

Hunching over is just about the worst thing you can do if you suffer from back pain. The entire spine is connected, and I have patients who are surprised when I explain how neck and upper back pain can manifest as low back pain. This is why it is especially important to be aware of your body while working in the kitchen. It is undeniable that we all hunch when leaning over a counter to chop or dice vegetables or a sink to wash dishes. If you have a deep sink, consider putting a plastic rack in it to raise the height so that you won't have to hunch over to get to the dishes and pots and pans.

The more you lean forward without support, the more it increases the stress and strain on your spinal erector muscles, which keep your head over your feet and within an area deemed "the cone of economy." For every inch you move out of this optimal alignment, your back is working overtime to keep you from falling on the floor. This stress and strain directly leads to low back pain and can be a meal and evening killer.

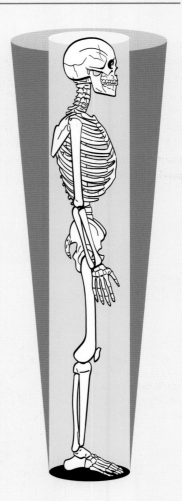

THE CONCEPT OF CONE OF ECONOMY

- **Normally when humans assume an erect posture, they stand within a certain zone of balance in which their torso remains within a certain distance from their pelvis.**
- **By doing this, energy expended by postural muscles is minimized.**
- **Beyond this zone, the cone of economy, energy expenditure rapidly increases and eventually spinal misalignment results, and external support (cane, crutch, or walker) may be necessary.**

An Easy Exercise that Helps Posture

This exercise, which helps both with posture and also strengthens the axial stabilizing muscles of the back, can be done anywhere, even while prepping or while seated on a stool in your kitchen. I recommend three sets of 15 reps. (If you're not able to do this easily, it's likely you are leaning and reaching too much and putting your back at risk.)

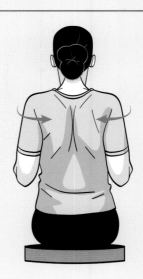

Shoulder Blade Squeeze Sit on an armless chair or stool. While maintaining good posture, pull your shoulder blades together. Hold for 5 seconds and then relax. Repeat three to five times, twice a day.

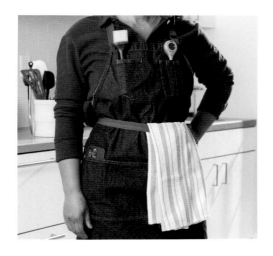

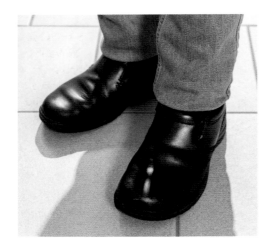

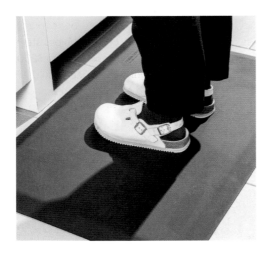

What You Need Beyond the Workstation

A GOOD APRON BRINGS THE KITCHEN TO YOU

Anything that keeps you more organized while cooking is a step towards lessening the labor involved, and that means time saved and energy conserved—a bonus if you have chronic pain that gets worse when you are tired. That's why a good apron is the ideal kitchen companion. Yes, it protects your clothes, but more important, an apron with multiple pockets and long ties that wrap around to the front provides places to stash things. Tuck your quick-read thermometer into a top pocket so it's there when you need to check that spatchcocked roast chicken for doneness; loop a dish towel around the front strings so it's at the ready for any prep messes (no need to walk to the sink and back), to wipe off a knife so that you can use it again, or to grab a hot skillet handle. Tuck a timer or your phone into a larger pocket.

INVEST IN GOOD SHOES FOR THE KITCHEN

The hospital operating room and the kitchen aren't as different as you might think. The time spent standing and moving around can wreak havoc on your back and your joints. Take a lesson from the medical and cooking professionals and get yourself a great pair of shoes. The gold standard is closed-toe clogs that are easy to slip on, have a great sturdy sole with excellent arch and heel support, and have built-in cushioning that conforms to your foot for a perfect, custom fit. My shoe of choice is the **Sanita Professional Clogs**, but there are other great options from Dansko, Crocs, and Birkenstocks. Be sure to check out their professional lines for the same shoes that surgeons wear in the operating room and chefs wear in the kitchen.

INVEST IN GOOD ANTI-FATIGUE FLOOR MATS

Anti-fatigue mats can reduce the negative impacts on joints and the spinal column caused by prolonged standing. The mats are also meant to encourage the muscles in our legs and feet to make microadjustments that stimulate blood flow, prevent blood from pooling in the lower body, and reduce the risk of leg swelling and cramps as well as more serious conditions like blood clots. Although the recipes in this book require a limited amount of standing time (that can be a potential back pain trigger), there is no way to completely avoid prep work and monitoring the stove, not to mention loading the dishwasher. These mats with their resilient surface reduce the stress on your lower back significantly. Our favorite is the **Williams Sonoma WellnessMat**.

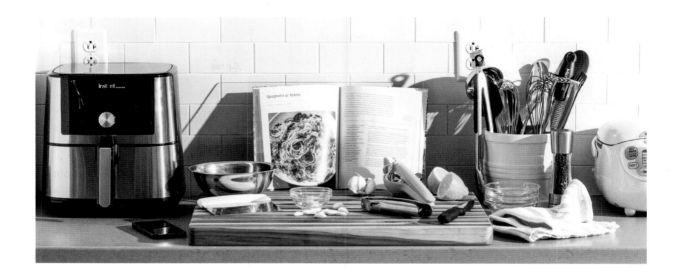

FIND A SPOT FOR YOUR COOKBOOK OR ELECTRONICS

If you're cooking recipes from this book, or indeed any cookbook, you're going to want a sturdy cookbook holder that will keep the book open and the pages protected from splatter. Our favorite is **Clear Solutions Deluxe Cookbook Holder**. If you prefer to use electronic recipes, set up your phone or tablet near your workstation for easy access and also so that you can listen to music or podcasts. Consider doing a deep dive into the settings to prevent your device from locking or going to sleep, increase the font size for ease of reading, and even change the contrast so that the instructions are easy to read even in bright sunlight.

STORE YOUR MOST-USED APPLIANCES ON YOUR COUNTERTOP

No one wants to clutter up their kitchen countertops with space-hogging appliances, but if there are some that you use again and again, having them handy reduces the chance that you will injure yourself lifting one out of the cabinet. Only you can decide which appliances deserve a spot on your countertop, since even in large kitchens this space is at a premium. Do you tend to use your big food processor a lot? If so, keep it handy or think about whether a smaller one would mostly suffice (see page 34). When it comes to larger things like a slow cooker, Instant Pot, and air fryer, it pays to keep them

on an accessible rack somewhere or, if you plan to use them frequently, perhaps in a cabinet at eye level if there isn't room on your counter. Reaching upward for something as heavy as a full-size slow cooker is not a good idea for anyone and especially for someone who has back issues. See page 45 for tips for moving heavy appliances safely.

INVEST IN A TOP-QUALITY TRASH CAN WITH A FOOT PEDAL

Nothing is more annoying than a trash can with a flimsy top, one you have to lift up by hand when you need to use it. Plus, every time you have to manually open and close the top you'll need to sanitize your hands to prevent cross-contamination. These days, your choices include sleek models in fingerprint-proof stainless steel with motion sensors that can set you back close to $200. No matter its cost, a well-designed trash can should combine a sturdy, spacious, and easy-to-clean frame with a lid that opens wide and then seals tight to trap in odors. It should also be easy to use. Since we often approach a trash can with both hands full, we prefer hands-free models. Our favorite is the **Simplehuman 50L Rectangular Step Can**, which has a lid that opens fully and quickly for complete access to its sturdy, roomy barrel and can be kept open with the flip of a small switch, and its lightweight liner can be removed for cleaning.

ORGANIZE STORAGE OF POTS AND PANS

There are many ways to organize your pots and pans so that you aren't either struggling to find them or reaching into deep cabinets to pull them out, when you are most likely to aggravate your back. First, think about the ones you use the most and which of those should simply live on your stovetop. Perhaps you want to keep a prized Dutch oven on the stovetop if you like to make stovetop meals or stews and braises. A large saucepan is also a good candidate for your stovetop, as is a 10-inch nonstick skillet (we use it quite often for many of the recipes in this book), which will fit on a stovetop without taking up too much space. Here are some storage ideas for everything else.

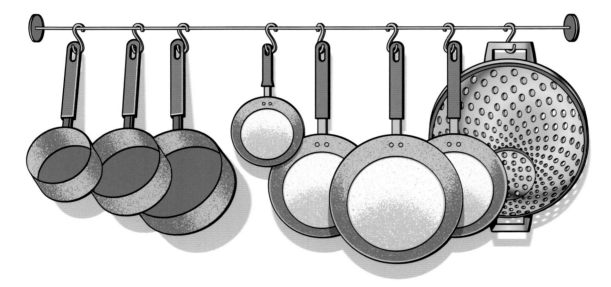

Use wall or ceiling-mounted pot racks. If you have the wall space, racks are a great way to customize access to a multitude of skillets and other pots, not to mention other often used items, such as colanders and strainers. The S hooks that come with these racks give you the flexibility to organize things however you wish and you can hang them at a height that works for you to minimize strain when reaching. Ceiling mounted pot racks are also great. Both options make a beautiful addition to your kitchen.

Buy racks and make your own storage system. There is no one-size-fits-all solution for store-bought racks for storing skillets, but you can buy inexpensive racks that come in many sizes to suit your needs. Just be sure the cabinet where you are putting them doesn't require you to practically get on the floor to have access to them.

Make the most of rolling cabinet shelves. If you are really lucky, cabinet shelves that roll out have already been built into your kitchen, making it easy to access all your pots and pans and lids. If not, you might consider hiring a carpenter to install these.

Consider the humble peg board. Take a cue from Julia Child and keep your pans on a peg board. You can have lots of ideas about size and color to make it the centerpiece of your kitchen.

Purchase an eye-catching standing rack. If you have the space, these tiered racks with shelves are not only a great way to have ready access to your most beloved pots and pans, but a beautiful way to display them—especially if you have colorful enameled pans.

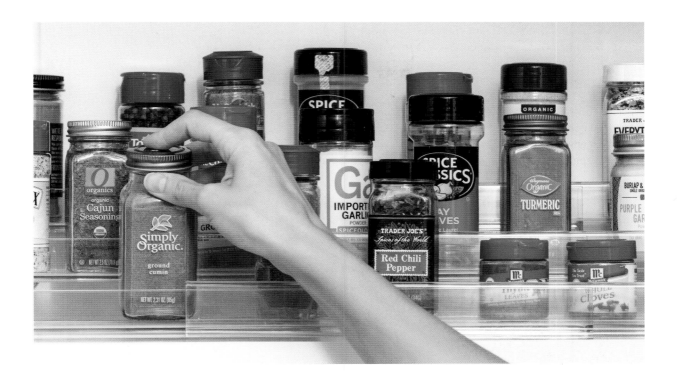

ORGANIZE YOUR SPICES

It's a problem that has plagued generations of cooks: What's the best way to store and organize spices so that they are visible and you don't waste time looking for them every time you make a recipe? Despite our best efforts, most of us have a drawer or a cabinet that's cluttered with mismatched spices. All too often, a jar or tin gets shoved to the back and is never seen again. Finding a system for organizing your spices will declutter your kitchen and make you a more efficient cook; it may also free up space in your cabinet or drawer so that you can expand your collection over time. There are a few methods for organizing your spices: wall racks, in-cabinet adjustable storage racks, lazy Susans, and in-drawer spice racks. If you have the space, it's best to opt for a device that can hold a lot of spices. We found smaller models to be disappointingly inefficient and find it's best to choose a spice storage device that can hold 50 or more spice containers. Because there is no one-size-fits-all solution, here are a few that we can recommend: **Spicy Shelf Deluxe**, **mDesign 3 Tier Expandable Spice Rack Organizer**, and **Lynk Professional 4-Tier Steel Spice Drawer Organizer**.

GIVE YOUR PANTRY A MAKEOVER

If your pantry is organized, you will feel more in control. Find a system for storing similar categories of things together in a way that makes them visible to you. For instance, devote a shelf or cabinet to categories of dry goods from canned tomato products and canned beans to sauces, rice, grains, and more. The key is to have a system that works for you and will keep you from searching endlessly for things when you are ready to cook; it will also keep you from buying items you already have simply because you cannot find them.

Use a Utensil Crock for Your Most-Used Cooking Implements

The beauty of a utensil crock is that it can corral your most-used prep and cooking utensils. How you organize utensils is a personal choice, but the value of a crock is undisputed in an ergonomic kitchen, simply because having the items you use most within reach and not buried in drawers streamlines the cooking process. We like to keep a utensil crock near the stove, so tools like silicone spatulas, metal spatulas, kitchen shears, wooden spoons, and tongs (it's a good idea to have two sets) are within arms' reach when you are cooking. One of our favorite larger crocks is the **Circulon Ceramic Tool Crock.** If you have a lot of these sorts of tools, you may want them organized logically in two crocks. Other smaller tools should be organized in smaller containers on your kitchen counter—things like pastry brushes, smaller rubber spatulas and whisks, and your quick-read thermometer. It is also super handy to have multiple sets of measuring spoons in a small crock since you will reach for them again and again while cooking, and it's nice not to have to wash a teaspoon before using it yet again.

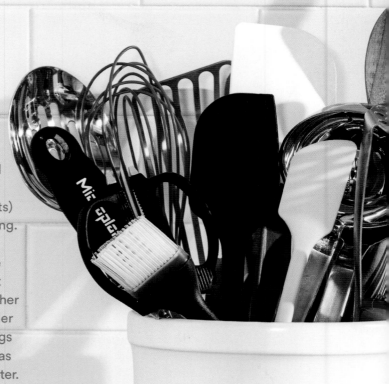

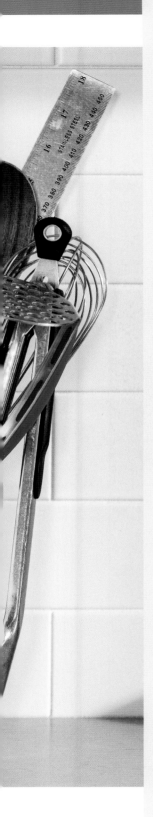

What's in Your Utensil Crock?

These are our favorites, the ones we keep reaching for while we're cooking. Every utensil on this list has been thoroughly tested by our editors and is the best in its category, so you'll always have the most reliable tools at hand.

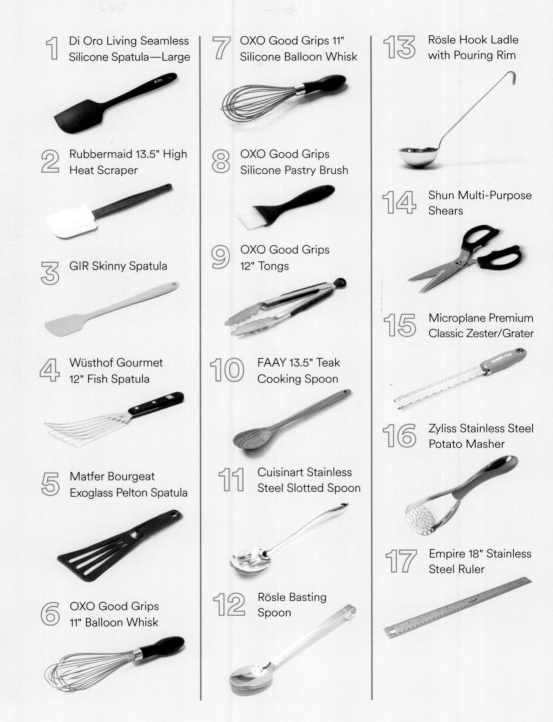

1 Di Oro Living Seamless Silicone Spatula—Large

2 Rubbermaid 13.5" High Heat Scraper

3 GIR Skinny Spatula

4 Wüsthof Gourmet 12" Fish Spatula

5 Matfer Bourgeat Exoglass Pelton Spatula

6 OXO Good Grips 11" Balloon Whisk

7 OXO Good Grips 11" Silicone Balloon Whisk

8 OXO Good Grips Silicone Pastry Brush

9 OXO Good Grips 12" Tongs

10 FAAY 13.5" Teak Cooking Spoon

11 Cuisinart Stainless Steel Slotted Spoon

12 Rösle Basting Spoon

13 Rösle Hook Ladle with Pouring Rim

14 Shun Multi-Purpose Shears

15 Microplane Premium Classic Zester/Grater

16 Zyliss Stainless Steel Potato Masher

17 Empire 18" Stainless Steel Ruler

Prep with Ease

In addition to standing and lifting, the biggest complaint about cooking that I hear from my patients is related to the amount of prep work required for recipes. Long ingredient lists and lots of knife work are not a good match for back pain sufferers. Prep for every recipe in this book takes no more than 25 minutes, and most are less. In addition, the test kitchen has come up with many tricks that streamline ingredient lists without shortchanging flavor, like super-simple stir-fry sauces, and recipes designed to use ingredients and equipment in new ways. In this section you will find tips and info on equipment that will make this process more efficient, along with easier ways to prep common ingredients, suggestions for buying prepped ingredients that work well, and more.

ASSEMBLE ALL YOUR INGREDIENTS AND TOOLS AT ONCE

Gathering everything you need to make a recipe is half the battle. If you get organized from the start, you won't be wandering around your kitchen with food-stained hands trying to find that jar of capers. It is also good to get out all the tools you will need to prep through the recipe, such as a Microplane, garlic press, juicer, and any knives. This is one of those simple strategies that is easy to execute and makes everything go more smoothly.

PREP AHEAD TO KEEP COOKING EASIER

It may sound obvious, but prepping your ingredients well before you start cooking is one of the best strategies to make the cooking process easier. Even simple things like opening and draining a can of beans, chopping an onion, and washing and chopping herbs will leave you free to enjoy the therapeutic benefits of actually cooking a meal because the most tedious parts have already been done. Throughout the book we have a Prep Ahead feature where we tell you exactly what can be done in advance, from simple ingredient prep, to recipe components, to dishes that can be made ahead in their entirety. For instance, for our Meaty Loaf Pan Lasagna (page 118) you could simply prep the ingredients, but you can also make the ricotta filling ahead and you can even assemble and refrigerate the entire lasagna several hours in advance.

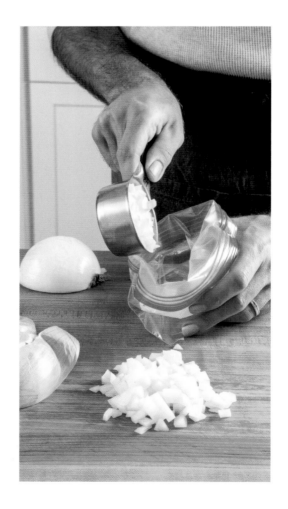

Standing for a long amount of time is the enemy of your back. There are a few ways to tackle this in the healthy back kitchen. The first is to lessen the amount of prep required with easier recipes by using already-prepped ingredients from the grocery store. But perhaps the biggest strategy is to set up a workstation on a kitchen counter and add a stool (see page 19). The relationship of your body to the counter while sitting will allow you the leverage to prep most things while sitting. If this is not a viable option for you, sit at your kitchen or dining room table and get some of the work done there.

There are many things you can prep from a table: Any ingredient prepped with your kitchen shears (trimming chicken, trimming green beans, snipping herbs, etc.) can be done at a table because you are usually holding the shears in one hand and the ingredient in the other. You can also use a Microplane from a sitting position and run it around a lemon or lime to zest, or run a knob of peeled ginger over it, which makes quick work of this normally tedious task. You can also wipe down and cut mushrooms and cut up small potatoes using a utility knife, among other simple tasks. Any small tasks using a paring knife can be done here too. But any prep work requiring the physics and leverage needed when cutting through an ingredient at a higher position, like chopping an onion, will have to be done at counter level (either sitting or standing). And some tasks, like cutting up a big piece of meat, have to be done standing to get enough leverage.

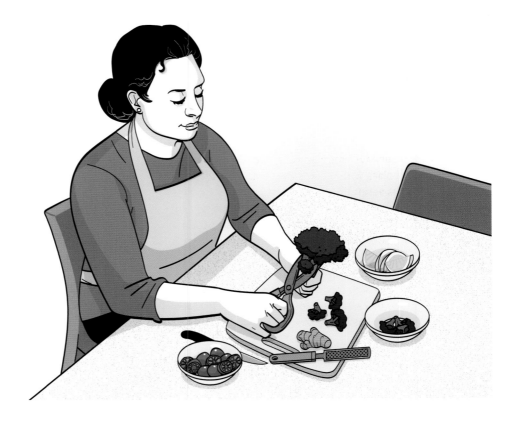

Make Sure You Have the Right Complement of Knives

Knives are perhaps the most important tool in any kitchen, not just the healthy back kitchen. Bad knives, dull knives, or the wrong knives are a real liability whether you have back issues or not, because they make every job harder. You will have to exert more force if you are using the wrong knife or a dull knife, and it is easy to strain the muscles in your back as a result. Also, some knives are heavier and longer than others, so they may be harder to handle. While a heavy knife can sometimes help with the leverage it provides when you need to cut through dense vegetables or meat, it may put undue stress on your upper arm and back. (And a knife that is too heavy for your hand could slip out of it and injure you.) Contrary to what many people seem to think, you don't need a lot of knives, just the right ones. Since this book is devoted to enhancing the cooking experience with less exertion, here are the knives we think you will use the most for prep work and the best ones to choose for each.

UTILITY KNIFE

I highly recommend that back patients buy a good utility knife. It is a cross between a chef's knife and a paring knife and what this means in practical terms is that it can function in almost any situation where you'd automatically reach for the bigger chef's knife. It has more power than a paring knife but gives you more control than a chef's knife. And its blade is short enough that you can use it sitting down—this is perhaps the most important reason to buy one. The winner of our testing is **Tojiro 150 mm Petty R-2 Powder Steel Knife**. We also like this somewhat less expensive utility knife: **MAC PKF-60 Pro Utility 6-inch Knife**.

CHEF'S KNIFE

There are some tasks where there are no substitutes for a chef's knife because of its size and the leverage it provides. For instance, if you are prepping a sweet potato or cutting a chuck roast into pieces for stew, there is no better knife than this one. Our favorite inexpensive chef's knife is the **Victorinox Swiss Army Fibrox Pro 8-inch Chef's Knife**.

PARING KNIFE

When you need to carefully cut wide strips of lemon peel (as you will if you make our Instant Pot Chicken Tagine on page 91) or remove the tendons from scallops (for the Seared Scallop Salad with Snap Peas and Radishes on page 73), you really need a small paring knife as its diminutive size makes it highly maneuverable and better able to hug curves than bigger knives. Plus, its light weight ensures that your hand doesn't get tired. It's also great for peeling fruits and vegetables and checking the doneness of fish. Our favorite? The inexpensive and super light **Victorinox Swiss Army Spear Point Paring Knife**.

SMALL SERRATED KNIFE

A small serrated knife makes some tasks even easier than using a paring knife. That is because even the best straight-edged blades squish soft tomatoes a tiny bit, and serrated blades are superior for nicking off tiny bits of orange pith. The **Wüsthof Classic 3.5-Inch Fully Serrated Paring Knife** is our favorite; it has slightly more heft than its competitors and razor-sharp serrations that glide through tomatoes and between citrus segments with ease.

Sharpening and Storing Your Knives

KEEP KNIVES SHARP

If your knives are dull, everything you try to do will take longer or just require more exertion than it should. And if you have back issues, dull knives will work against you. Think about cutting up even a small pork butt roast for Slow-Cooker Posole (page 163). A sharp knife will glide through the meat and feel like an extension of your hand. And your work will be over in short order. The same is true if you are cutting up raw chicken to make our Chicken Curry with Tomatoes and Ginger (page 174) or Chicken Lo Mein with Bok Choy (page 170). But try to do these tasks with a dull knife and making these streamlined recipes will take a lot more effort (and time). Even the most basic of prep tasks, like mincing an onion, can be problematic; try it with a less than sharp knife and not only are you apt to mash the onion (releasing even more of its eye-stinging vapors), you may also cut yourself since a dull blade requires more force to do the job and so has a higher chance of slipping and missing the mark. Plus, poorly cut food will not cook properly. A sharp knife will produce food that is evenly cut and therefore will cook at an even rate.

PUT THE BLADE TO THE PAPER TEST

Even the best knives will dull over time with regular use, so it is best to sharpen them regularly and hone them in between sharpenings. To determine if your knife needs sharpening, put it to the paper test: Hold a single sheet of basic printer/copy paper. Lay the blade against the top edge at an angle and slice outward. If the knife fails to slice cleanly, try steeling it. If it still fails, it needs sharpening.

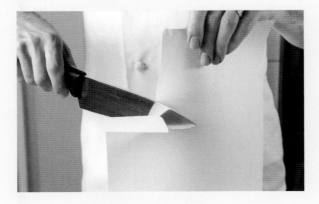

KNIFE HONING STEEL

A so-called sharpening steel, this is the metal rod sold with most knife sets. It doesn't really sharpen a knife, but rather hones the edge of a slightly dulled blade. Sweeping the blade along the steel realigns the edge. Whenever you feel that your knife is less sharp than it should be, try a honing rod. If you find that honing doesn't make much difference, it's time to get out the sharpener. Periodic honing will allow you to go longer between sharpening sessions, but it can't repair a very dull or damaged edge. While honing, make sure to maintain a 15-degree angle between the blade and the steel. Sweep your blade down the length of the rod four or five times on each side.

MANUAL AND ELECTRIC KNIFE SHARPENERS

The best manual knife sharpener is the **Chef's Choice Pronto Diamond Hone Knife Sharpener**. Tall walls hold the knife steady so that a 15-degree blade can be drawn through the chamber with even pressure. The slim body is easily stowed in a drawer.

Our winning electric model is the **Chef's Choice Trizor 15XV Knife Sharpener**. The aggressive first slot can quickly repair extensive damage and narrow a 20-degree Western knife to a sharper 15-degree edge. Use the fine slot to gently resharpen a slightly dull knife.

KEEP YOUR KNIVES ORGANIZED AND ACCESSIBLE

If you have the wall space, a heavy-duty magnetic rack will allow you to grab your knife swiftly in one easy movement and will hold knives of all shapes and sizes without taking up valuable drawer or counter space. Our favorite is the **Brooklyn Butcher Blocks 20-inch Knife Rack, Walnut**.

If you don't have the space to mount a rack, a knife block is the answer. Because conventional blocks hold only knives of specific sizes, we prefer universal blocks, which are designed to accommodate knives of all sizes in any configuration. Our winning block, the **360 Knife Block by Design Trifecta**, is a serious investment, but it will serve your knives well for years to come.

DON'T OVERLOOK KITCHEN SHEARS

You may only bring out your kitchen shears when trimming meat or cutting up a cooked chicken. If so, you are underestimating the power of this tool in the healthy back kitchen. Using shears requires less exertion than a knife (so less opportunity to aggravate your back), and you can easily do a multitude of prep tasks with them while sitting down—perhaps the biggest benefit they offer. They allow you to move your prep work to a kitchen or dining room table, taking the pressure off your back that standing exerts, to trim herbs and scallions or to cut up broccoli or a multitude of other ingredients. The ambidextrous, take-apart **Shun Multi-Purpose Shears** is our favorite.

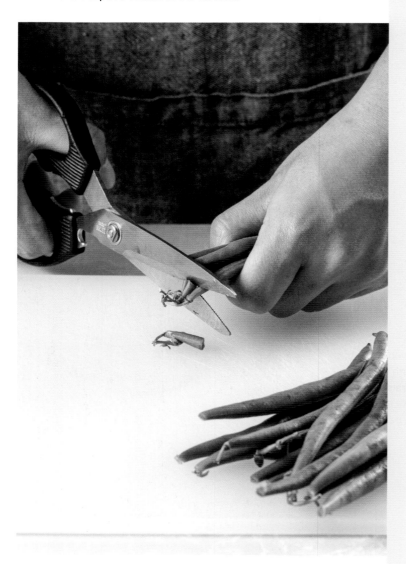

12 WAYS TO PUT YOUR KITCHEN SHEARS TO WORK

1   Trim fat from cuts of meat such as chicken thighs and pork roasts.

2   Cut whole or spatchcocked chicken into serving pieces.

3   Snip through the fat surrounding the loin muscle of pork chops to prevent buckling.

4   Snip bunches of chives and scallions into short lengths.

5   Slice basil with less bruising, and snip the leaves off parsley and cilantro.

6   Cut up bacon.

7   Chop whole peeled tomatoes in the can with less mess.

8   Trim the ends from handfuls of green or wax beans.

9   Remove florets from heads of broccoli and cauliflower.

10   Trim asparagus.

11   Chop up sticky dried fruit such as dates and figs.

12   Open those pesky packages of air-chilled chicken and boxes of all manner of ingredients like beans, diced tomatoes, and more.

Other Tools to Make Prep Easier

A SET OF SMALL, NESTING PREP BOWLS TO MISE EN PLACE LIKE A PRO

Organization in the kitchen equals efficiency, and the same is true when you are prepping ingredients. As we said earlier, this is known as mise en place, and getting all your ingredients measured out in prep bowls makes the process move more quickly, and often the prep can be done way in advance. A set of mini prep bowls will allow you to measure out, separate, and organize all your ingredients, making cooking tidier and more efficient. Furthermore, having all the ingredients organized will keep you from having to search for this spice or that herb, reducing repetitive movements that can put your back at risk for spasms and pain. Our favorite bowl set is **Anchor Hocking Custard Cups**. A small lip on the outside of the bowls makes them comfortable to grip. Lids for the bowls can be purchased separately.

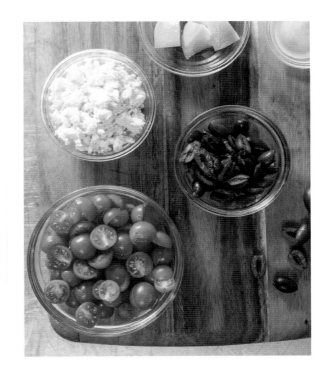

SMALL RIMMED BAKING SHEETS TO GET ORGANIZED (AND MORE)

In the test kitchen we use small rimmed baking sheets, also known as quarter sheet pans, to hold all our little bowls of prepped ingredients. In addition, these pans act as a convenient way for refrigerating prepped items like burgers and meatballs, resting cooked meats, and drying out herbs and greens on paper towels. If you are making a beefy stew or braise, it is also convenient to put the meat on a sheet pan to season it on both sides. We highly recommend the **Nordic Ware Naturals Quarter Sheet Pan**. For more important ways we use these pans while cooking the recipes in this book, see page 42.

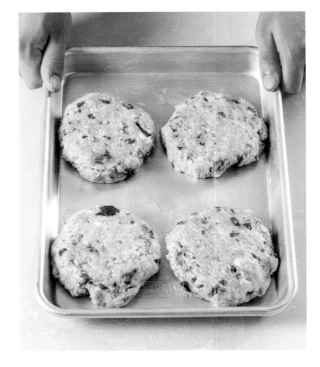

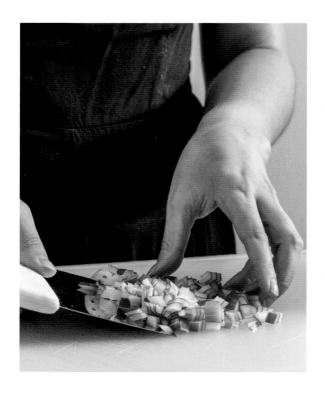

A BENCH SCRAPER TO TRANSFER INGREDIENTS EFFICIENTLY

Have you ever minced an onion and then tried to gather up the small bits and transfer them to your skillet? Or tried to collect chopped herbs and place them in a bowl for garnishing later? Maybe you've tried to use your chef's knife for this task—definitely not a good idea, as it will rapidly dull your blade or cause you to cut yourself. Enter the bench scraper, which is perfect for this task; it's a tool originally designed for bakers to lift dough off a cutting board or clean off a cutting board (also known as a "bench" by bakers) covered in flour. Why waste time and energy transferring ingredients to the stove or your mixing bowl when this simple tool makes it so much easier and more efficient? When we organize our workstation, we always make sure a bench scraper is right there. We also use it to clean off cutting boards and transfer prep remnants to a trash bowl or trash can. Our favorite is the **Dexter-Russell 6" x 3" Dough Cutter/Scraper—Sani-Safe Series**.

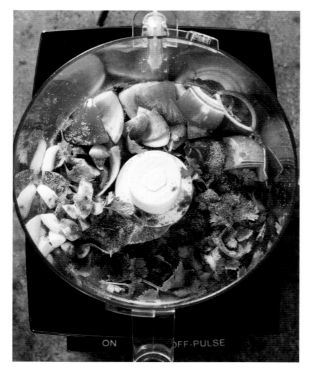

TWO FOOD PROCESSORS: YOUR ULTIMATE KITCHEN ASSISTANTS

A good food processor is like having a little motorized sous chef living in your cabinet. And two assistants are better than one, because in the healthy back kitchen, we recommend that you have both a large and a small food processor. Keep a small one on your counter for many small, easy tasks, such as making bread crumbs, chopping nuts, making mirepoix, or whipping up small recipes (like the Avocado Crema on page 217). But there are some recipes where you need the larger food processor, for instance for big batch pestos (pages 286–287) and making our Food Processor Gazpacho (page 143). Our winning 4-cup food processor is the **Cuisinart Elite Collection 4-Cup Chopper/Grinder**. Our winning large food processor is the **Cuisinart Custom 14-Cup Food Processor**.

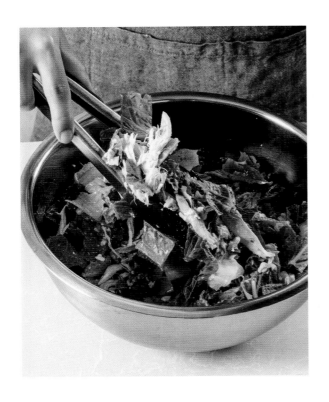

LIGHTWEIGHT MIXING BOWLS TO LIGHTEN YOUR LOAD

If you've been cooking for a long time, it's likely that you may find yourself with an assortment of glass, metal, and plastic mixing bowls. They are probably hard to store and, if they are glass, some of the larger bowls can weigh nearly 4 pounds. Lifting such bowls in and out of cabinets and the dishwasher is yet another strain on your back. At the very least, you need small, medium, and large bowls—by which we mean 1- to 1½-quart; 2½- to 3-quart; and 4- to 6-quart, respectively. Our favorite collection is **Vollrath Economy Stainless Steel Mixing Bowls**. The broad, shallow shape of these inexpensive bowls puts food within easy reach and allows for wide turns of a spatula. These are also the lightest bowls among those tested.

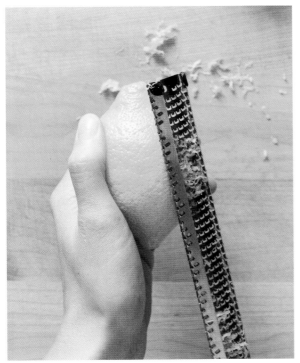

A MICROPLANE AND JUICER TO ZEST AND JUICE EASILY

If you have ever stood and pushed and twisted a halved lemon down on one of those stationary glass or metal juicers, you know that you have to put your weight behind it to extract a good amount of juice. You shouldn't have to twist your shoulder or throw your back out just to get a few tablespoons of lemon or lime juice. Our favorite manual juicer, the **Chef'n FreshForce Citrus Juicer**, makes the job far easier without the need to exert a lot of force. As for zesting citrus, the Microplane is great at efficiently removing the flavor-packed colored parts of citrus fruits. But it can do much more, such as grating ginger and garlic and finely grating Parmesan and Pecorino Romano cheese. Our winning Microplane is the **Microplane Premium Classic Zester/Grater**.

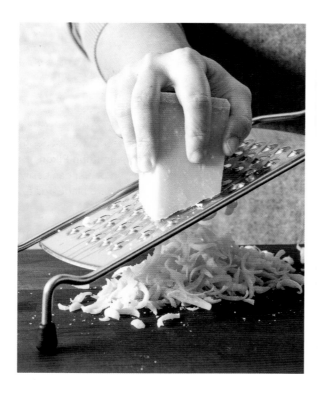

ERGONOMIC GRATERS FOR PREPPING CHEESE AND MORE

We use grated and shredded cheese a lot in the recipes throughout this book. Of course, to save time and effort you can buy many kinds of cheese already shredded or grated. But it's always handy to have a good grater around, not only for cheese that you can't buy grated, but for shredding carrots (great in a salad) or to coarsely grate a hard-boiled egg (as for Lemony Salmon and Roasted Beet Salad, page 68). And yes, you can grate cheese and vegetables in a food processor, but if you don't need a lot, it can be easier to just do it by hand. Our favorite box grater is the **Cuisinart Box Grater**; our favorite paddle grater is the **Rösle Coarse Grater**. Featuring big handles and rubber-tipped feet and bases, they are easy to hold and sit stably on a cutting board.

A QUALITY GARLIC PRESS (OR MICROPLANE) TO MINCE GARLIC EASILY

There are few recipes that don't require minced garlic. And honestly, there is no good substitution for the real deal. If you love knife work, you can certainly use a knife and mince it by hand. But there are easier ways that require little exertion or time:

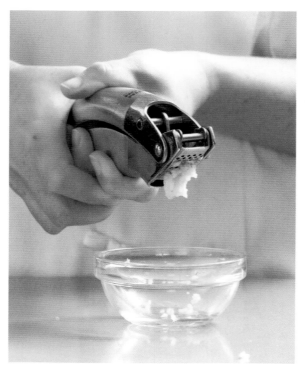

We recommend investing in a superior garlic press. Some presses are flimsy and don't shred all the garlic, require a lot of force to use, and are super-hard to clean. We recommend you go with the best, so we can fully recommend only one garlic press: the **Kuhn Rikon Stainless Steel Epicurean Garlic Press**. Its weighty, curved handles, stainless steel construction, and pop-out hopper make for a comfortable, easy-to-clean press that is smooth to operate—even with tricky unpeeled garlic cloves.

We are also fans of freezing peeled garlic and then using your Microplane to get a fine grate. You know those tubs of peeled garlic you find in the grocery store? One way to ensure that you always have peeled garlic on hand is to freeze a bunch of them in a zipper-lock bag. You'll always have garlic when you need it, and frozen cloves grate along the edge of a sharp Microplane like a dream.

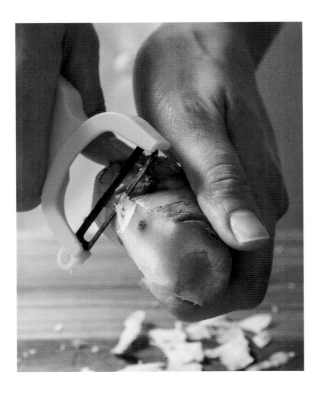

A SMALL BUT MIGHTY VEGETABLE PEELER TO PROTECT YOUR HANDS

A good peeler should be fast and smooth, shaving off just enough of the skin to avoid the need for repeat trips over the same section but not so much that the blade digs deeply into the flesh and wastes food. And when the work is done, your hand shouldn't feel worse for the wear. Don't be fooled by the featherweight design and cheap price tag of our winner, the **Kuhn Rikon Original Swiss Peeler**. This Y-shaped peeler can easily tackle every task, thanks to a razor-sharp blade and a ridged guide.

A MICROWAVE TO JUMP-START COOKING

The microwave can do more than reheat leftovers. It can really shorten up the time it takes to make a recipe—which means less time standing in the kitchen. We use it to "roast" the beets for our Lemony Salmon and Roasted Beet Salad (page 68), to cook the butternut squash that forms the buttery base in Seared Scallops with Sage Butter Sauce and Squash (page 197), and to parcook wedges of russet potatoes for Pan-Seared Strip Steaks with Crispy Potatoes (page 182) so that they can be browned quickly in the meaty juices left behind from cooking the steak (before the steak gets cold).

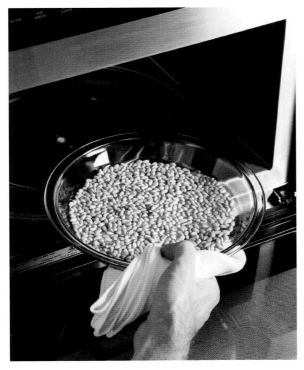

HOW TO TOAST NUTS IN THE MICROWAVE

We use toasted nuts throughout the book in many ways to add crunch and flavor to salads, vegetables, grains, and pestos. The process of toasting nuts can slow you down in the middle of prepping a recipe because it usually requires getting out a skillet or a baking sheet. Here is a far simpler way: Place the nuts in a shallow microwave-safe bowl or pie plate in a thin, even layer. Microwave on full power, stopping to check the color and stir every minute at first. As the food starts to take on color, microwave it in 30-second increments to avoid burning. You can toast larger batches of nuts this way and store them in the freezer. (They'll stay crunchy for up to a month.)

Prep School

TRICKS THAT MAKE COOKING EVEN EASIER

There are ingredients everyone ends up prepping constantly—think onions, shallots, bell peppers, and more. And some of the prep work can be tedious, like coring tomatoes and apples. Here in the test kitchen we like to teach people the absolute best way to prep everything, but for this book, we've developed a few radical tricks that make the job much faster and easier for anyone with back issues. Here are a few ideas to make prep work a little easier for you.

TOMATOES

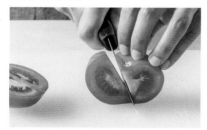 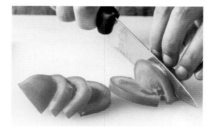

1 Simply cut planks at a slight diagonal all around circumference of tomato as close to core as you can until all you have left is the core.

2 Cut planks into desired size called for in recipe.

APPLES

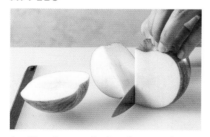 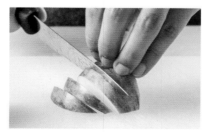

1 Simply cut planks all around circumference of apple.

2 Slice into thin attractive wedges. This is especially useful when cutting apples to incorporate into salad.

ROMAINE LETTUCE

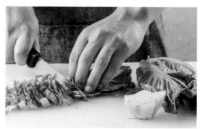

Cut off stem end of romaine heart. Slice through romaine heart lengthwise. Cut each section in half. Chop each of four sections into ½-inch pieces. Wash in salad spinner.

BELL PEPPERS

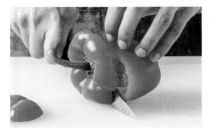

1 Chop off each end.

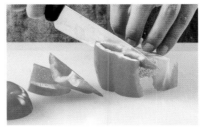

2 Slice edges from top to bottom so that you have four pieces. Remove any pith or seeds.

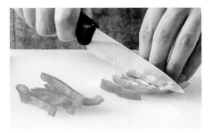

3 Cut pieces into desired size called for in recipe. Chop end pieces.

BROCCOLI

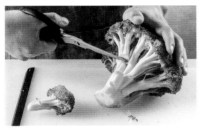

Hold broccoli head level with cutting board. Using kitchen shears, maneuver them so that you can simply cut off florets where stems meet larger stalk.

CELERY

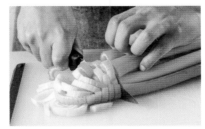

1 Instead of laboriously separating celery stalks and then chopping, simply slice off end of a bunch and proceed to chop celery until you have required amount.

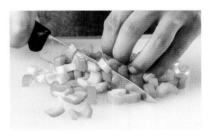

2 Chop or mince until pieces are size required for your recipe.

PARSLEY AND CILANTRO

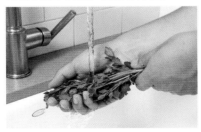

1 Wash bunch of herbs but do not cut stems.

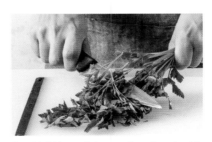

2 Hold bunch in one hand and with knife in other hand simply shave off leaves. Refrigerate what you do not need to use immediately.

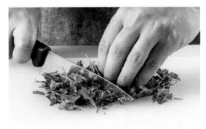

3 Mince leaves and any tender stems still attached.

ONION

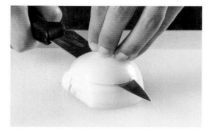

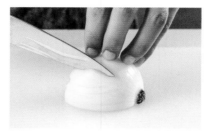

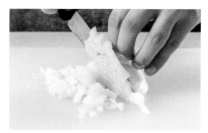

1   Halve onion through root end, then peel onion and trim top. Make several horizontal cuts from 1 end of onion to other but don't cut through root end.

2   Make several vertical cuts. Be sure to cut up to but not through root end.

3   Rotate onion so that root end is in back; slice onion thinly across previous cuts. As you slice, onion will fall apart into chopped pieces.

SHALLOT

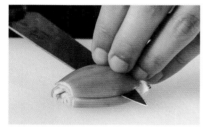

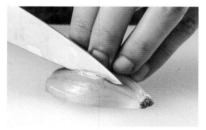

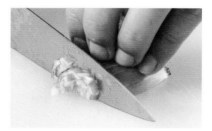

1   Halve shallot through root end, then make closely spaced horizontal cuts through peeled shallot, leaving root end intact.

2   Make several vertical cuts through shallot.

3   Finally, thinly slice shallot crosswise, creating fine mince.

LEEKS

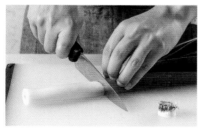

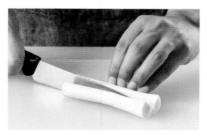

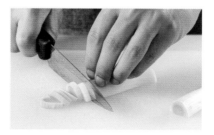

1   Trim root end and cut off upper portion of tough dark green layers.

2   Cut in half horizontally.

3   Cut each half crosswise into pieces, place in colander, and rinse thoroughly; alternatively, use salad spinner. Chop again if necessary.

KALE AND SWISS CHARD

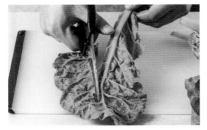

Use kitchen shears to remove leaves following line of stems. Flatten leaves and cut into strips or pieces according to recipe. Chop stems if being used in recipe.

CHUCK ROAST (FOR STEW)

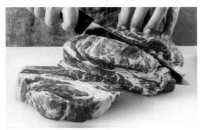

1   Remove twine if necessary. Cut roast into 1½-inch-thick slabs through diameter of roast. Trim away any chunks of hardened fat.

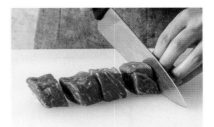

2   Cut each slab into 1½-inch strips, then cut each strip into 1½-inch pieces.

EMBRACE BUYING PREPPED INGREDIENTS

There are many ingredients available already prepped or cooked, and we call them out throughout the recipes in the book. Below is a list of some we think work well. But once you start noticing these ingredients, you may find even more in your local market, such as chopped herbs and other aromatics. If your store has a high-quality salad bar, feel free to raid it for washed and chopped ingredients you can use in your recipes or add to salad greens to make a simple salad feel more special.

- Peeled and cut up butternut squash
- Broccoli and cauliflower florets
- Trimmed asparagus spears
- Trimmed, ready-to-use green beans
- Sliced mushrooms
- Trimmed radishes
- Baby carrots
- Shredded and chopped carrots

- Carrot and celery sticks
- Sliced bell peppers
- Cooked beets; spiralized beets
- Washed romaine heart leaves and chopped romaine
- Baby kale
- Coleslaw mix
- Sliced zucchini; spiralized zucchini noodles
- Peeled garlic cloves
- Mirepoix mix

- Grated and shredded cheeses (Parmesan, Pecorino Romano, cheddar, mozzarella, goat cheese, feta, and more)
- Croutons
- Rotisserie chicken
- Chicken tenderloins
- Peeled and deveined shrimp
- Cooked salmon
- Stew meat
- Hard-boiled eggs

Cook with Ease

Pots and Pans and More

Now it's time to talk about cooking equipment. Just like it's not necessary to have a lot of knives, there is no need to have a huge arsenal of pots and pans. Case in point, all of the ergonomically designed and back-friendly recipes in this book use just the equipment in this section.

SMALL RIMMED BAKING SHEETS MAKE ROASTING POSSIBLE

Large rimmed baking sheets are off limits in the healthy back kitchen because transferring one full of meat or vegetables is a bit of a balancing act, and bending down to put one into and out of the oven is a back strain waiting to happen. We have already talked about the usefulness of small sheet pans when prepping (see page 33). But when you want to roast smaller quantities of food like One-Pan Steak Fajitas (page 228), they make the job eminently doable, and they also fit handily in a toaster oven. We also use them to roast smaller cuts of meat and chicken like Spatchcocked Roast Chicken with Rosemary and Garlic (page 88).

NONSTICK SKILLETS ARE THE WORKHORSE OF THE HEALTHY BACK KITCHEN

Throughout this book you will learn to use nonstick skillets in ways you may never have imagined. Their low sides mean food reduces quickly, so sauces reach the right consistency faster; and you can easily get a good sear on meat and fish as well. We press the advantages of the skillets to the max, using them to cook pasta in a brothy sauce, cook rice and other ingredients together, and rotate ingredients in and out in the course of a recipe to create one-dish meals (and in some cases, bypassing a casserole dish and the oven). Suddenly dishes such as Chicken and Chorizo Paella (page 222) and Skillet Penne alla Vodka (page 201) are one-dish wonders. Our favorite large nonstick skillet is the **OXO Good Grips Non-Stick Pro 12" Open Fry Pan**. All nonstick skillets will eventually wear out, so the OXO model's affordable price is an added bonus. But if you require an induction-compatible skillet, the **All-Clad Stainless 12" Nonstick Fry Pan** is an excellent, though considerably more

expensive, choice. It is important to buy one with a lid, as many recipes require one. Our favorite 10-inch nonstick skillet is the **OXO Good Grips Non-Stick Pro 10" Open Fry Pan**. We use it throughout the book for recipes that serve two, such as Modern Beef Pot Pie with Mushrooms and Sherry (page 98).

MULTIPLE SAUCEPANS ARE OUR UNSUNG HEROES

In the healthy back kitchen, we often turn to saucepans. They can stand in for larger, heavier pots; you can use them to make smaller-batch soups like our pantry-friendly Sun-Dried Tomato and White Bean Soup (page 138); and they are perfect for cooking hearty grains via the absorption method, no draining required—check out our Farro Risotto with Fennel and Radicchio (page 261). We also use them to make all manner of essential sides, such as rice pilaf, simple white rice, and cauliflower rice. The **All-Clad Stainless 4-Qt Sauce Pan** is our top pick. It's no featherweight, but its hefty frame hits the sweet spot between sturdy construction and easy handling; it also has a helper handle which makes lifting it far easier. The **Tramontina Tri-Ply Clad 4 Qt. Sauce Pan** (with helper handle) is our best buy.

Smaller nonstick saucepans have their place too. A small saucepan sees plenty of action—making smaller batches of rice, heating milk, melting butter, and warming up a little soup. It may be the smallest pan in the kitchen arsenal, but it's by no means the least important. Because most of these tasks don't involve browning (and many involve sticky foods), in the test kitchen we use nonstick 2-quart saucepans almost exclusively. Our favorite is the **Calphalon Contemporary Nonstick 2½ Quart Saucepan**.

A LIGHTWEIGHT DUTCH OVEN PUTS SOUPS, STEWS, AND BRAISES WITHIN REACH AGAIN

Every kitchen needs a good Dutch oven, but in the healthy back kitchen this time-honored pot is a liability. One of our favorites, the Le Creuset Dutch oven, weighs over 13 pounds *empty*. So not only are you faced with washing and putting away this heavy pot, you have to deal with it full of food, especially since many recipes require stovetop-to-oven cooking for best results. The solution is to buy a lightweight Dutch oven; our favorite is the 6-quart **All-Clad D3 Stainless Stockpot with Lid**, which weighs just 5 pounds. If you use this pot and bypass recipes that braise or stew in the oven, then a whole range of high-yield recipes are within reach, like our reengineered Stovetop Classic Pot Roast with Potatoes and Carrots (page 100); and it means you can make some big-batch recipes such as Tomato, Bulgur, and Red Pepper Soup (page 148). We recommend that you serve up these dishes at the stove using a good ladle to avoid ever having to lift the pot when it is full.

Weigh Your Options

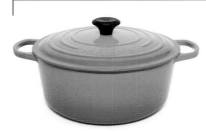

Le Creuset 7¼ Quart Round Dutch Oven
Weight: **13.7 LB**

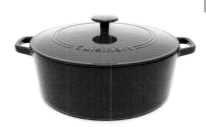

Cuisinart Chef's Enameled 7 Quart Cast Iron Casserole
Weight: **16.7 LB**

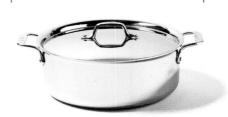

All-Clad D3 Stainless Stockpot with Lid, 6 Quart
Weight: **5 LB**

A SAFE WAY TO PUT SOMETHING IN THE OVEN

Placing something in a hot oven might be the most dangerous thing you do in the healthy back kitchen. Here is a strategy to keep your back safe. First, use a long pair of tongs to pull out the oven rack to reduce the distance you have to reach outside your "cone of economy" (page 21). Try coming to the rack from an angle or from the side of the oven. Place a stool or a rolling cart next to the oven to give yourself a place to put down the sheet pan or casserole dish en route from the counter to the oven.

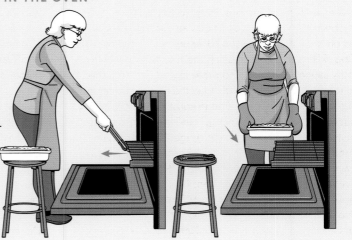

Use Convenience Appliances to Make Cooking Easier

Many of our favorite dinner recipes require standing for long stretches of time between prepping ingredients and adding them to a skillet or pot while cooking in increments. Not to mention the sorts of meaty braises that need to cook slowly in the oven. This is where the Instant Pot and the slow cooker are especially helpful and the ultimate ergonomic tools. The air fryer has its place for entirely different reasons (see page 46). What follows is specific information about how to use these appliances in the healthy back kitchen.

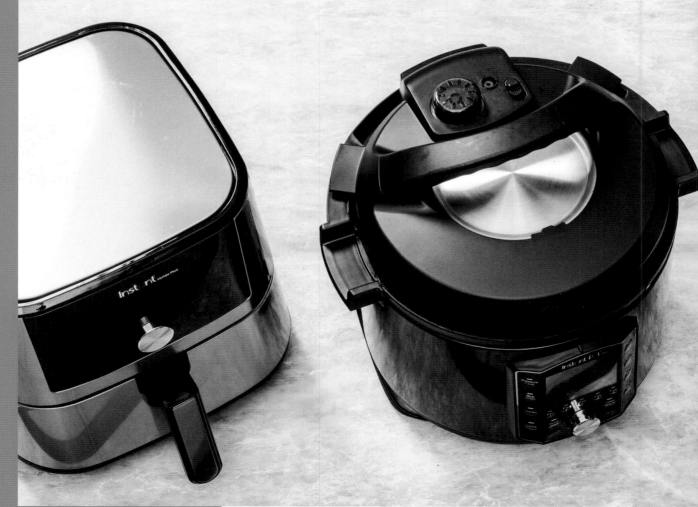

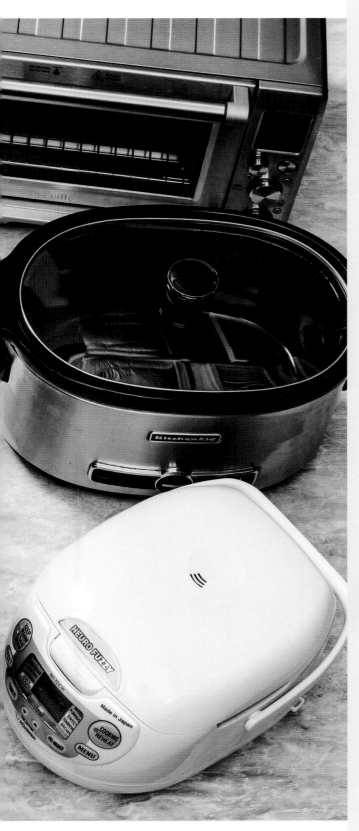

LIFTING AND PUTTING AWAY APPLIANCES

Just because we are lifting 5 to 15 pounds (of cooking equipment) while cooking instead of 50 to 150 pounds (of weights) doesn't mean we can't learn from extreme athletes like powerlifters. Technique and form are critical in the sport of weight lifting, and everything always revolves around the optimal alignment of the spine to ensure maximal biomechanical advantage when moving around enormous weights. When we are in the kitchen, it is important to remember that the further away from our bodies we hold a weight the more it will seem to weigh. This results in increased force on our spine, which works overtime to keep our head above our heels and prevent us from falling on our faces. If you keep the load as close to the body as possible, you can engage more of the bulk muscles instead of the spinal stabilizing muscles, which tire quickly and can go into spasm, ruining not only your whole day but potentially your whole week.

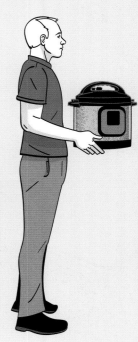

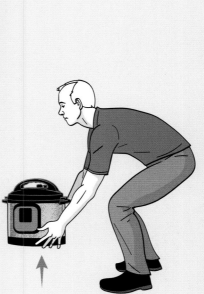

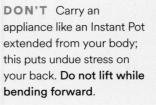

DON'T Carry an appliance like an Instant Pot extended from your body; this puts undue stress on your back. **Do not lift while bending forward**.

DO Use T-rex arms (tight to the body at 90-degree angles) and squat down with your legs as needed. **Hold load close to your body**.

Slow Cooker
THE KING OF WALKAWAY COOKING

The appeal of putting dinner in the slow cooker and walking away is easy to understand. And it is a godsend for those who cannot stand at the stove for extended periods of time or lift heavy pots or roasting pans. Look for these recipes that showcase the power of the slow cooker: Slow-Cooker Turkey Breast with Cherry-Orange Sauce (page 227) just might be your new Thanksgiving go-to centerpiece, as it delivers perfectly cooked meat and a delicious sauce. Slow-Cooker Citrus Braised Chicken Tacos (page 216) reinvents taco night with the clever use of aromatics and a little frozen orange juice that infuses boneless thighs with flavor. Slow-Cooker Bolognese (page 293) replaces the 3-hour bolognese you used to make, and no stovetop browning is required; it also delivers a large quantity of sauce (7 cups), so you can stock your freezer. Our winning slow cooker is the **KitchenAid 6-Quart Slow Cooker with Solid Glass Lid**.

Instant Pot
GREAT FOR ENTERTAINING (AND MORE)

The Instant Pot promises it can do it all, but we like to use it as a pressure cooker because everything, even pasta, goes into the pot to deliver a meal in short order. The pot also streamlines the cooking of meats that normally require lots of prep and a long cooking time and eliminates the need to lift a heavy Dutch oven full of food from the stovetop to the oven. The recipes in this book designed specifically for the Instant Pot make the most of this appliance, so the ingredients mingle, gain intensity, and are infused with flavor under pressure. And we love the way both vegetarian and meaty dishes are made easier: Instant Pot Bulgur with Spinach, Chickpeas, and Za'atar (page 245); Easy Instant Pot Beef Stew with Mushrooms and Bacon (page 159); and Instant Pot Braised Whole Cauliflower (page 271). You can brown food right in the insert, which saves steps (and dirty pans), and then simply add remaining ingredients and walk away until it's time to release the pressure. Our winning pot is the **Instant Pot Pro 8-Quart**. The **Instant Pot Pro 6-Quart** will work with all the recipes in this book.

Air Fryer
DELIVERS A SURPRISING RANGE OF ELEGANT AND EASY-PREP RECIPES

Air fryers are easy and convenient to cook in. Most don't need to be preheated, and those that do just need a few minutes; there's none of the splattering you get with traditional deep frying. It also allows you to bypass the oven. Best of all, it's a way to make easy-to-execute food with crisp and appealingly brown exteriors, such as Air-Fryer French Fries (page 281) and Air-Fryer Crispy Breaded Boneless Pork Chops (page 249). And it is exceptionally good at cooking fish perfectly, such as Air-Fryer Orange Mustard–Glazed Salmon (page 250). Air fryers come in different sizes as well, so you can choose one that works for your household. Our winning air fryer is the **Instant Vortex Plus 6-Quart Air Fryer**.

Toaster Oven
STANDS IN FOR A TRADITIONAL OVEN, NO BENDING REQUIRED

A good toaster oven functions as a small second oven, with the added benefit in the healthy back kitchen that it does not require you to bend over to put something in it because it is at counter height; also, you can easily see the progress of your food while it is cooking. All the recipes in this book that use the oven also can be made in a toaster oven, including Asparagus and Goat Cheese Tart (page 242). The best toaster ovens are incredibly accurate at regulating temperature, better than some traditional ovens. The rise of higher powered, function-clad, modern toaster ovens has paved the way for an appliance revitalization, with features like air-fry functions and touch-screen displays. Our winning toaster oven is the **Breville Smart Oven**.

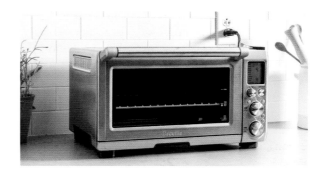

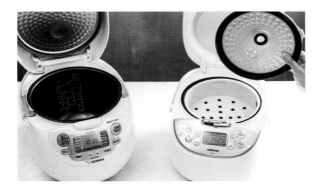

Rice Cooker
PERFECT RICE WITH THE PUSH OF A BUTTON

If you use a rice cooker, it's one more element of a meal that you can just check off your list and not think about until it's time to scoop up portions of perfectly steamed white or brown rice (and you can also use it to make quinoa and other grains). And rice cookers are inexpensive, too, so there is no reason not to add one to your arsenal of appliances that make cooking more convenient. We found two models that make exceptional rice and are also easy to use and clean. The **Zojirushi 5.5-Cup Neuro Fuzzy Rice Cooker & Warmer** is our top performer, followed closely by the **Toshiba 6-Cup Rice Cooker with Fuzzy Logic**.

Immersion Blender
THE FASTEST, EASIEST WAY TO PUREE

A standard blender is large, the glass jar makes it heavy, and it is hard to clean. Not to mention that if you are pureeing a soup, for instance, you have to get the soup into and out of the blender in batches. In short, using it requires multiple steps and a fair amount of lifting. The solution to all this work is an immersion blender. You can use it right in your pot, no transferring of hot liquids needed. It is compact and easy to store as well. We use it for multiple soups like Cauliflower Soup (page 144). And it has many uses beyond blending soups, such as blending frozen fruit for smoothies and even emulsifying mayonnaise or whipping egg whites or cream. You can also pulverize raw ingredients like frozen corn, as we do in Easy Corn Chowder with Bacon (page 151). Our winner, the **Braun MultiQuick 5 Hand Blender**, is lightweight and compact.

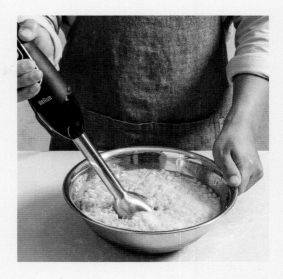

TIPS FOR USING AN IMMERSION BLENDER

1   Make sure the vessel you are using— whether it is a pot, saucepan, or bowl—is deep enough to use the blender properly and without splattering.

2   Keep the tip of the blender covered by at least an inch. Make sure the tip is not hitting the bottom of the vessel itself. Don't try to blend tiny amounts of ingredients.

3   Start blending on the slowest speed to first break up any large pieces and then switch to a higher speed to fully blend. Blending with too much force at the start can cause bits of ingredients to clog the blender mechanism. Keep the blender stick at an angle rather than straight up and down and move it around the vessel to blend efficiently.

4   If you are whipping cream or egg whites or making mayonnaise, move the blender around constantly to introduce air to provide lift.

5   Wash the blender by hand to preserve the sharpness of the blade.

Make Shopping Easier and More Pleasurable

Sometimes, if your pain is stealing your energy and motivation, using food shopping as a reason to get out of the house and to be active can be the jump start you need to get back on track. Whether it's a visit to your local supermarket or a chance to be outdoors at a local farmers' market, just being out in the world and accomplishing something practical is life affirming. If you're having a hard time getting started, remember something I always stress with my patients: Your pain is real. Pain is not just in your head, and it's not your fault. Everyone has pain at some point in their life, whether they want to admit it or not. When facing pain, remember to control what is controllable and let go of the rest. Living with pain requires compromises and new strategies, and this is especially true of shopping and cooking. Try some of these strategies and they will no doubt lessen the amount of time you need to spend walking around a grocery store and will limit the amount of heavy lifting on any given trip. You'll be less exhausted by the entire process and motivated to keep cooking.

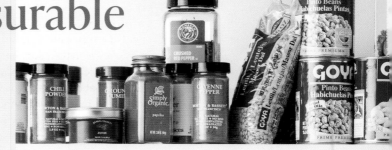

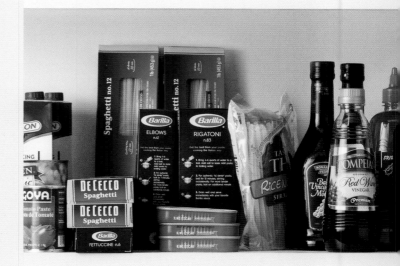

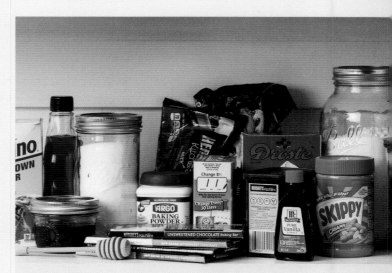

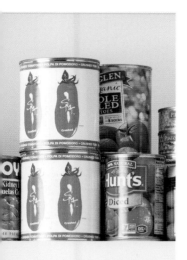

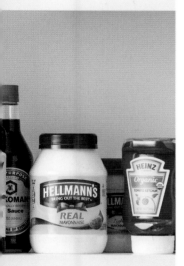

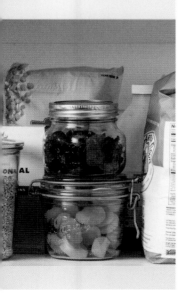

Buy Nonperishable Items Online

Nonperishables are generally heavy, and lugging them around is just not ideal. Plus, when you are in the store you should be focusing on picking out your own produce and meat because that is where a discerning eye really counts. And because nonperishable foods are easy to order reliably from various online sources or grocery stores that deliver, you can stock up, saving money and ensuring that you have a ready supply for those times when you don't feel like shopping.

Plan at Least Four Meals in Advance

A little careful planning will allow you to shop efficiently and minimize making multiple trips to the store. Aim to go to the store only once a week. Always have a back-pocket recipe in mind in the event the store doesn't have the cut of meat or a special ingredient you need for one of the meals you have planned.

Make a List and Shop Your Pantry First

A list is a great way to stay focused in the store, and if you check your pantry and fridge first, you won't spend time buying things you already have. If you have a solid list (and stick to it), you will spend vastly less time walking around the store thinking about what you might want to make and what you need to make it. A list will make you an efficient shopper.

Shop the Perimeter of the Store

If you keep your pantry stocked with nonperishable items, it will limit the need to walk up and down every aisle and allow you to focus instead on shopping the meat and fish counters and the produce section.

Unpack Carefully

No one likes unpacking and putting away a load of groceries, and if your back is compromised, it pays to be careful. Repetitive movements can be a pain trigger, so try to get all of your bags at a comfortable height on the counter or on your rolling cart so that you can get the ingredients organized and have to go into cabinets or the refrigerator only once or twice instead of over and over. Just as you might organize the ingredients before you start cooking, try to do the same when you are unpacking your groceries. If you have many nonperishable items like cans or boxes, load them onto your cart and wheel them to the pantry instead of lifting and carrying them one by one. The same applies to heavy refrigerated items like milk; load them up on your cart and roll it over to the fridge. Your back will thank you.

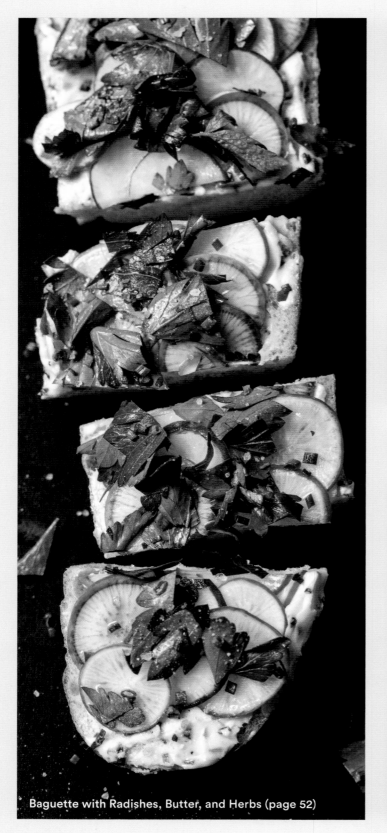

Baguette with Radishes, Butter, and Herbs (page 52)

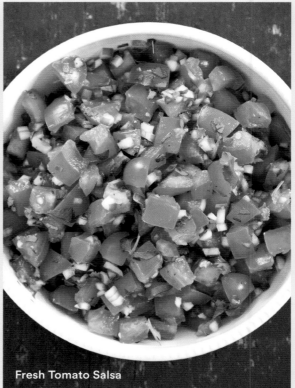

Fresh Tomato Salsa

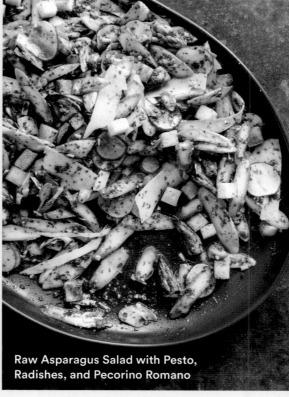

Raw Asparagus Salad with Pesto, Radishes, and Pecorino Romano

Get Inspired by the Produce at the Farmers' Market

I encourage my patients to keep moving and to get out of the house. And going to a local farmers' market is a great way to be outside, do a little walking, and buy some height-of-the-season produce. The freshness and colors of the ingredients are spectacular (and their flavors unbeatable). Even a simple ingredient like a gorgeous bunch of golden beets or the best looking heirloom tomatoes you've ever seen can be the inspiration for a meal. Many of these markets are in a park, so you will have the opportunity to sit down and rest when you need to and enjoy the scenery and the people watching. Here are some recipes to inspire you to visit a farmers' market soon.

Fresh Tomato Salsa

Makes about 3 cups

Place 1½ pounds chopped tomatoes in colander set over large bowl; layer ½ cup finely chopped red onion, ¼ cup chopped cilantro, 1 minced jalapeño, and 1 small minced garlic clove on top and let drain 30 minutes. Shake colander to drain excess juice. Discard juice, wipe out bowl, and transfer tomato mixture to bowl. Stir in 2 teaspoons lime juice, ½ teaspoon table salt, and pinch pepper. Season with sugar and extra lime juice to taste before serving.

Simple Tomato Salad with Capers and Parsley

Serves 4 to 6

Arrange 1½ pounds sliced tomatoes on large, shallow platter. Whisk 3 tablespoons extra-virgin olive oil, 1 tablespoon minced shallot, 1 tablespoon capers, 1 minced anchovy fillet, 1 teaspoon lemon juice, ½ teaspoon table salt, ¼ teaspoon pepper, and ⅛ teaspoon red pepper flakes together in bowl. Spoon dressing over tomatoes. Sprinkle with 1 tablespoon minced fresh parsley. Serve immediately.

Peach and Cucumber Salad with Mint

Serves 4 to 6

Combine 1½ tablespoons fish sauce, 1½ tablespoons sugar, 1 tablespoon grated lime zest and 3 tablespoons lime juice, 1½ teaspoons chili-garlic sauce, and 1½ teaspoons grated fresh ginger in large bowl. Add 1½ pounds chopped peaches, 1 thinly sliced cucumber, ½ cup chopped fresh mint, and 1 thinly sliced shallot and toss to combine. Let sit for 5 minutes so that flavors meld.

Raw Asparagus Salad with Pesto, Radishes, and Pecorino Romano

Serves 4 to 6

Cut tips from 2 pounds trimmed asparagus and slice spears ⅛ inch thick on bias. Add asparagus tips and spears, 5 thinly sliced radishes, and 2 ounces shaved Pecorino Romano cheese to ¾ cup Classic Basil Pesto (page 287) or store-bought pesto and toss to combine. Top with croutons, if desired. Season with salt and pepper to taste. Transfer salad to platter and serve.

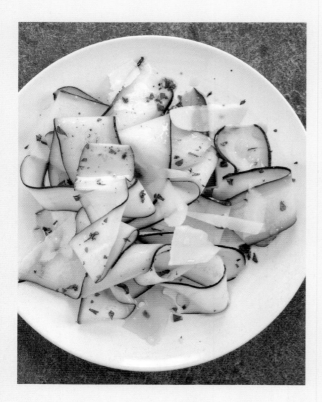

Zucchini Ribbon Salad with Shaved Parmesan

Serves 4 to 6

Using vegetable peeler, slice 3 (8-ounce) trimmed zucchini lengthwise into very thin ribbons. Gently toss zucchini ribbons in bowl with salt and pepper to taste, then arrange attractively on serving platter. Drizzle with ½ cup extra-virgin olive oil and ¼ cup lemon juice and sprinkle with 2 tablespoons minced fresh mint and 6 ounces shaved Parmesan.

Peach Caprese Salad with Raspberry Vinaigrette

Serves 4 to 6

Cut 1 pound ripe but slightly firm peaches into ½-inch wedges and toss with ¼ cup Raspberry Vinaigrette (page 85). Shingle peaches and 12 ounces fresh sliced mozzarella on serving platter. Drizzle any remaining dressing from bowl over top. Sprinkle with 6 torn basil or mint leaves. Season with salt and pepper to taste, and serve.

Baguette with Radishes, Butter, and Herbs

Serves 4 to 6 as an appetizer

Combine 5 tablespoons softened European-style unsalted butter, 2 tablespoons minced fresh chives, ⅛ teaspoon table salt, and ⅛ teaspoon pepper in bowl; set aside. Whisk 1 tablespoon minced fresh chives, ½ teaspoon lemon juice, and ½ teaspoon extra-virgin olive oil in second bowl. Add ½ cup coarsely chopped parsley and toss to coat. Season with salt and pepper to taste. Halve 1 (9-inch) baguette and spread butter mixture over cut sides. Shingle ½ cup thinly sliced radishes evenly over butter and top with parsley salad. Sprinkle with sea salt to taste. Cut baguette crosswise into 6 pieces.

Golden Beets with Tahini-Lemon Vinaigrette and Pepitas

Serves 4

Trim and peel 1½ pounds golden beets and cut into ½-inch pieces. Place in large bowl and sprinkle with ⅛ teaspoon table salt and pinch pepper. Microwave, covered, until tender, about 4 minutes; drain. Toss beets with ¼ cup Tahini-Lemon Dressing (page 85), top with ¼ cup toasted pepitas, and serve.

Green and Yellow Bean Salad with Sherry-Shallot Vinaigrette

Serves 4 to 6

Bring 2 quarts water to boil in large saucepan. Add 12 ounces trimmed green beans, 12 ounces trimmed yellow wax beans, and 2 teaspoons table salt and cook until beans are crisp-tender, about 5 minutes. Drain beans, add to bowl with ½ cup Make-Ahead Sherry-Shallot Vinaigrette (page 84) and 2 teaspoons minced fresh tarragon, and toss to combine. Refrigerate for at least 30 minutes or up to 3 days. Season with salt and pepper to taste. Serve cold or at room temperature.

Blistered Shishito Peppers with Chipotle Mayonnaise

Serves 4 as an appetizer

Heat 2 tablespoons vegetable oil in 12-inch skillet over medium-high heat until just smoking. Add 8 ounces shishito peppers and cook, without stirring, until skins are blistered, about 4 minutes. Using tongs, flip peppers and continue to cook until blistered on second side, about 4 minutes. Transfer to serving bowl and season with kosher salt to taste. Serve with Chipotle Mayonnaise (page 186) or lemon wedges.

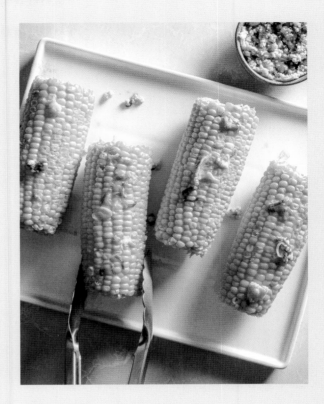

Steamed Corn with Miso-Honey Butter

Serves 4

Whip 3 tablespoons softened unsalted butter in bowl with fork until light and fluffy. Mix in 2 sliced scallions, 1 tablespoon honey, 1 tablespoon white miso, and 1 teaspoon soy sauce and season with salt and pepper to taste. Cover with plastic wrap and let rest so flavors meld, about 10 minutes, or roll into log and refrigerate. Meanwhile, set a steamer basket in a large pot with about 1 inch water. Bring to boil; carefully place 4 silked and husked ears of corn in basket. Cover and steam over high heat until tender, 7 to 10 minutes. Remove from basket with tongs and serve immediately with miso-honey butter.

Skillet-Roasted Sugar Snap Peas with Soy Sauce and Sesame Seeds

Serves 4

Heat 1 tablespoon vegetable oil in 12-inch skillet over high heat until shimmering. Add 1 pound trimmed sugar snap peas in single layer and cook, without stirring, for 30 seconds. Toss snap peas and spread into single layer. Continue to cook, tossing every 30 seconds, until snap peas are spotty brown and crisp-tender, 2 to 3 minutes. Add 1 minced garlic clove and cook, stirring constantly, until fragrant, about 30 seconds. Add 1 tablespoon soy sauce and cook until all liquid has evaporated, about 30 seconds. Off heat, add toasted sesame seeds, toss to combine, and serve.

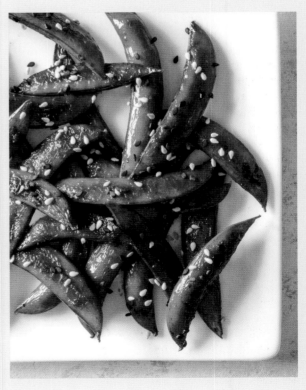

Keep Entertaining Simple and Enjoy It

Two of my core principles are to establish a routine and to be resilient, which can be hard to do. Your normal activities tend to go by the wayside when back pain or post-surgical recovery is in the picture. The key is to be resilient and to make adjustments along the way using new strategies (like shopping more efficiently and focusing on prepping ahead) and streamlined recipes. Spending time with family and friends is surely one of the most energizing activities there is, and cooking is one of the best ways to make this a routine. Another principle I talk about is the importance of giving and receiving, and of helping and serving others (literally, by preparing an amazing meal); this will bring you pain relief, happiness, and the resilience to keep going in the face of daily pain and disability. It's only natural that if you are having back problems you may be hesitant about entertaining. Here are some tips to entertain with ease without hurting your back.

BE STRATEGIC ABOUT YOUR MENU

The goal is to keep your menu simple. First, choose your main course and aim for either a fully make-ahead main course, such as Oven-Poached Side of Salmon (page 116), or a stew or a braise that will taste even better if made a day ahead, such as Slow-Cooker Brisket and Onions (page 106). Alternatively, choose a recipe that once prepped can be cooked quickly, such as Instant Pot Creamy Spring Vegetable Linguine (page 131). Avoid a menu where everything is on the stovetop at once and requires monitoring. Choose a simple side dish and an easy but elegant side salad.

DON'T STRESS OVER APPETIZERS

Buy the ingredients for a beautiful cheese and charcuterie board and round it out with nuts and fresh fruit. Let your imagination guide you here. With a beautiful wooden board and an array of fine cheeses and other ingredients, you can make a beautiful presentation. Everyone will be happy.

USE CONVENIENCE APPLIANCES TO YOUR ADVANTAGE

The Instant Pot, slow cooker, and air fryer can reduce the amount of time you need to stand at the stove. While your main course is in the oven or on the stovetop, use your slow cooker to make elegant and normally complex sides like risotto or polenta (pages 282–283); or use your air fryer to turn out perfectly cooked vegetables (pages 278–281). If you are making a simple curry or stir fry, make perfect rice in a rice cooker; it will stay warm while you are busy with everything else. And throughout the book you will find recipes making the most of an Instant Pot or slow cooker for hearty and company-worthy main courses.

SHARE THE WORK

Ask a family member or friend to help you with the prep work if you are feeling overwhelmed. Or ask someone coming to the gathering to make a side dish or a salad.

ORGANIZE YOUR HOUSE AND SET THE TABLE THE NIGHT BEFORE

There is no reason to wait until the last minute to get your living room in tip-top shape and your table set and dishes and platters organized. The dining room isn't the only place you can get a jump start on getting ready. You could even work on some of the ingredient prep or set out your tools and get your prep station ready. Check out some of the ways a rolling prep cart can help you get organized in the kitchen (see page 20).

KEEP SERVING SIMPLE (AND EASY ON YOUR BACK)

Whether you are entertaining or simply making dinner for your family, you need serving platters and bowls, and they can be heavy both to carry and to wash— not to mention hard to get into and out of a cabinet. A great alternative is melamine dishware. It is very popular now and quite beautiful (and inexpensive). And maybe rethink plating individual servings: Consider using serving dishes and letting each guest serve themself. Alternatively, repurpose your rolling cart to provide serving and plating tableside.

BE COMPASSIONATE ABOUT CLEARING AND CLEANING

After the meal, don't feel rushed to get everything cleared and cleaned before moving on to dessert or coffee. Your guests will likely be more than happy to bring their plates to the sink, which you could prefill with some hot water and dish soap to get a head start on the cleaning process. It will then be easy to load in the partially cleaned dishes and let the magic of the dishwasher do its thing. Alternatively, there is no rule that all the dishes have to be clean and put away. Feel free to let them soak overnight in the sink, and come back to tackle them in the morning, when you might have more energy, less pain, and more motivation. Remember, be compassionately imperfect. Go easy on yourself. Your guests won't know if the dishes were cleaned before bed, and they've likely been impressed by your meal and the fact that you did it all while suffering with pain.

EASY MENUS FOR ENTERTAINING

Many of these recipes have prep-ahead elements that make them perfect if you are entertaining because you can spread out the work and take breaks when you need to. Feel free to round out these menus with good crusty bread and a store-bought dessert.

- Easy Food-Processor Gazpacho (page 143) — *Serves 4*
- Arugula Salad with Steak Tips and Gorgonzola (page 64)

- Instant Pot Chicken Tagine (page 91) — *Serves 4 to 6*
- Couscous with Curry and Mint (page 260)

- Oven-Poached Side of Salmon with Fresh Tomato Relish (pages 116–117) — *Serves 8*
- Barley Salad with Pomegranate, Pistachios, and Feta (page 80)

- Air-Fryer Hoisin-Glazed Salmon (page 250); *recipe doubled* — *Serves 4*
- Braised Red Potatoes with Miso and Scallions (page 277)
- Simplest Green Salad (page 82)

- Stir-Fried Eggplant in Garlic-Basil Sauce (page 208) — *Serves 4*
- Sesame Sushi Rice (page 256)

- Marmalade-Glazed Pork Loin (page 111) — *Serves 4 to 6*
- Slow-Cooker Creamy Polenta (page 282)
- Radicchio, Endive, and Arugula Salad (page 83)

- Caramelized Black Pepper Chicken (page 173) — *Serves 4*
- Simple White Rice (page 255)

- Pork Tenderloin Stroganoff (page 112) — *Serves 4*
- Pan-Steamed Asparagus with Garlic (page 267)

Salad for Dinner

* Try these recipes first if today is not one of your better days and you need a soul-refilling meal with high return on your energy investment.

Blue Cheese, Walnut, and Chicken Chopped Salad

SERVES 4 — SUPER EASY

- ¼ cup extra-virgin olive oil
- 2 ounces blue cheese or Gorgonzola cheese, crumbled (½ cup), divided
- 3 tablespoons sherry vinegar or red wine vinegar
- 3 cups shredded chicken
- 1 large head romaine lettuce (14 ounces), cut into 1-inch pieces
- 1 cup walnuts or pecans, toasted and chopped

Why This Recipe Works Good cheese is one of life's great luxuries, and the star of this salad is the cheese. This version delivers big blue cheese flavor and tender, moist chicken. As an added bonus, not counting the olive oil, it has only five ingredients, so you can whip it together in 15 minutes if you have the cooked chicken on hand. What is also great is that the dressing is infused with the sharp bite of blue cheese: Microwaving a little of the oil and the cheese melds the two ingredients just enough. Then, whisking in sherry vinegar adds all the brightness the vinaigrette needs. And there is enough cheese left to toss with the salad so everyone gets their fill. You can use rotisserie chicken for this recipe or make Perfect Poached Chicken (page 61) or Easy Slow-Cooker Poached Chicken (below).

1   Microwave oil and ¼ cup blue cheese in large bowl until cheese is softened, about 30 seconds. Whisk in vinegar until combined.

2   Add chicken, lettuce, walnuts, and remaining ¼ cup blue cheese to bowl and toss gently to combine. Season with salt and pepper to taste. Serve.

MAKE IT YOURSELF
Easy Slow-Cooker Poached Chicken
Makes 3 to 4 cups chopped or shredded chicken

- 4 (6- to 8-ounce) boneless, skinless chicken breasts, trimmed
- ½ teaspoon table salt
- ¼ teaspoon pepper
- ⅔ cup chicken broth
- 1 bay leaf

Sprinkle chicken with salt and pepper and place in slow cooker insert. Add broth and bay leaf, then cover and cook until chicken registers 160 degrees, 2 to 3 hours on low. Transfer chicken to cutting board and let cool slightly. Slice, chop, or shred as desired. (Chicken can be refrigerated for up to 2 days. Let come to room temperature before using in salads.)

PREP AHEAD
You can shred the chicken, crumble the blue cheese, and toast and chop the nuts 1 day ahead and refrigerate separately.

MAKE IT EVEN EASIER
Toast the nuts in the microwave (see page 37). Buy bagged chopped romaine or raid your market's salad bar for it.

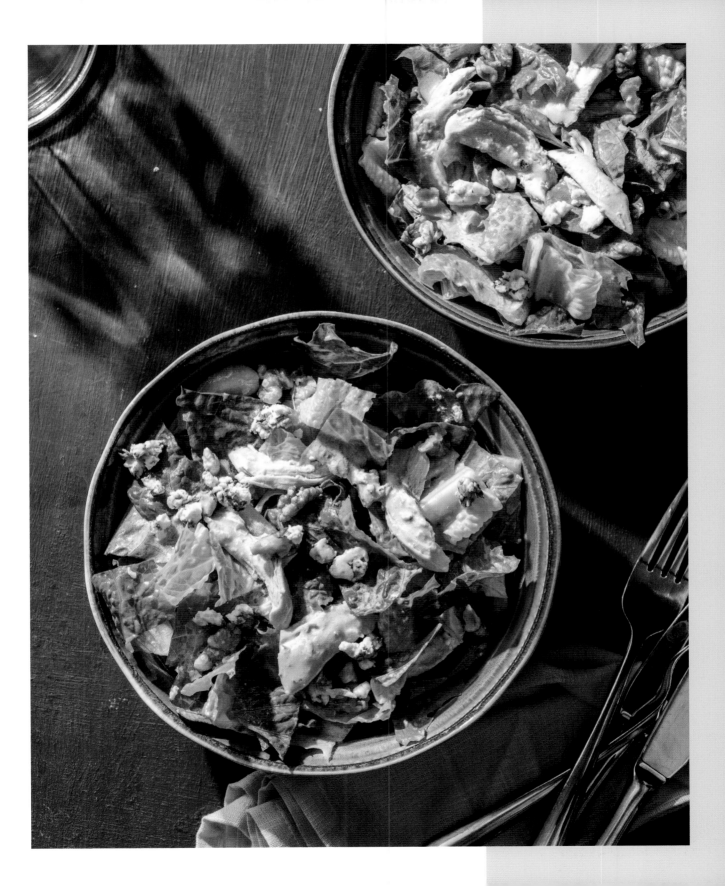

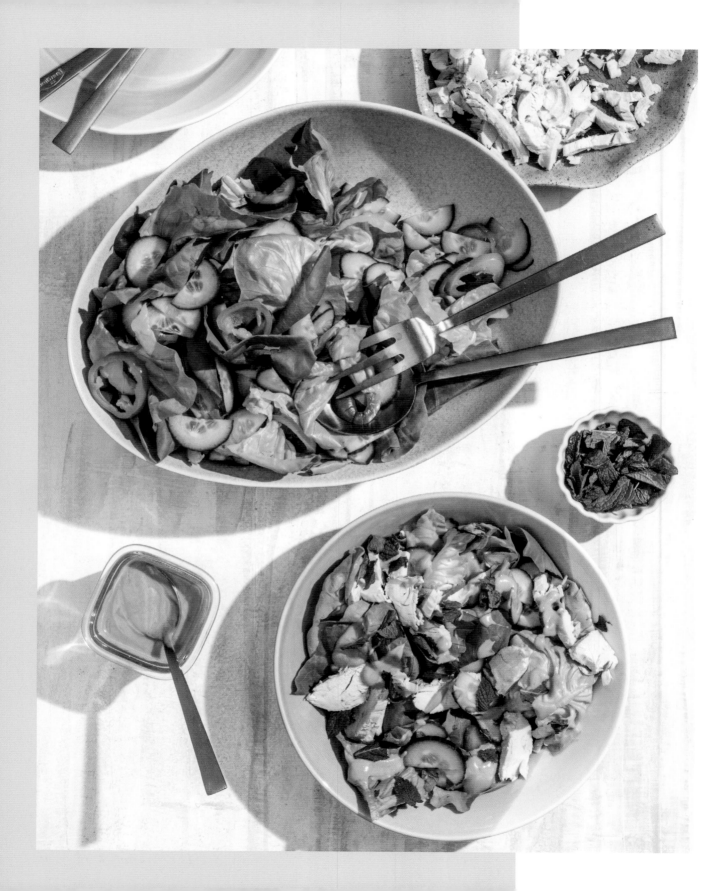

Bibb Lettuce and Chicken Salad with Peanut Dressing

SERVES 4 — SUPER EASY

Why This Recipe Works Tender Bibb lettuce and sliced chicken reach new heights with an easy-to-assemble and aromatic peanut dressing. Flavorings often seen in Thai cooking, from fish sauce and mint to rice vinegar and hot peppers, are the inspiration for this salad. Tossing these with Bibb lettuce, cucumber, and chicken in a peanut dressing creates a salad that is more than the sum of its parts. You can use rotisserie chicken for this recipe or make Perfect Poached Chicken (below), or Easy Slow-Cooker Poached Chicken (page 58).

1 For the Peanut Dressing Combine vinegar, peanut butter, and fish sauce in bowl. Microwave until peanut butter has just softened, about 15 seconds. Add oil and whisk until smooth and fully combined.

2 For the Salad Toss lettuce, cucumber, cherry peppers, and 3 tablespoons vinaigrette together in large bowl. Divide salad among 4 individual plates. Serve, topping individual portions with chicken. Drizzle with remaining vinaigrette and sprinkle with mint.

MAKE IT YOURSELF
Perfect Poached Chicken
Makes 3 to 4 cups shredded or chopped chicken

- 4 (6- to 8-ounce) boneless, skinless chicken breasts, trimmed
  Table salt for cooking chicken

1 Whisk 4 quarts cool water with 2 tablespoons salt in Dutch oven. Arrange chicken in steamer basket without overlapping. Submerge basket in pot. Heat over medium heat, stirring occasionally, until water registers 175 degrees, about 20 minutes.

2 Turn off heat, cover pot, remove from burner, and let sit until chicken registers 160 degrees, about 20 minutes. Transfer chicken to cutting board and let cool for 10 minutes. Slice, chop, or shred as desired. Serve. (Chicken can be refrigerated for up to 2 days. Let come to room temperature before using in salads.)

Peanut Dressing

- ¼ cup seasoned rice vinegar
- 3 tablespoons creamy peanut butter
- 1½ tablespoons fish sauce
- ¼ cup vegetable oil

Salad

- 2 heads Bibb or Boston lettuce (1 pound), leaves separated and torn into pieces
- 1 English cucumber, cut in half lengthwise then sliced thin
- ¼ cup thinly sliced jarred hot cherry peppers
- 1½ pounds cooked chicken, sliced thin
- ¼ cup fresh mint or cilantro leaves, torn

PREP AHEAD
You can slice the chicken, cucumber, and cherry peppers up to 2 days ahead and refrigerate separately. You can make the dressing up to 1 day ahead and refrigerate; bring to room temperature and whisk to recombine before using.

Zucchini Noodle Chicken Salad with Ginger and Garam Masala

SERVES 4

1 mango, peeled and cut into ¼-inch pieces

2 tablespoons chopped fresh cilantro or mint

2 teaspoons lemon juice

2 tablespoons vegetable oil, divided

4 garlic cloves, minced

4 teaspoons garam masala, divided

2 teaspoons grated fresh ginger

½ teaspoon table salt, divided

½ teaspoon pepper, divided

4 cups ½-inch pieces cooked chicken

1½ pounds zucchini noodles, cut into 6-inch lengths, divided

Why This Recipe Works I always viewed zucchini noodles with a healthy dose of skepticism—until I tried them. They have become one of my go-to ways to sneak vegetables and a healthy element into my favorite recipes. So this easy recipe pairs quick-cooking zucchini noodles (no boiling or heavy pot required) and chopped cooked chicken. Since spiralized noodles are available everywhere, there is no need to get out a spiralizer, if you even have one. Garam masala (a North Indian spice blend that contains cumin, coriander, cinnamon, bay leaf, and black pepper), garlic, and ginger—seasonings traditionally used in North Indian meat dishes—give the chicken deep flavor. And for hardly any extra work you can make an Herb-Yogurt Sauce to evoke a cooling raita. For bright color and a bit of sweetness, I love the addition of small pieces of mango (which can be hard to cut up, so feel free to use frozen mango, which is widely available). Cooking the zucchini noodles in two batches ensures that they don't overcook and turn mushy. Do cook them to your desired level of doneness, but be careful not to overcook them. You can use rotisserie chicken for this recipe or make Perfect Poached Chicken (page 61) or Easy Slow-Cooker Poached Chicken (page 58).

1 Combine mango, cilantro, and lemon juice in bowl; season with salt and pepper to taste and set aside until ready to serve. Whisk 2 teaspoons oil, garlic, 2 teaspoons garam masala, ginger, ¼ teaspoon salt, and ¼ teaspoon pepper together in medium bowl, then add chicken and toss to coat.

2 Heat 2 teaspoons oil in 12-inch nonstick skillet over medium-high heat until shimmering. Add 1 teaspoon garam masala, ⅛ teaspoon salt, ⅛ teaspoon pepper, and half of zucchini noodles and cook, tossing frequently, until crisp-tender, about 1 minute. Transfer to individual plates and repeat with remaining 2 teaspoons oil, remaining 1 teaspoon garam masala, remaining ⅛ teaspoon salt, remaining ⅛ teaspoon pepper, and remaining zucchini noodles. Top zucchini noodles with chicken and mango mixture. Serve.

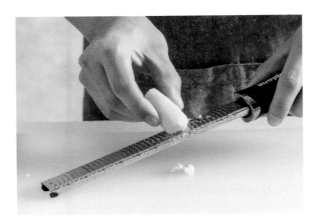

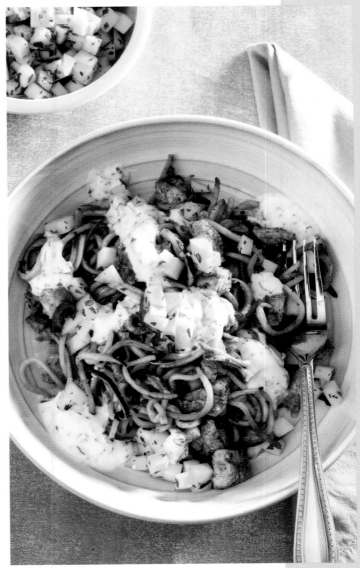

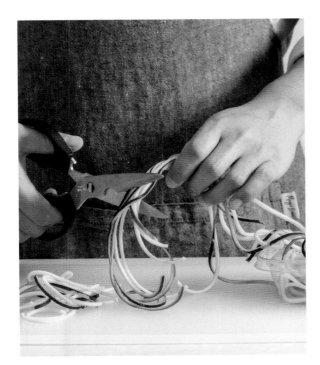

PREP AHEAD
You can cut up the chicken up to 2 days ahead and the mango up to 1 day ahead and refrigerate separately.

MAKE IT EVEN EASIER
You can use frozen mango chunks, thawed and cut into small pieces.

TAKE IT UP A NOTCH
Serve with Herb-Yogurt Sauce
Whisk 1 cup plain whole-milk yogurt; 1 teaspoon grated lemon zest; 2 tablespoons lemon juice; ¼ cup minced fresh cilantro, mint, or parsley; and 1 minced garlic clove together in bowl. Cover and refrigerate until flavors meld, at least 30 minutes. Season with salt and pepper to taste. Sauce can be refrigerated for up to 4 days. Makes 1 cup.

Arugula Salad with Steak Tips and Gorgonzola

SERVE 4

1 pound sirloin steak tips, trimmed

½ teaspoon table salt, divided

½ teaspoon pepper, divided

6 tablespoons extra-virgin olive oil, divided

1 shallot, minced

2 garlic cloves, minced

2 tablespoons cider vinegar

1 teaspoon Dijon mustard

1 teaspoon honey

12 ounces (12 cups) baby arugula

6 ounces Gorgonzola or blue cheese, crumbled (1½ cups)

PREP AHEAD
You can make the vinaigrette and crumble the Gorgonzola up to 1 day ahead and refrigerate separately. Bring the vinaigrette to room temperature and whisk to recombine before using. You can cook the steak tips up to 3 hours ahead and refrigerate. Bring to room temperature before using.

Why This Recipe Works When your brain is craving steak au poivre with pommes frites but your body needs a salad, this recipe is the perfect solution to satisfy brain, body, and soul. Dressing peppery arugula with a simple vinaigrette enlivened with blue cheese and then fortifying the salad with tender steak tips ensures a quick and elegant dinner salad when you don't have the energy to spend a lot of time in the kitchen. What makes this an easy entrée is that you can cook and refrigerate the steak tips up to three hours in advance. The supersimple vinaigrette features Dijon mustard to amp up the spiciness of the arugula, while cider vinegar and honey add a complementary fruity, sweet touch to the assertive greens. Sirloin steak tips, also known as flap meat, can be sold as whole steaks, cubes, and strips. To ensure uniform pieces, it is best to purchase whole steaks and cut them yourself after cooking. For optimal tenderness, make sure to slice the cooked steak against the grain (perpendicular to the fibers).

1   Pat steak dry with paper towels and sprinkle with ¼ teaspoon salt and ¼ teaspoon pepper. Heat 2 tablespoons oil in 12-inch nonstick skillet over medium-high heat until just smoking. Add steak and cook until well browned all over and beef registers 120 to 125 degrees (for medium-rare), about 9 minutes. Transfer to plate, tent with aluminum foil, and let rest for 15 minutes.

—   TAKE A 15-MINUTE BREAK   —

2   Whisk shallot, garlic, vinegar, mustard, honey, remaining ¼ teaspoon salt, and remaining ¼ teaspoon pepper together in large bowl. While whisking constantly, slowly drizzle in remaining ¼ cup oil until combined. Add arugula and Gorgonzola to vinaigrette and toss to combine. Season with salt and pepper to taste. Slice steak against grain ¼ inch thick. Divide salad among individual plates and top with sliced steak. Serve.

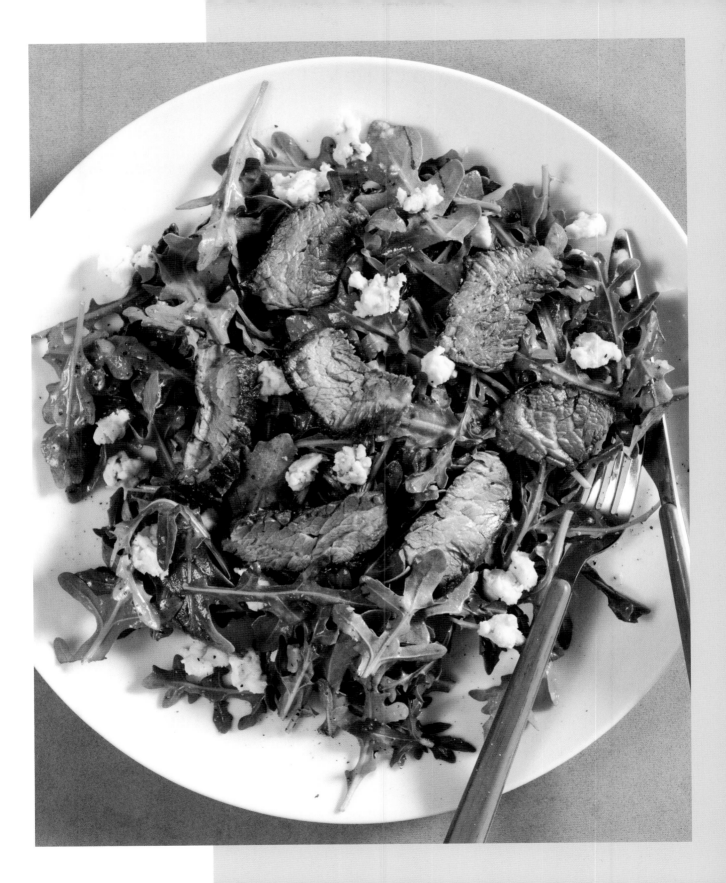

Chef's Salad with Turkey, Salami, and Asiago

SERVES 6 TO 8

2 heads romaine lettuce (1½ pounds), torn into bite-size pieces

4 ounces (4 cups) watercress, torn into 2-inch pieces, or baby arugula

½ cup torn basil leaves

9 ounces frozen artichokes, thawed and patted dry

½ cup Make-Ahead Balsamic-Fennel Vinaigrette (page 84)

8 ounces hard salami, cut into 2-inch-long matchsticks

8 ounces deli turkey, cut into 2-inch-long matchsticks

8 ounces Asiago cheese, crumbled (2 cups)

1½ cups croutons

½ cup pitted kalamata olives, chopped

Why This Recipe Works Whenever I'm out for lunch at a scientific meeting, my go-to is always the chef's salad. At home, you might think a chef's salad requires a huge amount of knife work and assembly time; but the truth is that with a little easy prep work, almost all of which can be done ahead, this salad comes together quickly. And since the prepped ingredients will keep for a day in your fridge, you can easily get a second meal out of the recipe with just a little last-minute work. For greens, sturdy romaine works best, but peppery watercress or baby arugula can also stand up to the strong flavors, so it's nice to add some to the mix. Thick slices of turkey and salami, and soft Asiago, complement the greens, and a make-ahead vinaigrette works with the rich components and will also give you enough left over for other salads during the week. For this salad, opt for a mild, soft Asiago cheese that crumbles easily; avoid aged Asiago that has a hard, dry texture. Frozen artichoke hearts are a convenient option, as they are usually already halved, but you can buy canned artichoke hearts packed in water and slice them yourself.

Gently toss romaine, watercress, basil, and artichokes with dressing in large serving bowl. Season with salt and pepper to taste. Arrange salami, turkey, and cheese over center of greens; top with croutons and olives. Serve immediately.

PREP AHEAD
You can prep all the ingredients (except the watercress and the basil) up to 1 day ahead and refrigerate separately. You can make the dressing up to a week ahead and refrigerate. Bring to room temperature and whisk or shake to recombine before using.

MAKE IT EVEN EASIER
Buy bagged chopped romaine or raid your market's salad bar for some.

TAKE IT UP A NOTCH
For additional color and flavor, add a cored and thinly sliced fennel bulb and a cup of jarred roasted red peppers, rinsed, dried, and sliced crosswise into ½-inch pieces. Toss them with an additional tablespoon of the vinaigrette and arrange around the perimeter of the salad.

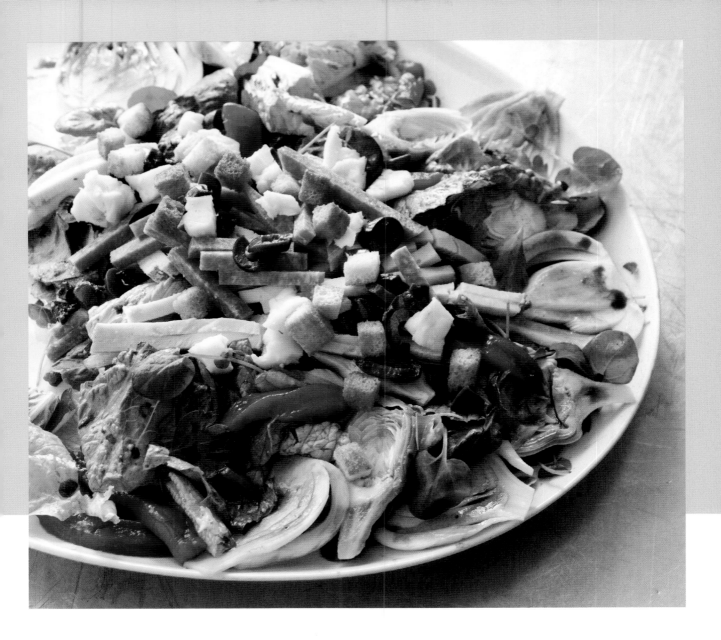

MAKE IT YOURSELF

Homemade Garlic Croutons

Preheat oven to 350 degrees. Combine 3 tablespoons extra-virgin olive oil, 3 minced garlic cloves, and ¼ teaspoon table salt in small bowl; let stand 20 minutes, then pour through fine-mesh strainer into medium bowl. Discard garlic. Add 3 cups fresh bread cubes to bowl with oil and toss to coat. Spread bread cubes in even layer on two small rimmed baking sheets and bake, on middle rack, stirring occasionally, until golden, about 15 minutes. Cool on baking sheets to room temperature. Croutons can be stored in an airtight container for up to 2 days. Makes about 3 cups. Note that you need only 1½ cups croutons for this salad.

Lemony Salmon and Roasted Beet Salad

SERVES 4

3 (6 to 8-ounce) skin-on salmon fillets, 1 to ½ inches thick

½ teaspoon plus ⅛ teaspoon table salt, divided

¼ teaspoon plus pinch pepper, divided

1 teaspoon grated lemon zest plus 7 tablespoons juice (3 lemons), divided

½ pound beets, trimmed, peeled, and cut into ½-inch pieces

⅓ cup extra-virgin olive oil

1 shallot, minced

2 tablespoons capers, rinsed

3 tablespoons minced fresh dill or parsley, divided

2 ounces (6 cups) baby arugula

2 hard-cooked eggs, grated

Why This Recipe Works I have to give credit to my mother-in-law for introducing me to the magic of beets. The sweet, earthy flavor of roasted beets is especially nice when paired with rich salmon and a bright lemon-caper dressing. But roasting beets in the oven takes an hour, so here the beets are peeled and cut and then "roasted" in the microwave, which reduces their cooking time to just 4 minutes. Poaching the salmon fillets in barely simmering water is the key to fish that is moist and perfectly cooked. Taking the time to dress each ingredient of this composed salad separately ensures that it is properly seasoned. I recommend using a handheld citrus juicer (see page 35), as it requires a lot less effort to extract juice than glass or metal citrus juicers.

1   Pat salmon dry with paper towels and sprinkle with ½ teaspoon salt and ¼ teaspoon pepper. Bring 4 cups water to boil in 12-inch skillet. Add ¼ cup lemon juice, reduce heat to medium-low, and gently slip salmon into water. Cover and simmer until center is still translucent when checked with tip of paring knife and salmon registers 125 degrees (for medium-rare), 4 to 6 minutes. Transfer salmon to plate. Using 2 forks, flake salmon into 1-inch pieces. Transfer to medium bowl and cover with foil.

—   **TAKE A 20-MINUTE BREAK**   —

2   Place beets in second medium bowl, sprinkle with remaining ⅛ teaspoon salt and remaining pinch pepper and add 1 tablespoon water. Microwave, covered, until tender, about 4 minutes.

3   Meanwhile, for dressing, whisk oil, shallot, capers, 1 tablespoon dill, and lemon zest and remaining 3 tablespoons juice together in large bowl.

4   Add 2 tablespoons dressing to bowl with beets, toss to combine, and let cool slightly. Add 2 tablespoons dressing to bowl with salmon and toss gently to combine. Add arugula to bowl with remaining dressing and toss to coat; season with salt and pepper to taste. Arrange arugula on serving platter or individual plates and top with eggs, salmon, beets, and remaining 2 tablespoons dill. Serve.

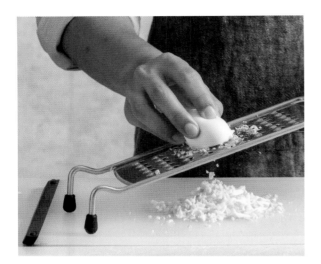

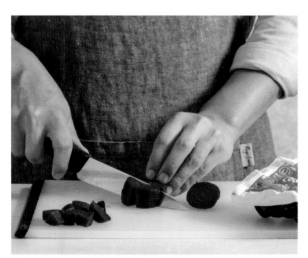

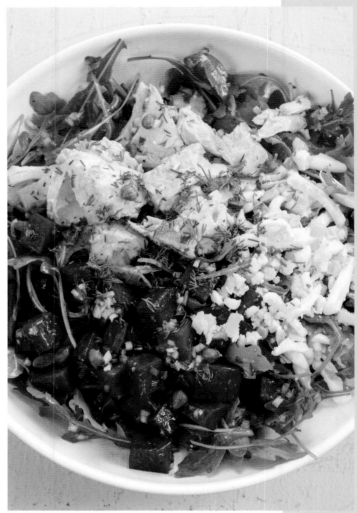

Easy-Peel Hard-Cooked Eggs
Makes 2 to 6 eggs

Bring 1 inch water to rolling boil in medium saucepan over high heat. Place 2 to 6 large eggs in steamer basket. Transfer basket to saucepan. Cover, reduce heat to medium-low, and cook eggs for 13 minutes. When eggs are almost finished cooking, combine 2 cups ice cubes and 2 cups cold water in medium bowl. Using tongs or spoon, transfer eggs to ice bath; let sit for 15 minutes. Peel before serving. Eggs can be refrigerated in their shells in airtight container for up to 5 days.

MAKE IT EVEN EASIER
Buy vacuum-sealed cooked beets, hard-boiled eggs, and cooked salmon. Most stores sell hard-boiled eggs in the refrigerated section, but you can often find them in salad bars too.

PREP AHEAD
You can poach the salmon and microwave the beets and refrigerate separately up to 1 day ahead. You can make the dressing up to 1 day ahead and refrigerate; bring to room temperature and whisk to recombine before using.

Smoked Salmon Niçoise Salad

SERVES 4

Dressing

- ⅔ cup sour cream or plain Greek yogurt
- 2 tablespoons lemon juice
- 2 tablespoons water
- 1 tablespoon chopped fresh dill or parsley
- ¼ teaspoon table salt
- ⅛ teaspoon pepper

Salad

- 1 pound small red potatoes, unpeeled, halved

  Table salt for cooking vegetables
- 8 ounces green beans, trimmed
- 10 ounces (10 cups) mesclun greens
- 4 hard-boiled eggs (page 69), halved
- 8 ounces sliced smoked salmon
- ½ cup pitted olives, halved

Why This Recipe Works In my dreams, I spend six months eating my way through the French countryside. When my mind snaps back to reality, I'm on the hunt for a classic French salad to enjoy, and it is almost always a niçoise salad from my local bistro. Here is a great no-fuss way to make this salad at home that bypasses the traditional process of cooking each component separately. Using rich, flavorful smoked salmon keeps things easy—no need stand at the stove poaching fresh salmon. The dressing has a nice twist, as it features sour cream and dill, ingredients traditionally paired with smoked salmon, which give the salad a certain richness. But the beloved salade niçoise ingredients are still here: hard-boiled eggs, green beans, potatoes, and olives. To save on effort, the vegetables cook together in a single pot of water, starting with the potatoes and then the green beans later, ensuring that both finish cooking at the same time. Small red potatoes are easy to prep and perfect here. For even cooking, use potatoes measuring 1 to 2 inches in diameter.

1   For the Dressing Combine sour cream, lemon juice, water, dill, salt, and pepper in small bowl.

2   For the Salad Bring 2 quarts water to boil in large saucepan over medium-high heat. Add potatoes and 1½ tablespoons salt; return to boil and cook for 10 minutes.

— TAKE A 10-MINUTE BREAK —

3   Add green beans to boiling water and continue to cook until both vegetables are tender, about 4 minutes. Drain.

4   Toss mesclun and ¼ cup dressing together in large bowl. Divide dressed mesclun, potatoes, green beans, and eggs evenly among individual plates. Top each portion with salmon and olives. Drizzle salads with remaining dressing. Serve.

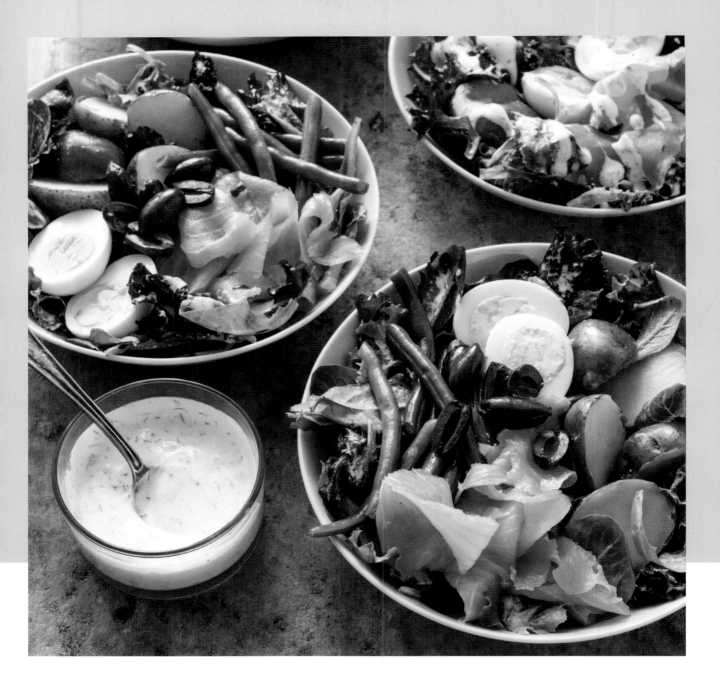

PREP AHEAD

You can make the dressing and refrigerate it for up to 4 days. Bring to room temperature and whisk to recombine before using. You can halve the potatoes up to 1 day ahead and refrigerate stored in a bowl covered with water. You can also halve the olives and refrigerate for up to 1 day ahead.

MAKE IT EVEN EASIER

Buy hard-boiled eggs. Most stores sell them in the refrigerated section, and you can often find them in salad bars too. Buy bagged trimmed green beans.

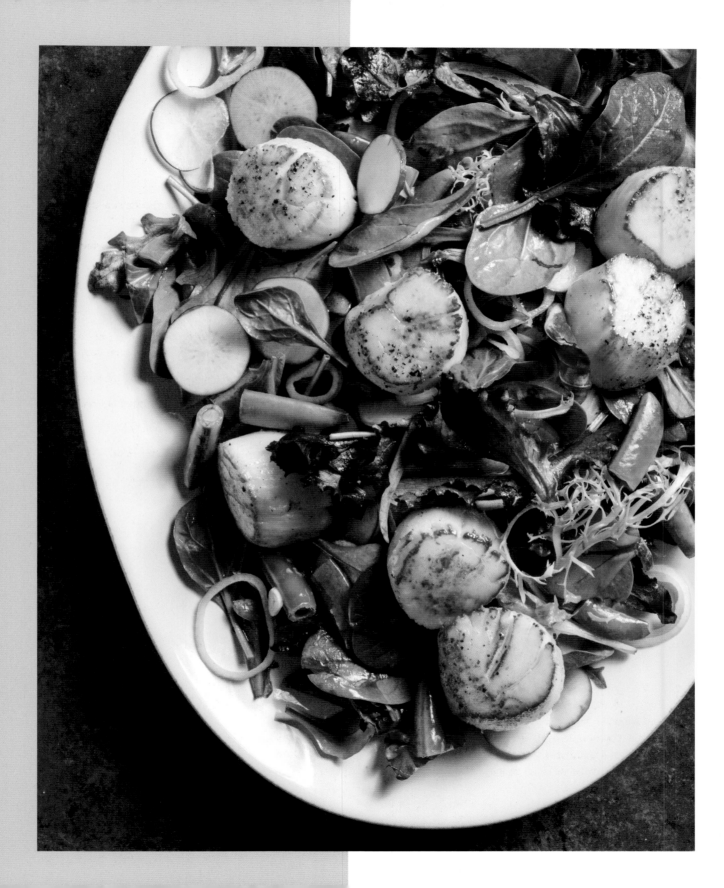

Seared Scallop Salad with Snap Peas and Radishes

SERVES 2

Why This Recipe Works Seafood is a great protein option for healthy, fast dinners, but it's easy to get trapped in the salmon, white fish, shrimp, and repeat cycle of meal planning. Scallops are the perfect way to shake up your rotation and are supereasy to prepare. If all your ingredients are prepped in advance, this elegant salad can be on the table in 10 minutes flat. Sandwiching the scallops between paper towels and letting them drain for 10 minutes before cooking rids them of excess moisture that would prevent them from developing a burnished crust in the skillet. Once they are ready to cook, just season them with salt and pepper and sear them in a hot skillet for a few minutes, until their centers are just opaque and their exteriors are well browned and flavorful. For the salad, simply toss delicate mesclun greens; fresh sugar snap peas; and thinly sliced, peppery radishes with an easy vinaigrette and arrange the scallops on top. Be sure to buy "dry" scallops, which don't have chemical additives and taste better than "wet." Dry scallops will look ivory or pinkish; wet scallops are bright white.

1   Place scallops on large plate lined with paper towels. Place paper towels on top of scallops and press gently to blot liquid. Let scallops sit at room temperature for 10 minutes while towels absorb moisture.

— TAKE A 10-MINUTE BREAK —

2   Combine vinegar and mustard in large bowl. Whisking constantly, drizzle 2 tablespoons oil into vinegar mixture in slow, steady stream. Add snap peas, mesclun, radishes, and shallot and toss gently to coat. Season with salt and pepper to taste. Divide salad among individual plates or transfer to serving platter.

3   Sprinkle scallops with salt and pepper. Heat remaining 1 tablespoon oil in 12-inch nonstick skillet over high heat until just smoking. Add scallops in single layer, flat side down, and cook, without moving, until well browned, 1½ to 2 minutes. Flip scallops and continue to cook until sides of scallops are firm and centers are opaque, 30 to 90 seconds (remove smaller scallops as they finish cooking). Arrange scallops over salad. Serve.

12 ounces large sea scallops, tendons removed

 1 tablespoon red wine vinegar

 ½ teaspoon Dijon mustard

 3 tablespoons extra-virgin olive oil, divided

 6 ounces sugar snap peas, strings removed, halved crosswise

 4 ounces (4 cups) mesclun

 4 radishes, trimmed and sliced thin

 1 shallot, sliced thin

 ¼ teaspoon table salt

 ⅛ teaspoon pepper

MAKE IT EVEN EASIER
Buy trimmed snap peas and trimmed and sliced radishes.

Warm Spiced Pearl Couscous Salad with Chorizo

SERVES 4

2 cups pearl couscous

12 ounces Spanish-style chorizo sausage, cut into ½-inch pieces

4 carrots, peeled and chopped

5 tablespoons extra-virgin olive oil, divided

½ teaspoon table salt

2⅔ cups chicken or vegetable broth

2 teaspoons smoked paprika

1 teaspoon ground cumin

2 (15-ounce) cans chickpeas, rinsed and patted dry

1⅓ cups chopped fresh parsley or cilantro

1 cup raisins, chopped dried apricots, chopped dates, or chopped dried figs

2½ tablespoons lemon juice, plus lemon wedges for serving

Why This Recipe Works I'm a big fan of Spanish chorizo, a highly seasoned and cured smoked sausage, because it adds complexity and bold flavor to any dish it is used in. And that is exactly the case in this hearty make-ahead salad. As an added bonus, with the exception of the chorizo, you likely have most of the ingredients in your pantry. The first step is to toast pearl couscous with the chorizo and carrots and then simmer them in broth seasoned with smoked paprika and cumin (for even more smoky flavor). Canned chickpeas add heft, and parsley delivers freshness. Dried fruit gives additional textural contrast and a hint of sweetness, while a squeeze of lemon juice brightens up this gorgeous entrée salad. Do not substitute regular couscous, as it requires a different cooking method and will not work in this recipe.

1 Combine couscous, chorizo, carrots, 1 tablespoon oil, and salt in large saucepan and cook over medium heat, stirring frequently, until half of grains are golden, about 5 minutes. Stir in broth, paprika, and cumin and bring to simmer. Cover and cook over low heat until broth is absorbed and couscous is tender, about 18 minutes.

— TAKE AN 18-MINUTE BREAK —

2 Let couscous sit off heat, covered, for 5 minutes. Stir in chickpeas, parsley, raisins, lemon juice, and remaining ¼ cup oil. Season with salt and pepper to taste. Serve with lemon wedges.

PREP AHEAD
You can peel and chop the carrots and cut up the chorizo and dried fruit up to 1 day ahead and refrigerate separately. You can make the salad and refrigerate it for up to 2 days.

MAKE IT EVEN EASIER
Buy shredded carrots instead of chopping your own.

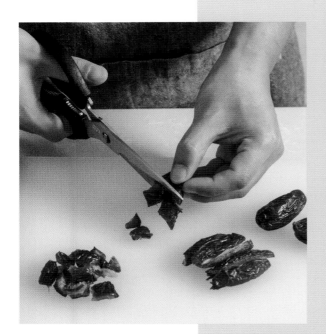

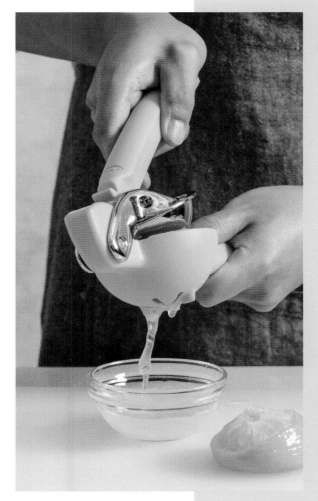

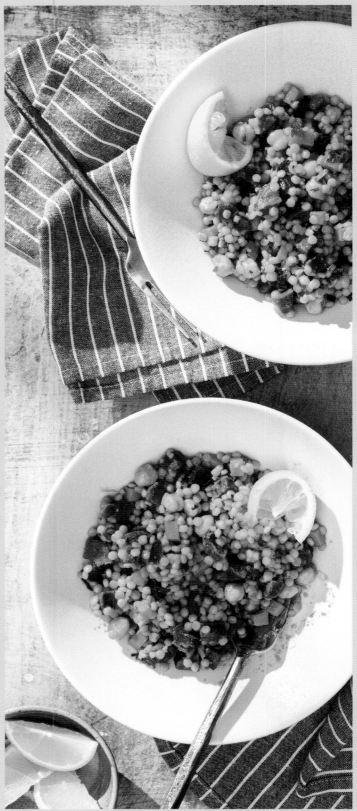

Lentil Salad with Pomegranate and Walnuts

SERVES 4 — SUPER EASY

3 tablespoons extra-virgin olive oil

1½ tablespoons lemon juice

¼ teaspoon table salt

¼ teaspoon pepper

2 (15-ounce) cans lentils, rinsed

¼ cup chopped fresh parsley

6 radishes, trimmed, halved, and sliced thin

¼ cup walnuts, toasted and chopped coarse, divided

½ cup pomegranate seeds, divided

Why This Recipe Works I've suddenly started seeing canned lentils stacked up on display at my supermarket and for good reason: They are recipe-ready and supernutritious. Here is a recipe that makes the most of them, turning out a delicious and elegant main course salad with minimal effort, perfect for those days when a more involved meal would be out of the question. It is also fantastic as a side for simply prepared fish or chicken. This impressive dish pairs the firm-on-the-outside, creamy-on-the-inside canned legume with a tart vinaigrette and adds pomegranate seeds for juicy pops of sweetness and walnuts for crunch. Sliced radishes and chopped parsley bring welcome freshness to the complexly flavored, beautifully textured, good-for-you salad that's not much more difficult than opening a can.

Whisk oil, lemon juice, salt, and pepper together in large bowl. Add lentils, parsley, radishes, half of walnuts, and half of pomegranate seeds to dressing and toss to combine. Season with salt and pepper to taste. Transfer to serving dish and sprinkle with remaining walnuts and pomegranate seeds. Serve.

PREP AHEAD

You can toast and chop the walnuts up to 1 day ahead. You can make the dressing up to 1 day ahead and refrigerate; bring to room temperature and whisk to recombine before using. You can make the salad and refrigerate up to 1 day ahead; add the walnuts and pomegranate seeds just before serving.

MAKE IT EVEN EASIER

Buy trimmed and sliced radishes. Toast the walnuts in the microwave (see page 37).

VARIATION
Lentil Salad with Spiced Carrots and Cilantro

Omit the parsley, radishes, walnuts, and pomegranate seeds. Combine 3 carrots, peeled and grated, 1 teaspoon cumin, ½ teaspoon cinnamon, and ⅛ teaspoon cayenne pepper (optional) in bowl. Cover and microwave until carrots are crisp-tender, 2 to 4 minutes. To the dressing, add the carrot mixture, lentils, and ¼ cup chopped cilantro and toss to combine.

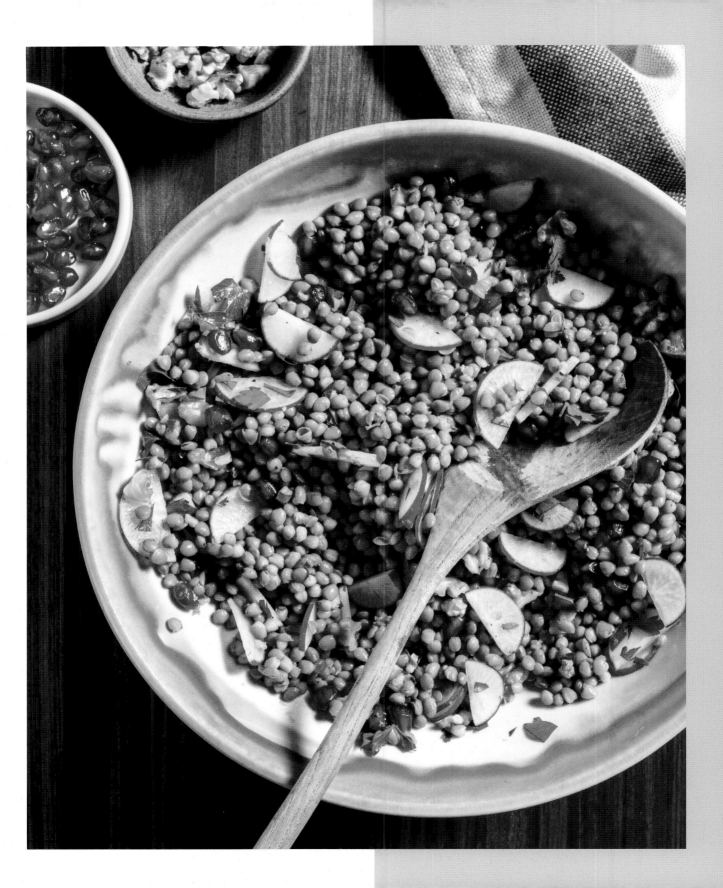

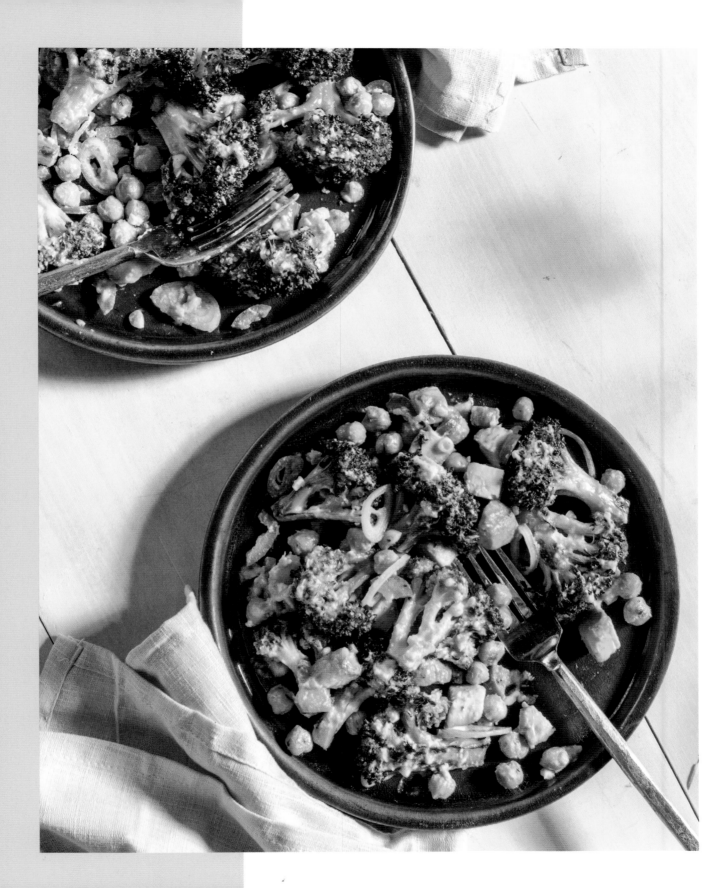

Warm Broccoli, Chickpea, and Avocado Salad

SERVES 4

Why This Recipe Works I love that in this recipe you can get broccoli and chickpeas nice and crispy in a skillet, delivering roasted flavor without having to turn on the oven. And while I usually think of serving avocados sliced or in guacamole, here they form the base for an ingenious dressing, no mayonnaise required. Simply mash together avocado, olive oil, and some of the pickled jalapeño brine for a supersimple dressing. Just before serving, toss more avocado with the crispy broccoli and chickpeas, along with the pickled jalapeños and thinly sliced shallots, to add a sharp bite that cuts through the richness of the dressing.

2 avocados, halved, pitted, and cut into ½-inch pieces, divided

½ cup drained pickled jalapeños, chopped, plus ¼ cup brine

7 tablespoons extra-virgin olive oil, divided

1½ pounds broccoli florets, cut into 1- to 1½-inch pieces

1 teaspoon table salt, divided

¾ teaspoon pepper, divided

2 (15-ounce) cans chickpeas, rinsed

1 large shallot, sliced thin

1 Mash ½ cup avocado, jalapeño brine, and 2 tablespoons olive oil in serving bowl with fork until combined; set dressing aside. Heat 3 tablespoons oil in 12-inch nonstick skillet over medium heat until shimmering. Add broccoli, ¾ teaspoon salt, and ½ teaspoon pepper. Cook, stirring occasionally, until broccoli is dark brown and crispy in spots, about 15 minutes. Transfer broccoli to bowl with reserved dressing and cover with foil. Toss remaining avocado with pickled jalapeños in small bowl and set aside.

— TAKE A 15-MINUTE BREAK —

2 Add remaining 2 tablespoons oil to now-empty skillet and heat over medium-high heat until shimmering. Add chickpeas, remaining ¼ teaspoon salt, and remaining ¼ teaspoon pepper and cook until lightly browned, about 8 minutes. Add to bowl with broccoli and dressing.

3 Add avocado mixture and shallot to bowl and stir to combine. Season with salt and pepper to taste. Serve.

PREP AHEAD
You can cut up the broccoli and slice the shallot up to 1 day ahead and refrigerate separately.

MAKE IT EVEN EASIER
Buy bagged broccoli florets.

Barley Salad with Pomegranate, Pistachios, and Feta

SERVES 4 — SUPER EASY

1½ cups pearl barley

½ teaspoon table salt, plus salt
for cooking barley

2 tablespoons pomegranate
molasses

½ teaspoon ground cinnamon

¼ teaspoon ground cumin

3 tablespoons extra-virgin olive oil,
plus extra for drizzling

½ cup coarsely chopped fresh
cilantro or mint

⅓ cup golden raisins or chopped
dried apricots

¼ cup shelled pistachios or
whole almonds, toasted and
chopped coarse

3 ounces feta or goat cheese,
cubed or crumbled (¾ cup)

6 scallions, green parts only,
sliced thin

½ cup pomegranate seeds

Why This Recipe Works This is one of those recipes that is so stunningly beautiful that you might think it is complicated to make. But it is not. In fact, it is quite simple to put together, and the hardest part of it is cooking the barley—but that can be done days in advance (and really is not hard at all). So if you are ever struggling to come up with a delicious vegetarian main dish or company-worthy side dish, look no further than this Mediterranean salad with its layers of flavorful and beautiful ingredients. To cook the barley, the trusty pasta method is easiest, since you simply boil the grains in salted water in an easy-to-lift saucepan until they're tender and then drain and spread out on a small rimmed baking sheet to dry (rather than allowing them to clump in the pot). For flavor, toasty pistachios and cilantro, balanced by warm, earthy spices and sweet golden raisins, raise the level of the salad, while salty feta cheese, scallions, and pomegranate seeds adorn the top. Do not substitute hulled barley or hull-less barley in this recipe. If using quick-cooking or presteamed barley (read the package carefully to determine this), you will need to decrease the barley cooking time in step 1. While you may be tempted to eat all your pistachios and pomegranate seeds while prepping, resist the temptation! The colors and the flavors they add will make the wait worth it.

1 Bring 2 quarts water to boil in large saucepan. Add barley and 1½ teaspoons salt, return to boil, and cook until tender, about 25 minutes.

— TAKE A 25-MINUTE BREAK —

2 Drain barley. Spread onto small rimmed baking sheet and let cool completely, about 15 minutes.

— TAKE A 15-MINUTE BREAK —

3 Whisk pomegranate molasses, cinnamon, cumin, salt, and oil together in large bowl. Add barley, cilantro, raisins, and pistachios and toss gently to combine. Season with salt and pepper to taste. Spread barley salad evenly on serving platter and top with feta, scallions, and pomegranate seeds in separate diagonal rows. Drizzle with extra oil and serve.

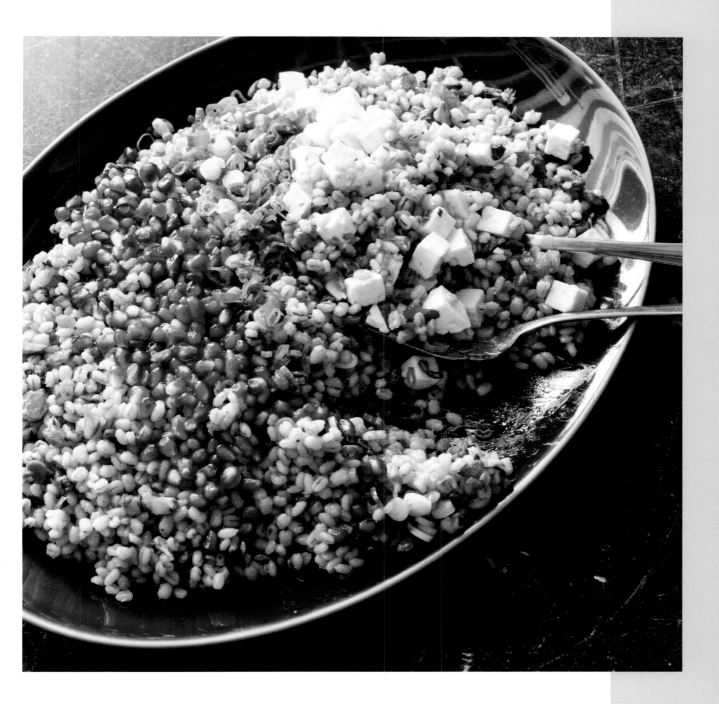

PREP AHEAD

You can cook the barley up to 3 days ahead and refrigerate. You can crumble the cheese, toast and chop the pistachios, and slice the scallions up to 1 day ahead and refrigerate separately.

MAKE IT EVEN EASIER

Buy crumbled feta cheese and toasted chopped pistachios. You can also toast the pistachios in the microwave if you buy them untoasted (see page 37).

Side Salad Inspiration

Unless I'm making a one-dish meal, I tend to serve a side salad alongside a main course each night. It's a healthy way to round out the meal, and it takes little effort. And when I'm cooking for friends and family, the same is also true. So here are a few of my favorites from the test kitchen that are sure to inspire you to get your wooden bowl out of the cabinet and give salads the attention they deserve. Feel free to scale down the ingredients if you are serving just 2 people.

Simplest Green Salad

Serves 4

This salad makes an elegant pairing with just about any dish. The dressing requires no measuring, no whisking, and (virtually) no thought. For the salad, all you need is lettuce, good quality oil, vinegar, half a garlic clove, salt, and pepper. It's vital to use high-quality ingredients—you can't camouflage wilted lettuce, flavorless oil, or too-harsh vinegar. Try interesting and flavorful leafy greens, such as mesclun, arugula, or Bibb lettuce. This is a great way to make the most of the mixed salad greens at the farmers' market during the summer. Add toppings of your choice, if you wish.

½ garlic clove, peeled
8 ounces (8 cups) lettuce, torn into
   bite-size pieces if necessary
   Oil
   Vinegar

Rub inside of salad bowl with garlic. Add lettuce. Slowly drizzle oil over lettuce, tossing greens very gently, until greens are lightly coated and just glistening. Season with vinegar, salt, and pepper to taste and toss gently to coat. Serve.

Arugula Salad with Fennel and Shaved Parmesan

Serves 4 to 6

Arugula is a cruciferous green with a lively, peppery bite, so it's important to choose accompaniments that can stand up to its assertive character. In this salad, the sweet anise flavor of fresh fennel tempers the peppery sharpness of arugula, making for a delicate and flavorful salad that is quick and easy. Shaved Parmesan adds a pleasant salty note. To make things even easier, buy shaved Parmesan at the market.

6 ounces (6 cups) baby arugula
1 large fennel bulb, stalks discarded,
   bulb halved, cored, and sliced thin
1½ tablespoons lemon juice
1 small shallot, minced
1 teaspoon Dijon mustard
1 teaspoon minced fresh thyme or rosemary
1 small garlic clove, minced
⅛ teaspoon table salt
   Pinch pepper
¼ cup extra-virgin olive oil
1 ounce shaved Parmesan cheese

Gently toss arugula and fennel together in large bowl. Whisk lemon juice, shallot, mustard, thyme, garlic, salt, and pepper together in small bowl. Whisking constantly, slowly drizzle in oil until emulsified. Drizzle dressing over salad and toss gently to coat. Season with salt and pepper to taste. Serve, topping individual portions with Parmesan.

Mâche Salad with Cucumber and Mint

Serves 6 to 8

Pretty mâche lettuce makes an elegant salad with its rosette-like leaves and nutty taste. The crisp, fresh flavor of thinly sliced cucumber is a nice contrast, chopped mint adds brightness, and crunchy pine nuts reinforce the mâche's buttery notes. A simple dressing of lemon juice, fresh parsley, fresh thyme, and minced garlic is all that is needed, but capers add some welcome briny contrast. Mâche is a very delicate green, so be sure to handle it gently and make sure that it is thoroughly dry before tossing it with the vinaigrette. You can use baby spinach or mesclun instead of the mâche.

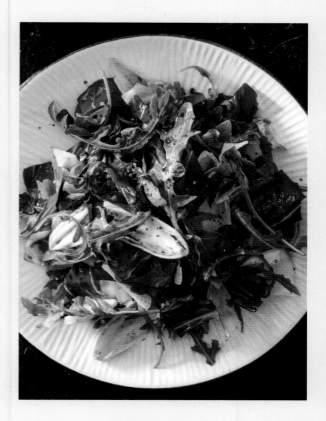

- 12 ounces (12 cups) mâche
- 1 English cucumber, sliced thin
- ½ cup chopped fresh mint or parsley
- ⅓ cup pine nuts, toasted
- ¼ cup extra-virgin olive oil
- 1 tablespoon lemon juice
- 1 tablespoon capers, minced
- 1 tablespoon minced fresh parsley or cilantro
- 1 teaspoon minced fresh thyme or rosemary
- 1 garlic clove, minced
- ¼ teaspoon table salt
- ¼ teaspoon pepper

Gently toss mâche, cucumber, mint, and pine nuts together in large bowl. Whisk oil, lemon juice, capers parsley, thyme, garlic, salt, and pepper together in small bowl. Drizzle dressing over salad and toss gently to coat. Season with salt and pepper to taste. Serve.

Radicchio, Endive, and Arugula Salad

Serves 4 to 6

If you are entertaining and want a simple salad that is a little bit out of the ordinary, this one fits the bill perfectly. It's a beautiful salad with its red, white, and green hues, and it is complex in flavor, with bitter and spicy tastes of different greens contrasting perfectly with a slight sweetness from balsamic in the vinaigrette. By definition, a vinaigrette contains oil, vinegar, and salt and pepper.

This is an ultra vinaigrette, balancing the sweet complexity of balsamic vinegar with the tartness of red wine vinegar. To keep the greens fresh, toss them with the bold dressing just before serving.

- 1 small head radicchio (6 ounces), cored and cut into 1-inch pieces
- 1 head Belgian endive (4 ounces), cut into 2-inch pieces
- 3 ounces (3 cups) baby arugula
- 3 tablespoons extra-virgin olive oil
- 1 tablespoon plus 1 teaspoon balsamic vinegar
- 1 teaspoon red wine vinegar
- ⅛ teaspoon table salt
  Pinch pepper

Gently toss radicchio, endive, and arugula together in large bowl. Whisk oil, balsamic vinegar, red wine vinegar, salt, and pepper together in small bowl. Drizzle vinaigrette over salad and toss gently to coat. Season with salt and pepper to taste. Serve.

Vinaigrettes That Jazz Up Everyday Side Salads

A vinaigrette or dressing is the conductor of a salad, the element that brings ingredients together cohesively, binding them with flavor, richness, and aroma, and showing them off with gloss. Here are just a few of the test kitchen's favorites. To dress a salad, you will need about 1 tablespoon vinaigrette per 2 cups washed and dried greens.

Make-Ahead Vinaigrette

Makes about 1 cup

It is superhandy to stash a flavorful vinaigrette in your fridge that will keep for a week. To prevent the oil and vinegar from separating, this dressing includes mustard and mayonnaise, two natural emulsifiers, and a surprising ingredient—molasses—as a third stabilizer. Just a tablespoon molasses works wonders without imparting a strong flavor. Cutting the olive oil with some vegetable oil ensures that the refrigerated dressing is always pourable. Do not use blackstrap molasses. This vinaigrette pairs well with nearly any green.

- 1 tablespoon regular or light mayonnaise
- 1 tablespoon molasses
- 1 tablespoon Dijon mustard
- ½ teaspoon table salt
- ¼ cup white wine vinegar
- ½ cup extra-virgin olive oil, divided
- ¼ cup vegetable oil

1 Combine mayonnaise, molasses, mustard, and salt in 2-cup jar with tight-fitting lid. Stir with fork until mixture is milky in appearance and no lumps of mayonnaise or molasses remain. Add vinegar, seal jar, and shake until smooth, about 10 seconds.

2 Add ¼ cup olive oil. Seal jar and shake vigorously until combined, about 10 seconds. Repeat with remaining ¼ cup olive oil and vegetable oil in separate additions, shaking until combined after each addition. Vinaigrette should be glossy and lightly thickened after all oil has been added. Season with salt and pepper to taste.

VARIATIONS

Make-Ahead Sherry-Shallot Vinaigrette

Add 2 teaspoons minced shallot and 2 teaspoons minced fresh thyme to jar with mayonnaise. Substitute sherry vinegar for white wine vinegar.

Make-Ahead Balsamic-Fennel Vinaigrette

Toast 2 teaspoons fennel seeds in a skillet and crack them using a mortar and pestle.

Add toasted and cracked fennel seeds to jar with mayonnaise. Substitute balsamic vinegar for white wine vinegar.

Make-Ahead Cider-Caraway Vinaigrette

Toast 2 teaspoons caraway seeds in a skillet and crack them using a mortar and pestle.

Add toasted and cracked caraway seeds to jar with mayonnaise. Substitute cider vinegar for white wine vinegar.

PREP AHEAD

You can make these vinaigrettes up to 1 week in advance and refrigerate; shake to recombine before using.

Raspberry Vinaigrette
Makes about ⅓ cup

This recipe works nicely when you want a slightly sweet vinaigrette. The combination of jam, red wine vinegar, and Dijon mustard keeps the sweetness in check and gives the vinaigrette its bright flavor. It pairs especially well with salads topped with berries or other fruit, but is equally good with simple mixed greens. Avoid chunky preserves and supersweet jams.

- 2 tablespoons seedless raspberry jam
- 2½ teaspoons red wine vinegar
- 1 teaspoon Dijon mustard
- ⅛ teaspoon table salt
- ⅛ teaspoon pepper
- 3 tablespoons extra-virgin olive oil

Whisk jam in medium bowl until smooth. Add vinegar, mustard, salt, and pepper, whisking until combined. Whisking constantly, slowly drizzle in oil until emulsified. (Dressing can be refrigerated for up to 4 days; whisk to recombine before using.)

Tahini-Lemon Dressing
Makes ½ cup

The rich sesame flavor of tahini pairs perfectly with lemon juice and garlic in a dressing that's best with mild greens.

- 2½ tablespoons lemon juice
- 2 tablespoons tahini
- 1 tablespoon water
- 1 garlic clove, minced
- ½ teaspoon table salt
- ⅛ teaspoon pepper
- ¼ cup extra-virgin olive oil

Whisk lemon juice, tahini, water, garlic, salt, and pepper together in bowl. Whisking constantly, slowly drizzle in oil until emulsified. (Dressing can be refrigerated for up to 4 days; whisk to recombine before using.)

Maple-Mustard Vinaigrette
Makes about ½ cup

The combination of cider vinegar and maple syrup is an unexpected one, but captures the essence of fall in a jar. A little minced shallot gives it a savory note, while Dijon mustard cuts the sweetness of the maple syrup. This vinaigrette is especially good on chopped romaine. But feel free to improvise and drizzle it on roasted vegetables too.

- 2 tablespoons cider vinegar
- 2 tablespoons maple syrup
- 1 teaspoon minced shallot
- 1 teaspoon Dijon mustard
- ¾ teaspoon table salt
- ½ teaspoon pepper
- 3 tablespoons extra-virgin olive oil

Whisk vinegar, maple syrup, shallot, mustard, salt, and pepper together in medium bowl. Whisking constantly, slowly drizzle in oil until emulsified. (Dressing can be refrigerated for up to 4 days; whisk to recombine before using.)

Yogurt-Dill Dressing
Makes about ⅔ cup

Yogurt and dill are a match made in cucumber heaven. Pair this with a salad topped with cucumbers and cherry tomatoes. The dressing is also great drizzled over roast salmon or blanched green beans.

- ⅓ cup plain whole-milk yogurt
- 2 tablespoons chopped fresh dill, parsley, or chives
- 1½ tablespoons whole-grain mustard
- ⅛ teaspoon table salt
- ⅛ teaspoon pepper
- 1 tablespoon extra-virgin olive oil

Whisk yogurt, dill, mustard, salt, and pepper together in large bowl. Whisking constantly, slowly drizzle in oil until emulsified. (Dressing can be refrigerated for up to 4 days; whisk to recombine before using.)

Streamlined

Comfort Classics

* Try these recipes first if today is not one of your better days and you need a soul-refilling meal with high return on your energy investment.

Spatchcocked Roast Chicken with Rosemary and Garlic

SERVES 4 — SUPER EASY

2 tablespoons extra-virgin olive oil, divided

1 teaspoon minced fresh rosemary

1 garlic clove, minced

1 (3½- to 4-pound) spatchcocked chicken, trimmed

1 teaspoon table salt

½ teaspoon pepper

Lemon wedges

Why This Recipe Works When your back is acting up or you are trying to avoid triggering pain, a whole roast chicken is usually not on the menu: You have to lift it into and out of the oven in a roasting pan or large skillet, and then when it's done, carve it into pieces for serving. A spatchcocked chicken (otherwise known as a butterflied chicken), however, is far easier to manage (and way easier on the back) and easier to cut up. They are usually small enough (4 pounds or less) to fit perfectly on a small, lightweight rimmed baking sheet, and many stores now sell them already spatchcocked. (If not, ask the butcher to do it for you.) Another plus is that they cook faster and more evenly, and they are easier to flavor. For this recipe, a very hot oven helps brown the skin, which is first simply rubbed with oil, salt, and pepper. Brushing it partway through cooking with a mixture of more oil, chopped fresh rosemary, and minced garlic adds a big hit of flavor. Do not use a chicken larger than 4 pounds. Note that you can also make this recipe in your toaster oven.

1   Preheat oven to 500 degrees. Meanwhile, combine 1 tablespoon oil, rosemary, and garlic in bowl; set aside.

2   Pat chicken dry with paper towels, then rub with remaining 1 tablespoon oil and sprinkle with salt and pepper. Place chicken on small rimmed baking sheet, tucking wings under breasts.

3   Roast chicken, on lower-middle rack, until just beginning to brown, about 20 minutes.

— TAKE A 20-MINUTE BREAK —

4   Remove chicken from oven and brush with oil mixture. Rotate pan and continue to roast chicken until breast registers 160 degrees and thighs register 175 degrees, about 22 minutes.

— TAKE A 22-MINUTE BREAK —

5   Transfer chicken to carving board and let rest for 10 minutes. Carve chicken and serve with lemon wedges.

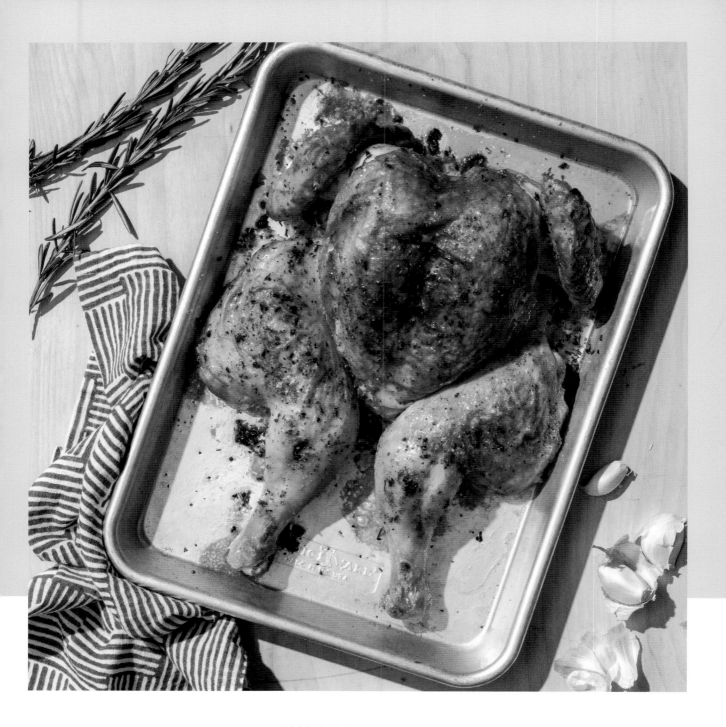

VARIATION

Spatchcocked Roast Chicken with Sesame and Ginger

Combine 1 tablespoon toasted sesame oil, 1 tablespoon extra-virgin olive oil, 1 teaspoon grated fresh ginger, ½ teaspoon five-spice powder, and pinch red pepper flakes in bowl; substitute for oil, rosemary, and garlic in step 1.

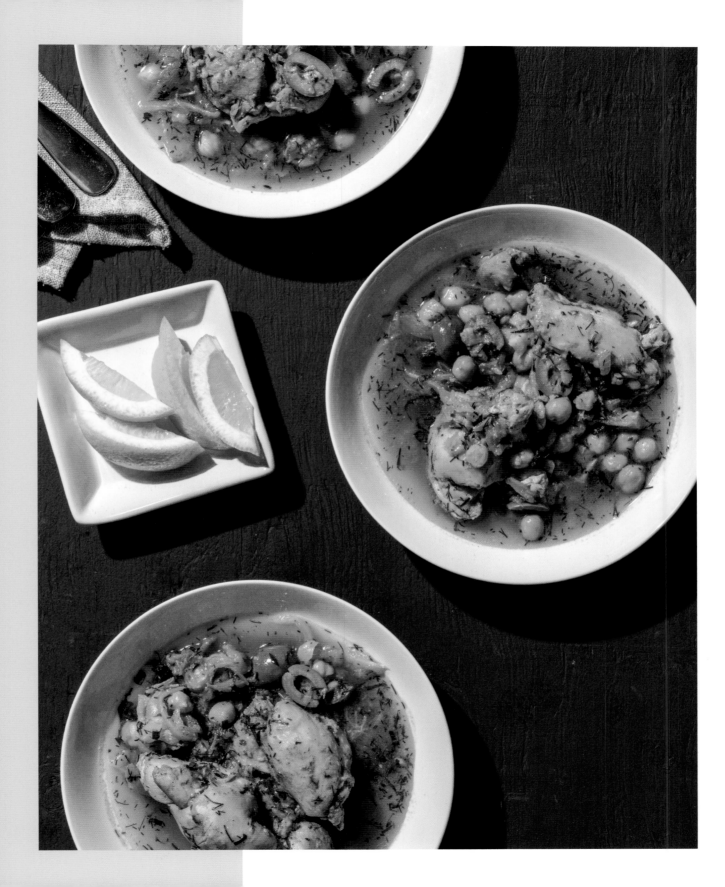

Instant Pot Chicken Tagine

SERVES 4 TO 6 — SUPER EASY

Why This Recipe Works This cornerstone of Moroccan cuisine, heady with spices, salty with olives, and bright with lemon, is a balancing act of flavors ready-made for the Instant Pot: The enclosed environment ensures that none of that flavor escapes and, even better, it intensifies them. The broth that results from cooking this tagine in the Instant Pot is like none other I've tasted—make sure you have a soup spoon or a hunk of crusty break to get every last drop. A mix of fresh fennel and readily available canned chickpeas gives the meal heft, while paprika, cumin, and ginger lend depth and a little sweetness. Cayenne adds subtle heat, and aromatic turmeric colors the broth a deep, attractive yellow. Raisins lend a pleasant floral flavor, as do a couple of wide strips of lemon zest. Finally, brine-cured olives provide a salty counterpart to the sweet and complex broth. Don't core the fennel before cutting it into wedges; the core helps hold the wedges together during cooking. Note that it will take the Instant Pot about 10 minutes to come up to pressure and start the cook cycle.

1 Using highest sauté function, cook oil, garlic, paprika, turmeric, cumin, ginger, and cayenne in electric pressure cooker until fragrant, about 1 minute. Turn off electric pressure cooker, then stir in chickpeas, fennel wedges, broth, and zest.

2 Sprinkle chicken with salt. Nestle chicken into pot and spoon some of cooking liquid over top. Lock lid in place and close pressure release valve. Select high pressure cook function and cook for 10 minutes.

— TAKE A 20-MINUTE BREAK —

3 Turn off electric pressure cooker and quick-release pressure. Carefully remove lid, allowing steam to escape away from you. Discard lemon zest. Stir in olives, raisins, parsley, and fennel fronds. Season with salt and pepper to taste. Serve with lemon wedges.

PREP AHEAD
You can combine the spices up to 1 week ahead. You can trim the chicken up to 1 day ahead and refrigerate, covered, until using. You can cut up the fennel and halve the olives up to 1 day ahead and refrigerate separately.

1 tablespoon extra-virgin olive oil

5 garlic cloves, minced

1½ teaspoons paprika

½ teaspoon ground turmeric

½ teaspoon ground cumin

¼ teaspoon ground ginger

¼ teaspoon cayenne pepper

1 (15-ounce) can chickpeas, rinsed

1 fennel bulb, 1 tablespoon fronds minced, stalks discarded, bulb halved and cut lengthwise into ½-inch-thick wedges

1 cup chicken broth

3 (2-inch) strips lemon zest, plus lemon wedges for serving

2 pounds boneless, skinless chicken thighs, skin removed, trimmed

½ teaspoon table salt

½ cup pitted large brine-cured green or black olives, halved

⅓ cup raisins

2 tablespoons chopped fresh parsley

Green Chicken Enchiladas

SERVES 4 TO 6

2 (10-ounce) cans green enchilada sauce

1¼ cups chopped fresh cilantro, divided

3 cups shredded chicken

2½ cups shredded Mexican cheese blend or mild cheddar cheese, divided

12 (5½-inch) corn tortillas

Lime wedges

Why This Recipe Works At our house, enchiladas are in the comfort meal rotation, but preparing them can be a multi-hour, labor-intensive endeavor that involves making the sauce, poaching the chicken, and more—but it doesn't have to be that way. Starting with a rotisserie chicken and canned enchilada sauce makes this comforting meal more accessible for back pain suffers and shortens the dish's prep time to minutes. And instead of using a heavy casserole dish, you can arrange the enchiladas on a small rimmed baking sheet. Pureeing cilantro with the enchilada sauce creates a fresh alternative to an otherwise standard sauce. When rolling the enchiladas, place roughly the same amount of filling right down the center of each tortilla. Placing the enchiladas seam-side down ensures that they don't fall apart in the oven. You can use rotisserie chicken for this recipe or make Perfect Poached Chicken (page 61) or Easy Slow-Cooker Poached Chicken (page 58).

1   Preheat oven to 400 degrees. Grease small rimmed baking sheet. Puree enchilada sauce and 1 cup cilantro in food processor. Combine 1 cup enchilada sauce mixture, chicken, and 1½ cups cheese in large bowl and toss to combine. Season with salt and pepper to taste.

2   Wrap tortillas in clean dish towel and microwave until pliable, about 1 minute. Top each tortilla with ¼ cup chicken mixture and roll tightly. Arrange, seam-side down, on prepared baking sheet. Spray lightly with cooking spray, then top with additional 1 cup enchilada sauce mixture and remaining 1 cup cheese. Place sheet pan on middle rack and bake until cheese is melted and enchiladas are heated through, about 20 minutes.

—   TAKE A 20-MINUTE BREAK   —

3   Sprinkle remaining ¼ cup cilantro over enchiladas. Serve with lime wedges, passing remaining sauce at table.

PREP AHEAD

You can make the sauce up to 1 day ahead and refrigerate. You can shred the chicken up to 2 days ahead and refrigerate.

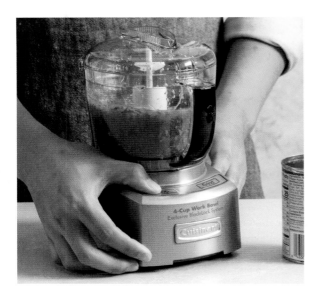

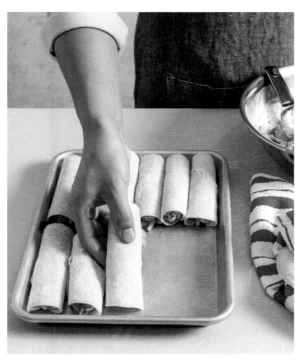

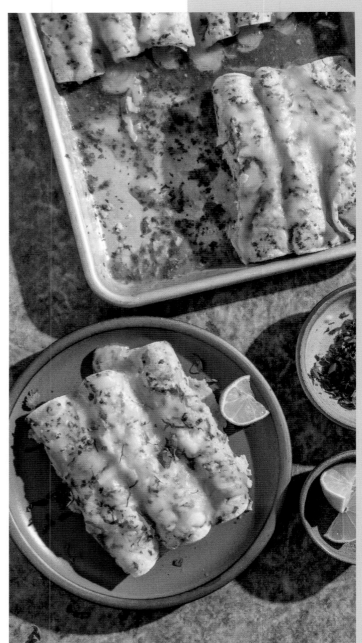

TAKE IT UP A NOTCH
Serve with Quick Pickled Shallots and Radishes

Whisk ¼ cup lime juice, 1 teaspoon sugar, and ¼ teaspoon table salt in medium bowl until sugar and salt have dissolved. Stir in 6 large trimmed and sliced radishes and 1 sliced shallot. Let sit for 15 minutes for flavors to blend or refrigerate for up to 1 hour. Drain before serving. Makes 1 cup.

Chicken, Spinach, and Artichoke Pot Pie

SERVES 4

1¼ pounds frozen spinach, thawed and squeezed dry

1 (5.2-ounce) package Boursin Garlic & Fine Herbs cheese

1 cup jarred whole artichoke hearts packed in water, halved

2 carrots, peeled and shredded

¾ cup chicken broth

½ cup heavy cream

¼ cup capers, rinsed

1 tablespoon Wondra flour

12 ounces boneless, skinless chicken breasts, trimmed and sliced thin

1 teaspoon grated lemon zest

¼ teaspoon table salt

⅛ teaspoon pepper

1 (9½ by 9-inch) sheet puff pastry, thawed

1 large egg, lightly beaten with 2 tablespoons water

Why This Recipe Works I would argue that a pot pie is the pinnacle of comfort food—because who doesn't love cracking into a rich, flaky pastry dough to get at a heady mixture of chicken and vegetables in a creamy sauce? But if you are having back issues, you've no doubt put this recipe in cold storage due to the extensive prep work involved and the need to stand at the stove poaching chicken, making a roux, and building the sauce. Now you can put this dish on the table again by using a few tricks that streamline it but don't skimp on the comfort factor. And since this recipe is scaled down to serve 4, you can use a smaller casserole dish: an 8-inch square pan instead of a heavy 9 x 13-inch dish. Thawed frozen spinach and jarred artichokes pack in a serving of vegetables with very little prep work. Boursin cheese is the other key to the recipe's ease, melting into an exceptionally lush sauce when combined with broth and cream and thickened with finely ground Wondra flour. Last, a buttery sheet of store-bought puff pastry makes the perfect top crust. You can substitute 6 ounces frozen artichoke hearts, thawed and patted dry, for the jarred artichokes. To thaw frozen puff pastry, let it stand either in the refrigerator for 24 hours or on the counter for 30 to 60 minutes. You can substitute all-purpose flour for the Wondra flour, if necessary; however, the sauce will have a pasty, slightly gritty texture.

1   Preheat oven to 425 degrees. Spray 8-inch square baking dish with vegetable oil spray. Stir spinach, Boursin, artichokes, carrots, broth, cream, capers, and flour together in bowl, then transfer to prepared dish.

2   Toss chicken with lemon zest in second bowl, sprinkle with salt and pepper, and spread in even layer over spinach mixture. Cut puff pastry into 8-inch square and place over top of chicken. Cut four 2-inch slits in center of dough, then brush dough with egg wash.

3   Bake, on middle rack, until crust is golden brown and filling is bubbling, about 30 minutes, rotating dish halfway through baking.

— TAKE A 30-MINUTE BREAK —

4   Remove pot pie from oven and let cool for 10 minutes before serving.

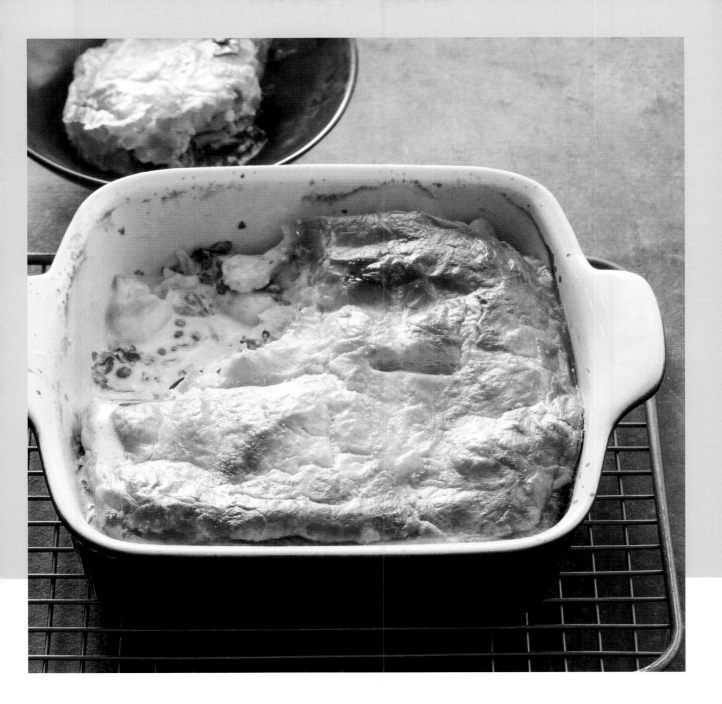

PREP AHEAD

You can trim and slice the chicken and shred the carrots up to 1 day ahead and refrigerate separately. The assembled pie, prepared through step 2, can be refrigerated for up to 1 day; bake as directed in step 3.

MAKE IT EVEN EASIER

Buy shredded carrots. Buy chicken tenderloins, which will be easier to slice.

Tuscan Steak with Garlicky Spinach

SERVES 2

12 ounces (12 cups) baby spinach

2 tablespoons water

1 (1¾-pound) porterhouse or T-bone steak, 1 to 1½ inches thick, trimmed

3 garlic cloves, 1 halved, 2 sliced thin

¼ teaspoon table salt

⅛ teaspoon pepper

2 tablespoons plus 1 teaspoon extra-virgin olive oil, divided

⅛ teaspoon red pepper flakes

Lemon wedges

Why This Recipe Works Tuscan-style steak is a Florentine specialty that marries a grilled thick porterhouse steak with garlic, olive oil, and lemon and a side of garlicky spinach or arugula. To keep this special meal simple for just two, it is easier to bring it indoors. Rubbing the steak with a garlic clove before browning it in a skillet perfumes it with subtle garlic flavor. Parcooking the spinach in the microwave helps rid it of excess liquid. You can then cook the spinach in the same skillet used for the steak with even more garlic (sliced rather than minced to keep it from burning). For a finishing touch in keeping with this meal's Italian roots, drizzle the steak with olive oil and serve it and the spinach with lemon wedges. The acidic notes of the lemon juice sharpen the flavors of the beef and cut its richness. If you don't have a microwave-safe bowl large enough to accommodate the entire amount of spinach, cook it in a smaller bowl in two batches; use 1 tablespoon water per batch and cook each batch for 1 to 2 minutes.

1 Microwave spinach and water in covered bowl, stirring occasionally, until spinach is beginning to wilt and has decreased in volume by half, about 2 minutes. Remove bowl from microwave and keep covered for 1 minute. Carefully uncover spinach, allowing steam to escape away from you, and transfer to colander. Squeeze spinach between tongs to release excess liquid; set aside.

— TAKE A 15-MINUTE BREAK —

2 Pat steak dry with paper towels, rub halved garlic clove over bone and meat on each side, and sprinkle with salt and pepper. Heat 2 teaspoons oil in 10-inch skillet over medium-high heat until just smoking. Place steak in skillet and cook, without moving, until well browned on first side, about 6 minutes. Flip steak, reduce heat to medium, and continue to cook until meat registers 120 to 125 degrees (for medium-rare), about 8 minutes. Transfer steak to carving board, tent with aluminum foil, and let rest for 10 minutes.

— TAKE A 10-MINUTE BREAK —

3 Add 2 teaspoons oil, pepper flakes, and sliced garlic to now-empty skillet and cook over medium heat until fragrant, about 2 minutes. Add spinach and cook until heated through, about 2 minutes. Season with salt and pepper to taste.

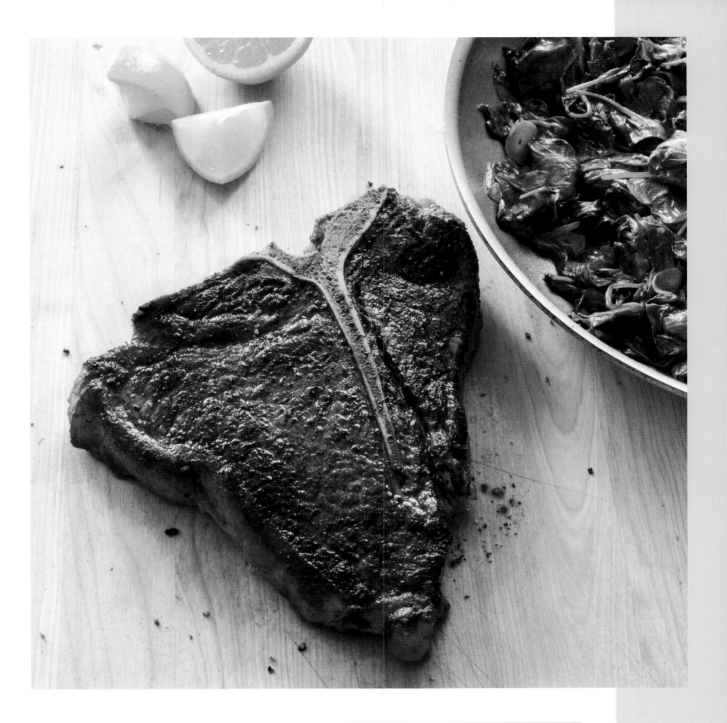

4 Cut strip and tenderloin pieces off bone, then slice each piece ¼ inch thick. Transfer steak to serving platter and drizzle with remaining 1 tablespoon oil. Serve with spinach and lemon wedges.

PREP AHEAD
You can trim the steak up to 1 day ahead and refrigerate.

Modern Beef Pot Pie with Mushrooms and Sherry

SERVES 2

1 pound boneless beef short ribs, trimmed and cut into ¾-inch pieces

¼ teaspoon table salt

⅛ teaspoon pepper

2 tablespoons vegetable oil, divided

12 ounces cremini mushrooms, trimmed and quartered

1 small onion, chopped fine

1 tablespoon tomato paste

¼ teaspoon dried thyme

1½ tablespoons all-purpose flour

¼ cup dry sherry

1¼ cups beef broth

1 (8-inch) baguette, sliced ½ inch thick, ends discarded

1 ounce shredded Gruyère cheese (¼ cup)

2 tablespoons minced fresh chives

Why This Recipe Works This rich and luxurious dish is exactly the kind of cooking I believe is good for the soul. But generally, the litany of pots and pans required to make both the filling and the crust for pot pie makes this comforting dish unrealistic for anyone who wants to avoid standing for an hour in the kitchen. This simplified version puts it within reach, and the bit of stovetop-to-oven juggling it requires is well worth the effort. (And using a small skillet makes this so much easier.) Browning flavorful boneless short ribs (which are easier to prep than a chuck roast) for deeper flavor is a must; you then use the leftover fat to cook the mushrooms and onion. A little flour helps thicken the filling to a rich consistency. Slices of crusty bread brushed with oil and sprinkled with nutty Gruyère cheese ramp up the comfort food quotient with very little work. You will need a 10-inch broiler-safe skillet with a tight-fitting lid for this recipe.

1 Preheat oven to 400 degrees. Pat beef dry with paper towels and sprinkle with salt and pepper. Heat 2 teaspoons oil in 10-inch broiler-safe skillet over medium-high heat until just smoking. Brown beef on all sides, about 9 minutes; transfer to bowl and cover to keep warm.

— TAKE A 15-MINUTE BREAK —

2 Add mushrooms, onion, and 1 teaspoon oil to fat left in skillet and cook over medium heat until mushrooms have released their liquid and vegetables are softened and lightly browned, about 8 minutes. Stir in tomato paste and thyme and cook until fragrant, about 30 seconds. Stir in flour and cook for 1 minute.

3 Stir in sherry, scraping up any browned bits, and cook until almost completely evaporated, about 2 minutes. Slowly stir in broth, smoothing out any lumps. Bring to simmer, then stir in beef along with any accumulated juices. Cover, transfer skillet to oven, and cook on middle rack until beef is tender, about 1 hour, stirring once halfway through cooking.

— TAKE A 1-HOUR BREAK —

4 Using pot holder, remove skillet from oven. Adjust oven rack 8 inches from broiler element and heat broiler. Being careful of hot skillet handle, season beef with salt and pepper to taste.

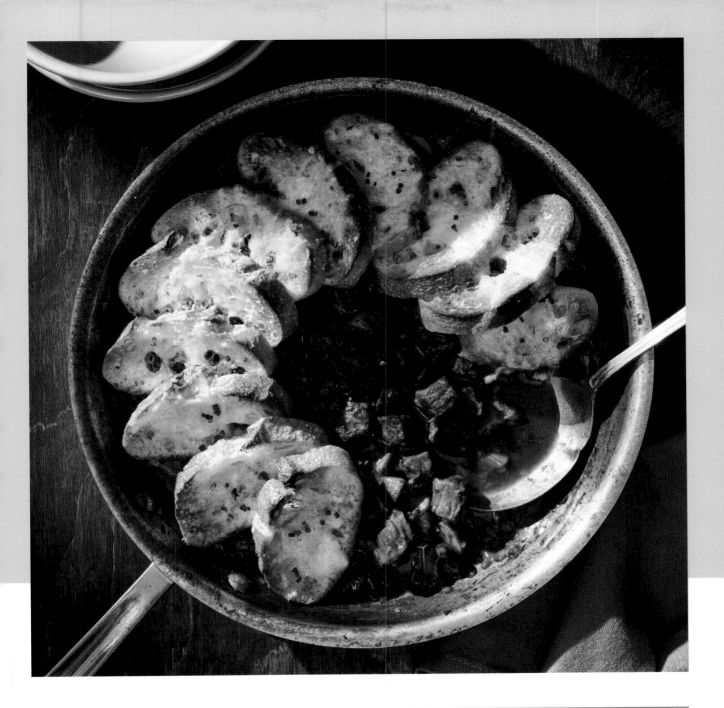

5 Brush bread with remaining 1 tablespoon oil and shingle around edge of skillet, leaving center open. Sprinkle Gruyère over bread. Broil until cheese is melted and bread is browned, about 2 minutes. Remove skillet from oven and let casserole cool for 5 minutes. Sprinkle with chives and serve.

PREP AHEAD

You can prep all the ingredients up to 1 day ahead and refrigerate separately. You can make the filling up to 1 day ahead and reheat before adding the bread and cheese and finishing the recipe.

Stovetop Classic Pot Roast with Potatoes and Carrots

SERVES 6 TO 8

1 (4-pound) boneless beef chuck-eye roast, pulled into 2 pieces at natural seam and trimmed

2 teaspoons table salt, divided

1¼ teaspoons pepper, divided

1 tablespoon vegetable oil

1 onion, chopped fine

2 celery ribs, chopped fine

2 tablespoons all-purpose flour

1 tablespoon tomato paste

3 garlic cloves, minced

¼ teaspoon dried thyme

1½ cups dry red wine

1½ cups beef broth

1 tablespoon soy sauce

1 pound small Yukon Gold potatoes, unpeeled

2 bay leaves

1 pound baby carrots

2 tablespoons minced fresh parsley

Why This Recipe Works When a beautiful and well-marbled piece of chuck roast simmers in a fragrant braising liquid for hours, it is magically transformed into hunks of meltingly tender fork-ready beef packed with deep flavor. But in the healthy back kitchen, making pot roast comes with a few intractable issues. Most notably, it usually requires transferring the beef, along with the liquid and vegetables, to the oven to cook gently, so depending on the heft of your Dutch oven, you may need to lift a nearly 20-pound pot. A stovetop-only recipe for this ultimate comfort classic solves the problem. The first step here is to break the roast into two even pieces, allowing you to remove any big chunks of fat as well as reduce the cooking time. And if you are wondering why there is a full tablespoon of soy sauce in this recipe, it adds umami flavor to braises such as this, especially when you skip the browning step. To keep things easy on the prep side, whole, unpeeled small potatoes are added right to the pot with the beef. After 2 hours of cooking on the stovetop, prep-free baby carrots join the mix to cook until they are fork tender and the meat is falling apart. If it is hard for your stove to maintain a truly low heat, consider using a flame tamer (see opposite page). Use potatoes measuring 1 to 2 inches in diameter.

1   Pat beef dry with paper towels and sprinkle with 1½ teaspoons salt and 1 teaspoon pepper.

2   Heat oil in Dutch oven over medium-high heat until shimmering. Add onion, celery, remaining ½ teaspoon salt, and remaining ¼ teaspoon pepper and cook over medium heat until vegetables are softened and browned, 8 to 10 minutes. Stir in flour and tomato paste and cook for 1 minute. Stir in garlic and thyme and cook until fragrant, about 30 seconds. Slowly stir in wine, broth, and soy sauce, scraping up any browned bits and smoothing out any lumps.

3   Nestle beef into liquid and add potatoes and bay leaves. Bring to a simmer, cover, reduce heat to low, and cook for 2 hours.

— TAKE A 2-HOUR BREAK —

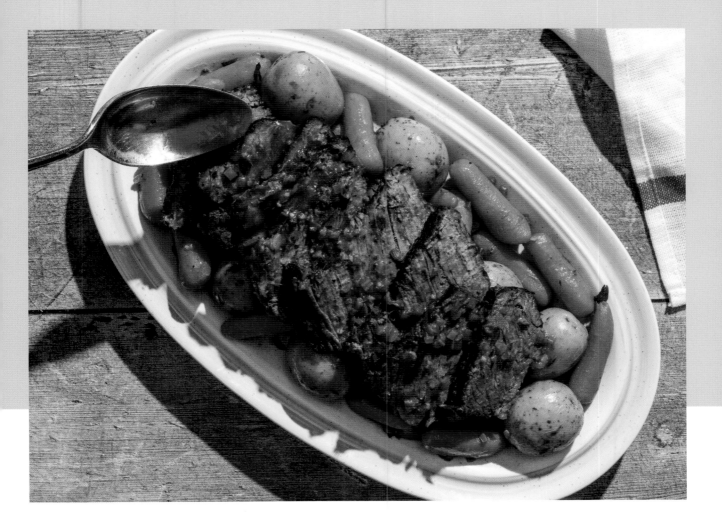

4   Turn roasts, add carrots, cover, and cook until beef is tender and fork slips easily in and out of meat, 1½ to 2 hours.

— TAKE A 1½- TO 2-HOUR BREAK —

5   Transfer roasts to carving board, tent with aluminum foil, and let rest for 20 minutes.

— TAKE A 20-MINUTE BREAK —

6   Discard bay leaves. Transfer vegetables to serving dish and tent with foil. Using large spoon, skim fat from surface of sauce. Stir parsley into sauce and season with salt and pepper to taste.

7   Slice meat against grain ½ inch thick and arrange on serving dish with vegetables. Spoon 1 cup sauce over meat and serve, passing remaining sauce separately.

PREP AHEAD
You can prep the meat, onion, and celery up to 1 day ahead and refrigerate separately. The cooked pot roast and vegetables can be refrigerated for up to 3 days; reheat in a 12-inch skillet over medium-low heat adding additional broth as needed.

HOW TO IMPROVISE A FLAME TAMER
Take a long sheet of heavy-duty aluminum foil and shape it into a 1-inch-thick ring. Make sure the ring is of an even thickness so that the pot will rest flat on it.

Slow-Cooker Shredded Beef Tacos

SERVES 4 TO 6 — SUPER EASY

½ onion, chopped fine

3 garlic cloves, minced

1 tablespoon tomato paste

1 tablespoon vegetable oil

1–2 tablespoons minced canned chipotle chile in adobo sauce

½ teaspoon ground cinnamon

¾ cup water

1 tablespoon honey

2 pounds boneless beef chuck-eye roast, pulled apart at seams, trimmed, and cut into 1½-inch pieces

½ teaspoon table salt

¼ teaspoon pepper

12–18 (5½-inch) corn tortillas, warmed

Crumbled queso fresco

Lime wedges

Why This Recipe Works This easy-to-prepare slow-cooker filling makes shredded beef tacos a great weeknight meal. It uses a chuck roast, with its big, beefy flavor, as the basis for the filling because chuck becomes meltingly tender and shreddable in the slow cooker—plus it's inexpensive and easy to find. Cutting the roast into 1½-inch pieces helps it cook faster and, as a result, become even more tender than when left whole. For the sauce, a mixture of convenient canned chipotle chiles, tomato paste, and a hint of cinnamon ensures an ultraflavorful mix. First blooming the aromatics with oil in the microwave brings out their full flavor. They are then added to the slow cooker with a little honey to balance the heat, while water helps distribute the spices evenly. Once the beef is pull-apart tender, just mash it to the right shredded consistency for tacos. To complement the warm spices of the beef, it's nice to serve the tacos with a cool and tangy cabbage slaw.

1   Microwave onion, garlic, tomato paste, oil, chipotle, and cinnamon in bowl, stirring occasionally, until onion is softened, about 5 minutes; transfer to slow cooker. Stir in water and honey. Sprinkle beef with salt and pepper and stir into slow cooker. Cover and cook until beef is tender, 7 to 8 hours on low or 4 to 5 hours on high.

—   TAKE A BREAK   —

2   Transfer beef to bowl and, using potato masher, smash until coarsely shredded. Cover to keep warm. Meanwhile, turn slow cooker to high and cook until sauce is slightly reduced, about 10 minutes. Add ½ cup sauce to meat and combine.

3   Serve beef with additional sauce, as desired; tortillas; queso fresco; and lime wedges.

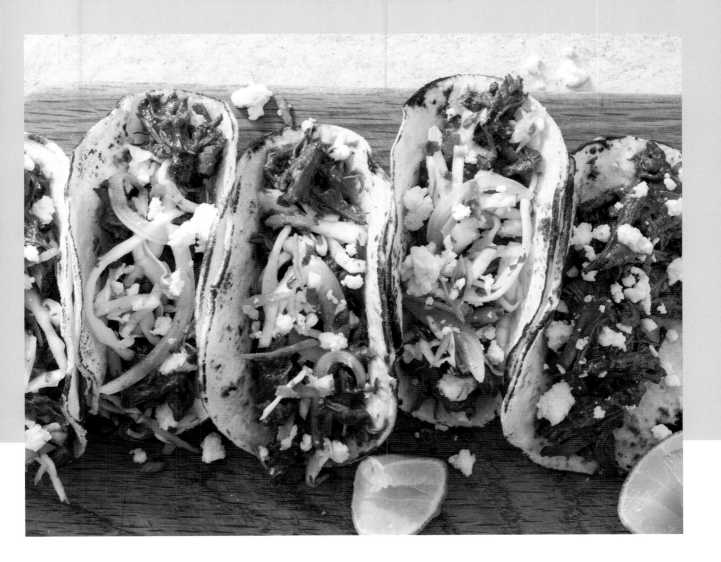

PREP AHEAD

You can chop the onion, cut up the beef, and crumble the queso fresco up to 1 day ahead and refrigerate separately. You can make the shredded beef up to 1 day ahead and refrigerate (store extra sauce separately); rewarm beef and sauce in a skillet over medium heat before using.

MAKE IT EVEN EASIER

Ask the butcher at your local market to cut up the meat for you.

TAKE IT UP A NOTCH

Serve with Tangy Coleslaw

Combine one (14-ounce) bag coleslaw mix, ½ cup minced onion, and 1 peeled and shredded carrot in large bowl. Bring 1 cup distilled white vinegar, ½ cup sugar, 1 tablespoon vegetable oil, 1 teaspoon salt, and ½ teaspoon pepper to simmer in small saucepan over medium heat, stirring to dissolve sugar. Once simmering, pour hot vinegar mixture over coleslaw mixture and toss to combine. Refrigerate until fully chilled and coleslaw mix is wilted, about 2 hours. Season with salt and pepper to taste. Serve, using slotted spoon. Coleslaw can be refrigerated up to 2 days ahead. Makes 4 cups.

Glazed Meatloaf with Root Vegetables

SERVES 2

10 square saltines

¼ cup grated Parmesan cheese

1 large egg

2 tablespoons water

2 teaspoons soy sauce

⅛ teaspoon dried thyme

½ teaspoon garlic powder

½ teaspoon pepper, divided

12 ounces 85 percent lean
ground beef

3 tablespoons ketchup

½ pound baby carrots

6 ounces parsnips or turnips,
peeled and cut into
1-inch pieces

2 teaspoons extra-virgin olive oil

¼ teaspoon table salt

2 teaspoons minced fresh chives

Why This Recipe Works There's something nostalgic about a classic meatloaf supper, but doing all the dishes afterward—not so much. For a mostly hands-off one-pan meal of meatloaf and roasted vegetables for just two, this recipe uses straightforward meatloaf ingredients that don't require precooking. A panade of crushed saltines, egg, and water keeps the ground beef moist in the oven, while soy sauce and Parmesan cheese add savory depth. The addition of fresh thyme and garlic powder adds pep, and an egg holds the meatloaf together. Finally, a coating of ketchup contributes a sweet and tangy glaze that nicely complements the meat. Hearty carrots and parsnips (or turnips) are the perfect vegetables to roast alongside the meatloaf because they only get better the longer they cook. To brighten the vegetables' deep, roasted flavor, sprinkle with chives just before serving. Note that you can also make this recipe in a toaster oven.

1 Preheat oven to 400 degrees. Line small rimmed baking sheet with aluminum foil and spray with vegetable oil spray.

2 Pulse saltines in food processor until finely ground. Combine saltine crumbs, Parmesan, egg, water, soy sauce, thyme, garlic powder, and ¼ teaspoon pepper in large bowl. Mix until all crumbs are moistened and mixture forms paste. Add beef and mix with your hands until thoroughly combined.

3 Transfer meatloaf mixture to center of prepared sheet. Using your wet hands, shape into 7 by 3½-inch rectangle; top should be flat and meatloaf should be an even 1½ inches thick.

4 Brush top and sides of meatloaf with ketchup. Toss carrots, turnips, oil, salt, and remaining ¼ teaspoon pepper together in bowl. Place vegetables cut sides down on sheet around meatloaf. Bake, on lower rack, until meatloaf registers 160 degrees, about 30 minutes.

— TAKE A 30-MINUTE BREAK —

5 Remove sheet from oven. Using 2 spatulas, transfer meatloaf to cutting board. Tent with foil and let rest while vegetables finish roasting. Return vegetables to oven and continue to roast until tender and beginning to brown, about 7 minutes. Slice meatloaf, sprinkle vegetables with chives, and serve.

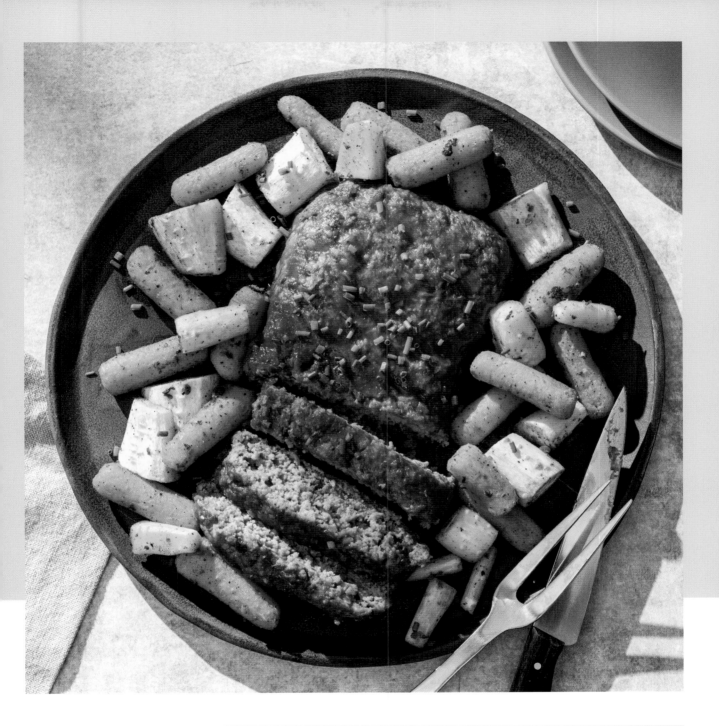

Slow-Cooker Brisket and Onions

SERVES 10 TO 12 — SUPER EASY

1 tablespoon paprika

2 teaspoons onion powder

1 teaspoon table salt

1 teaspoon garlic powder

⅛ teaspoon cayenne pepper

1 (5-pound) beef brisket, flat cut, fat trimmed to ¼ inch

1 tablespoon vegetable oil

2 large onions, halved and sliced ½ inch thick

3 tablespoons all-purpose flour

1 tablespoon tomato paste

3 garlic cloves, minced

1 cup chicken broth

2 tablespoons plus 1 teaspoon red wine vinegar, divided

1 tablespoon packed brown sugar

3 sprigs fresh thyme

3 bay leaves

Why This Recipe Works There are many things about this brisket recipe that make it perfect for the healthy back kitchen repertoire. First, it is a make-ahead recipe by necessity, as brisket benefits greatly from a spice rub and at least 8 hours of time in the fridge. Second, when made in the slow cooker, there is no need to brown this unwieldy cut. You do have to get out a skillet to brown the onions and build an aromatic sauce, but that is a small price to pay for a centerpiece roast that becomes meltingly tender during the long cooking time. Finally, it feeds a crowd and also makes great leftovers. Building the sauce on top of the onions is easy: Simply add flour, tomato paste, and garlic and deglaze the mixture with broth. A hefty dose of red wine vinegar, a little brown sugar, and fresh thyme plus bay leaves, added right to the slow cooker, finishes the base for the sauce. Once the spice-rubbed meat is added to the slow cooker, its juices can slowly mingle with all the other ingredients. Be sure to buy the brisket "first cut" or "flat cut," not "point cut," which is thicker and fattier. You will need a 5- to 7-quart oval slow cooker for this recipe.

1   Combine paprika, onion powder, salt, garlic powder, and cayenne in bowl. Using fork, prick brisket all over. Rub spice mixture over brisket, wrap tightly in plastic wrap, and refrigerate for 8 to 24 hours.

2   Heat oil in 12-inch skillet over medium heat until shimmering. Add onions and cook until softened and lightly browned, about 9 minutes. Stir in flour, tomato paste, and garlic and cook until fragrant, about 1 minute. Slowly stir in broth, scraping up any browned bits and smoothing out any lumps; transfer to slow cooker.

3   Stir 2 tablespoons vinegar, sugar, thyme sprigs, and bay leaves into slow cooker. Unwrap brisket and nestle fat side up into slow cooker. Spoon portion of onion mixture over brisket. Cover and cook until beef is tender, 9 to 10 hours on low or 6 to 7 hours on high.

— TAKE A BREAK —

4   Transfer brisket to carving board, tent loosely with aluminum foil, and let rest for 20 minutes.

— TAKE A 20-MINUTE BREAK —

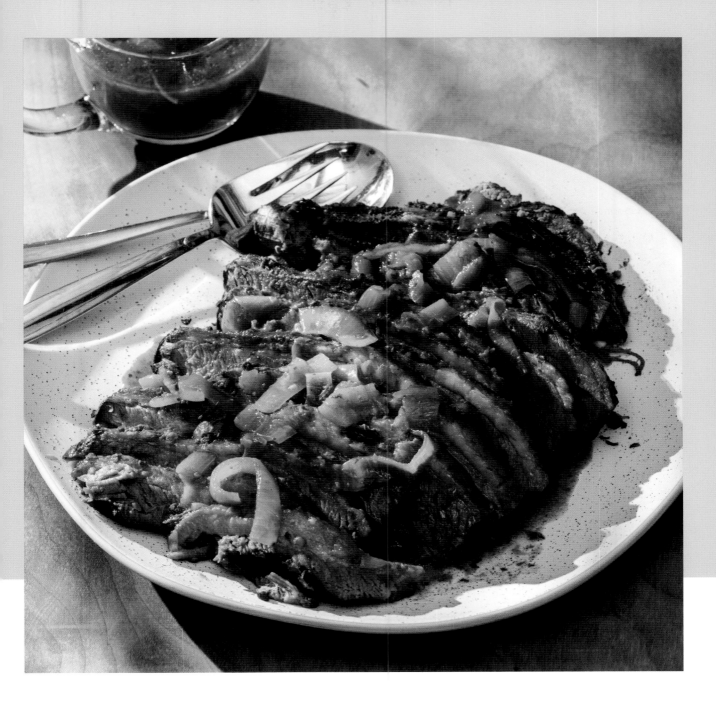

5 Discard thyme sprigs and bay leaves. Using large spoon, skim fat from surface of sauce. Stir in remaining 1 teaspoon vinegar and season with salt and pepper to taste. Slice brisket against grain into ½-inch-thick slices and arrange on serving dish. Spoon 1 cup sauce over brisket and serve, passing remaining sauce separately.

PREP AHEAD

You can make the spice rub up to 1 day ahead. You can slice the onions up to 1 day ahead and refrigerate. You must refrigerate the spice-rubbed brisket for at least 8 hours or up to 24 hours ahead.

Instant Pot Wine-Braised Short Ribs and Potatoes

SERVES 4

1½ pounds boneless short ribs, trimmed

¾ teaspoon table salt, divided

¼ teaspoon pepper

1 tablespoon extra-virgin olive oil

1 onion, chopped fine

6 garlic cloves, minced

2 tablespoons tomato paste

1 teaspoon dried oregano

1 (14.5-ounce) can diced tomatoes

½ cup dry red wine

1 pound small red potatoes, unpeeled, halved

2 tablespoons minced fresh parsley

PREP AHEAD
You can trim the short ribs and chop the onion up to 1 day ahead and refrigerate. You can cut the potatoes and refrigerate, covered with water in a bowl, for up to 1 day.

Why This Recipe Works This elegant meal is perfect for a small dinner party, but easy enough to make almost anytime. You do have to rotate things in and out of the Instant Pot, but that is not difficult, and once the ribs are under pressure, you can step away for a significant amount of time. When I was testing recipes in this book, this one was so appealing that it instantly became part of our regular dinner rotation. The first step is to brown just half of the easy-prep boneless short ribs and then set them aside to build the base of the sauce, which is complex with red wine, tomato paste, tomatoes, and aromatics. All of the ribs then go into the pot to cook for an hour under pressure, giving you a solid amount of time to do something else. As the ribs rest, it's time to cook the potatoes in the delicious fat and juices left in the pot, which takes just 4 minutes under pressure. Use small red potatoes measuring 1 to 2 inches in diameter. Note that it will take the Instant Pot about 10 minutes to come up to pressure and start the cook cycle.

1   Pat short ribs dry with paper towels and sprinkle with ½ teaspoon salt and pepper. Using highest sauté function, heat oil in electric pressure cooker for 5 minutes (or until just smoking). Brown half of short ribs on all sides, about 7 minutes; transfer to plate.

2   Add onion and remaining ¼ teaspoon salt to fat left in pot and cook, using highest sauté function, until onion is softened, about 3 minutes. Stir in garlic, tomato paste, and oregano and cook until fragrant, about 30 seconds. Stir in tomatoes and their juices and wine, scraping up any browned bits. Nestle browned short ribs (with any accumulated juices) and the remaining uncooked short ribs into pot. Lock lid in place and close pressure release valve. Select high pressure cook function and cook for 60 minutes.

—   TAKE A 70-MINUTE BREAK   —

3   Turn off instant pot and let pressure release naturally for 15 minutes.

—   TAKE A 15-MINUTE BREAK   —

4   Quick-release any remaining pressure, then carefully remove lid, allowing steam to escape away from you. Transfer short ribs to serving dish, tent with aluminum foil, and let rest while cooking potatoes.

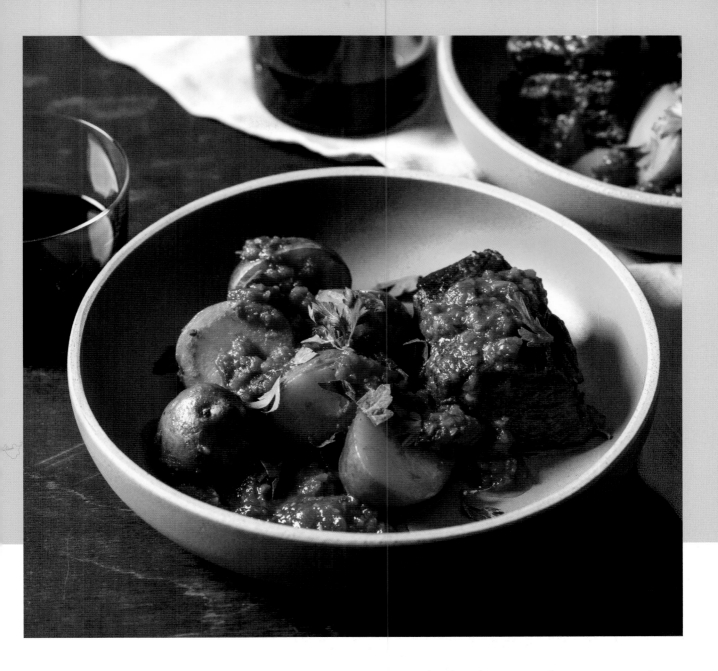

5 Add potatoes to liquid in pot. Lock lid in place and close pressure release valve. Select high pressure cook function and cook for 4 minutes.

— TAKE A 14-MINUTE BREAK —

6 Turn off instant pot and quick-release pressure. Carefully remove lid, allowing steam to escape away from you.

7 Using slotted spoon, transfer potatoes to serving dish. Simmer liquid on highest sauté function until reduced to 1½ cups, about 5 minutes. Using spoon, skim excess fat from surface of sauce. Season sauce with salt and pepper to taste. Spoon sauce over short ribs and potatoes and sprinkle with parsley. Serve.

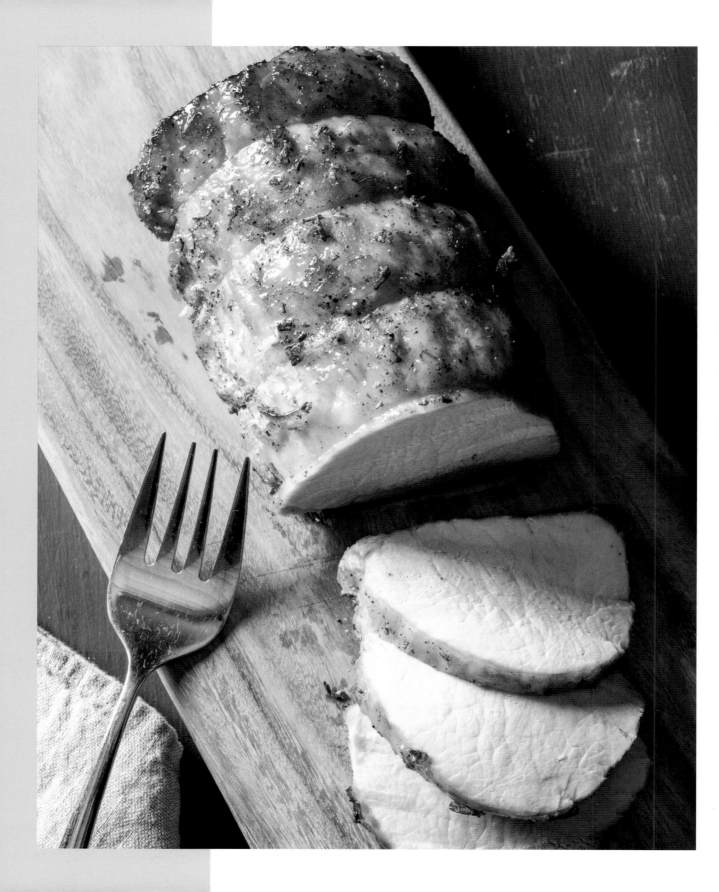

Marmalade-Glazed Pork Loin

SERVES 4 TO 6 — SUPER EASY

Why This Recipe Works It's good to have a trusty recipe for roasting a pork loin in your back pocket, because not only does it make a great entrée, a three-pound roast fits on a small rimmed baking sheet and is easy to maneuver into your oven or toaster oven. It's also a recipe that takes just minutes to prep and gives you lots of walkaway time. Glossing the roast with a bittersweet marmalade-rosemary glaze adds plenty of flavor to the rather mild pork. Letting the roast rest before slicing allows the juices to redistribute through the meat. A well-marbled pork loin roast from the blade is ideal for this recipe. For best results, avoid using enhanced pork (pork injected with a solution of water, salt, and chemicals); it causes the pork to exude excess liquid as it cooks.

1 (3-pound) boneless pork loin roast, trimmed and tied at 1½-inch intervals

1 teaspoon table salt

½ teaspoon pepper

3 tablespoons orange marmalade

1½ teaspoons extra-virgin olive oil

1½ teaspoons chopped fresh rosemary

1   Preheat oven to 375 degrees. Place pork in center of small rimmed baking sheet and sprinkle with salt and pepper.

2   Combine marmalade, oil, and rosemary in bowl. Spread mixture on pork. Roast, on middle rack, until instant-read thermometer inserted in thickest part of meat registers 135 to 140 degrees, about 50 minutes.

— TAKE A 50-MINUTE BREAK —

3   Transfer roast to carving board and let rest for 10 minutes.

— TAKE A 10-MINUTE BREAK —

4   Remove twine from roast and slice pork. Serve.

PREP AHEAD
You can trim and tie the pork up to 1 day ahead and refrigerate.

Pork Tenderloin Stroganoff

SERVES 4

3 ounces pancetta, cut into
¼-inch pieces

1 tablespoon extra-virgin olive oil

1 (12-ounce) pork tenderloin,
trimmed, halved lengthwise,
and sliced crosswise ¼ inch
thick

3 tablespoons all-purpose flour,
divided

1 teaspoon table salt, divided

1 teaspoon pepper, divided

3 tablespoons unsalted butter,
divided

12 ounces cremini mushrooms,
sliced

1 large onion, chopped fine

4 teaspoons chopped fresh
sage, divided

3 garlic cloves, minced

2 teaspoons tomato paste

4 cups chicken broth

¼ cup dry white wine

8 ounces (4 cups) egg noodles

½ cup sour cream

2 tablespoons minced
fresh chives

Why This Recipe Works I grew up in the Midwest, where hearty, meaty dishes like stroganoff were always on the menu, especially during the cold winter months. I have to admit that I had never had a stroganoff made with pork tenderloin, but with its faintly sweet flavor and relatively low price, the pork makes for an excellent riff on this supercomforting dish of creamy noodles and meat. This recipe requires a bit of work, but much of the prep can be done in advance. It also makes great leftovers if you are cooking for just two. Crisping up a bit of diced pancetta first makes a big difference, as it adds a layer of salty, intense pork flavor to enhance the tenderloin's relatively mild flavor. From there, dredging thin slices of pork tenderloin in seasoned flour ensures that the pork remains tender and adds body and creaminess to the sauce. After quickly browning the pork and creating a flavorful fond in the pot, adding earthy cremini mushrooms, floral sage, and concentrated tomato paste creates a savory underpinning. A bit of white wine adds brightness, and cooking the noodles in the saucy mix of wine and chicken broth ensures that they soak up lots of flavor.

1 Cook pancetta and oil in Dutch oven over medium heat until pancetta is lightly browned and crispy, about 10 minutes. Using slotted spoon, transfer pancetta to large plate, leaving fat in pot.

— TAKE A 10-MINUTE BREAK —

2 Toss pork, 2 tablespoons flour, ½ teaspoon salt, and ½ teaspoon pepper together in bowl. Add 1 tablespoon butter to fat left in pot and melt over high heat. Add pork in single layer, breaking up any clumps, and cook without stirring until browned on bottom, about 2 minutes. Stir and continue to cook until pork is no longer pink, about 1 minute. Transfer to plate with pancetta.

3 Melt remaining 2 tablespoons butter in now-empty pot over medium heat. Add mushrooms, onion, remaining ½ teaspoon salt, and remaining ½ teaspoon pepper and cook until any liquid has evaporated and vegetables have just begun to brown, about 8 minutes. Add 1 tablespoon sage, garlic, tomato paste, and remaining 1 tablespoon flour and cook until fragrant, about 30 seconds. Turn off heat and cover pot.

— TAKE A 15-MINUTE BREAK —

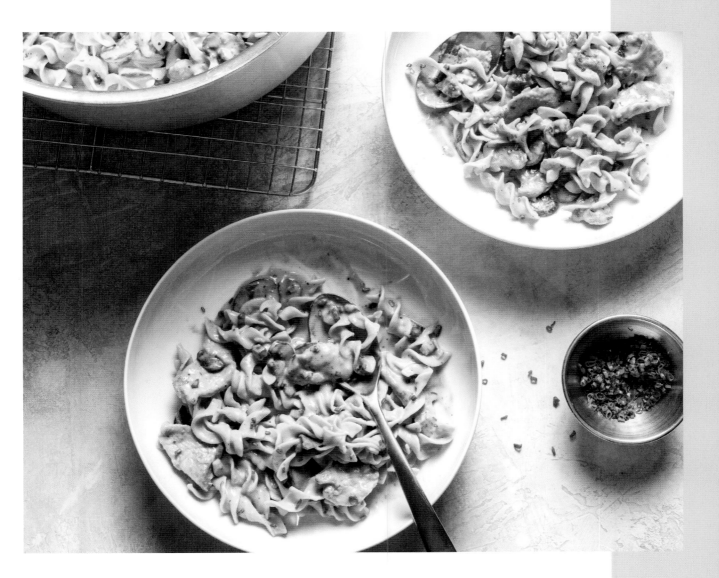

4   Add broth and wine to pot and bring to simmer over medium heat, scraping up any browned bits. Stir in noodles and cook, uncovered, until noodles are just tender, about 10 minutes.

— TAKE A 10-MINUTE BREAK —

5   Add pork and pancetta and cook until warmed through, about 1 minute. Off heat, stir in sour cream and remaining 1 teaspoon sage until thoroughly combined. Season with salt and pepper to taste. Sprinkle with chives and serve.

PREP AHEAD

You can prep the pancetta, pork, mushrooms, and onions and refrigerate separately up to 1 day ahead. You can refrigerate the stroganoff for up to 1 day; reheat in a 12-inch skillet over medium-low heat, adding additional broth as needed.

MAKE IT EVEN EASIER

Buy sliced mushrooms and chopped pancetta.

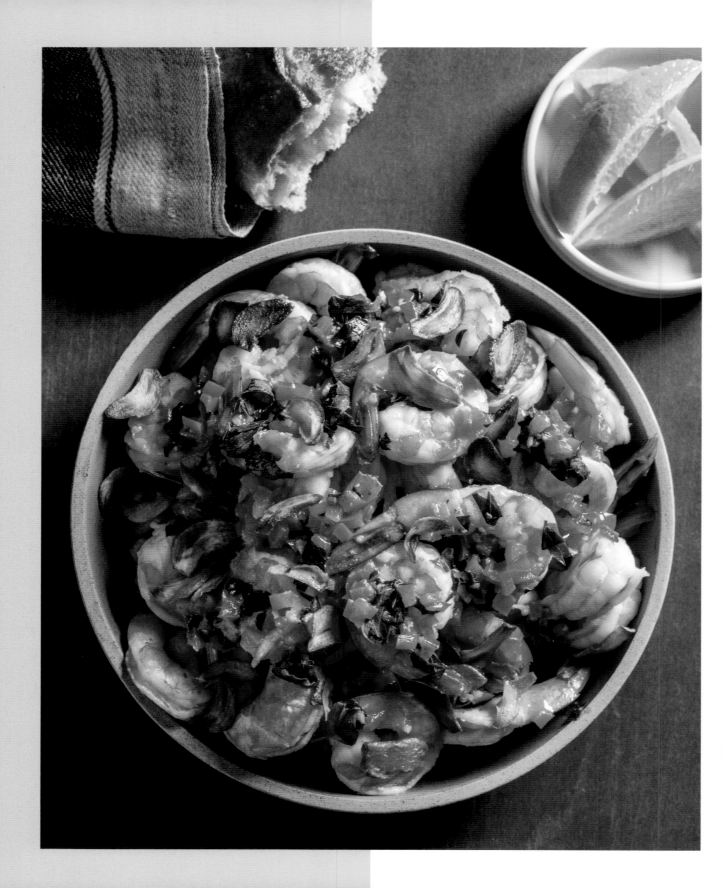

Sizzling Garlic Shrimp

SERVES 4 — SUPER EASY

Why This Recipe Works A cousin of shrimp scampi, this rendition of garlic shrimp is a real treat and super easy to make. Served with crusty bread to mop up the buttery juices, it is an indisputable comfort classic. And while it is a great weeknight dinner, you could also serve it as an appetizer at a dinner party. The first step in building flavor is to heat sliced garlic in olive oil until the garlic is slightly browned and crisp (these garlic chips are then added just before serving). The garlic-infused oil left behind is used to quickly cook diced bell pepper and the shrimp. A splash of dry sherry on the shrimp instantly elevates the flavor. Then you move the shrimp to a serving platter and make a very quick sauce in the pan with more garlic (this time minced), parsley, butter, and lemon juice to complete the satisfying dish. Make sure you have all your ingredients prepped before you start cooking, as the recipe moves very quickly once started.

1 Pat shrimp dry and sprinkle with salt and pepper.

2 Cook oil and sliced garlic in large skillet over medium heat, stirring often, until garlic is golden and crisp, about 3 minutes. Using slotted spoon, transfer garlic to small bowl. Add bell pepper and pepper flakes to skillet and cook until bell pepper is soft, about 3 minutes. Increase heat to high, add shrimp, and cook until edges turn pink, about 1 minute. Flip shrimp, add sherry, and simmer until shrimp are just cooked through, about 1 minute. Using slotted spoon, transfer shrimp to serving platter.

3 Add minced garlic, parsley, butter, and lemon juice to skillet and simmer until thickened, about 1 minute. Adjust seasonings, pour sauce over shrimp, and scatter browned garlic chips on top. Serve with lemon wedges.

1½ pounds peeled and deveined large shrimp (26 to 30 per pound)

¼ teaspoon table salt

¼ teaspoon pepper

¼ cup extra-virgin olive oil

6 cloves garlic, sliced thin lengthwise, plus 1 clove minced

1 red bell pepper, seeded and diced

¼ teaspoon red pepper flakes

¼ cup dry sherry

2 tablespoons chopped fresh parsley leaves

2 tablespoons unsalted butter, softened

1 tablespoon fresh lemon juice, plus lemon wedges for serving

---

PREP AHEAD
You can dice the pepper up to 1 day ahead and refrigerate.

Oven-Poached Side of Salmon

1 (4-pound) center-cut skin-on salmon fillet, pin bones removed

1 teaspoon table salt

2 tablespoons cider vinegar

6 sprigs fresh tarragon or dill, plus 2 tablespoons minced

2 lemons, sliced thin, plus lemon wedges for serving

Why This Recipe Works I'm a firm believer that socializing with friends is key to everyone's well-being, and that a great way to do that is to entertain, but entertain simply. What I love about this classic salmon recipe is that it is easy to assemble and eliminates both the need to use a heavy fish poacher and standing at the stove for half an hour making sure the salmon doesn't overcook. The low, gentle heat of the oven steam-cooks the foil-wrapped side of salmon that is topped with lemon slices and fresh tarragon or dill to infuse it with flavor. This moist, gentle cooking method produces soft, supple salmon from end to end. The foil-wrapped salmon is placed directly on the oven rack—no heavy baking sheet required. Just pull out the oven rack a few inches and carefully place the salmon right on it. However, this is a case where you might ask a family member or friend to help you take it out of the oven when it is done, as it will be hot and a bit awkward. Use heavy-duty aluminum foil measuring 18 inches wide.

1 Preheat oven to 250 degrees. Cut 3 pieces of heavy-duty aluminum foil 12 inches longer than side of salmon. Working with 2 pieces of foil, fold up 1 long side of each by 3 inches. Lay sheets side by side with folded sides touching, fold edges together to create secure seam, and press seam flat. Center third sheet of foil over seam. Spray foil with vegetable oil spray.

2 Pat salmon dry with paper towels and sprinkle with salt. Lay salmon, skin side down, in center of foil. Sprinkle with vinegar, then top with tarragon sprigs and lemon slices. Fold foil up over salmon to create seam on top and gently fold foil edges together to secure; do not crimp too tightly.

3 Lay foil-wrapped salmon directly on middle oven rack (without baking sheet). Cook until center registers 135 to 140 degrees, 45 to 60 minutes. (To check temperature, poke thermometer through foil and into fish.)

— TAKE A 45-MINUTE BREAK —

4 Remove salmon from oven and carefully open foil. Let salmon cool for 30 minutes.

— TAKE A 30-MINUTE BREAK —

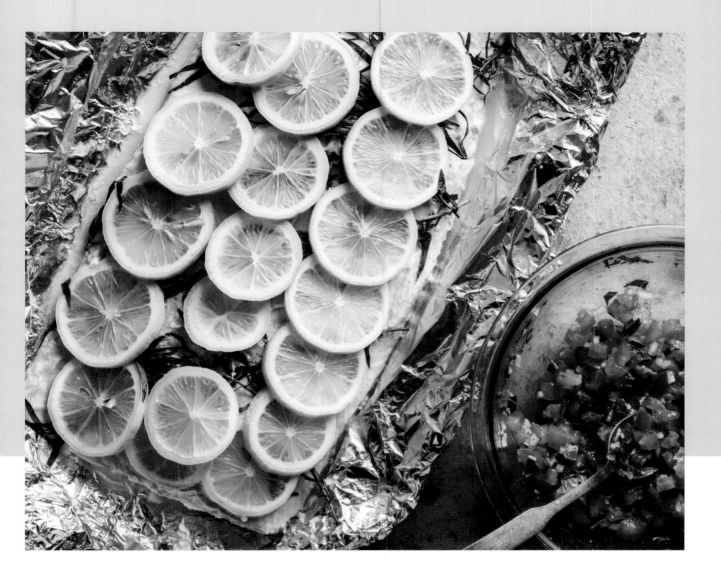

5 Pour off any accumulated liquid, then reseal salmon in foil and refrigerate until cold, at least 1 hour or up to 24 hours.

— TAKE A BREAK —

6 Unwrap salmon and brush away lemon slices, tarragon sprigs, and any solidified poaching liquid. Transfer fish to serving platter, sprinkle with minced tarragon, and serve with lemon wedges.

PREP AHEAD

After the salmon has cooled for 30 minutes in step 4, it must be refrigerated for at least 1 hour or up to 24 hours before serving.

TAKE IT UP A NOTCH
Serve with Fresh Tomato Relish

Combine 4 finely diced plum tomatoes, ½ minced small shallot, 1 minced garlic clove, 2 tablespoons chopped fresh basil, 1 tablespoon extra-virgin olive oil, and 1 teaspoon red wine vinegar in medium bowl. Season to taste with salt and pepper. Relish can be made up to 3 hours ahead and refrigerated. Makes 1½ cups.

Meaty Loaf Pan Lasagna

SERVES 2 TO 3

- 1 tablespoon extra-virgin olive oil
- 8 ounces meatloaf mix
- ¼ teaspoon plus ⅛ teaspoon table salt, divided
- 1 (16-ounce) jar tomato sauce
- 1 tablespoon heavy cream
- 4 ounces (½ cup) whole-milk or part-skim ricotta cheese
- 1 ounce grated Parmesan cheese (½ cup) plus 2 tablespoons, divided
- 3 tablespoons chopped fresh basil
- 1 large egg, lightly beaten
- ⅛ teaspoon pepper
- 4 no-boil lasagna noodles
- 4 ounces shredded whole-milk mozzarella cheese (1 cup), divided

PREP AHEAD

You can make the ricotta mixture up to 1 day ahead and refrigerate. The fully assembled lasagna can be refrigerated for up to 2 hours before baking; increase baking time by 10 minutes.

Why This Recipe Works Nothing satisfies like a big square of cheesy, meaty, homemade lasagna. But this timeless classic usually feeds a crowd and takes some time to put together. Made in a loaf pan, this petite lasagna is better suited for a couple (with leftovers) and puts lasagna back in the rotation of anyone suffering from back pain because it is easier to assemble and requires far less standing time. In addition, no-boil lasagna noodles make assembly go quickly; plus, the noodles fit perfectly into the loaf pan. And finally, instead of making a from-scratch sauce, jarred tomato sauce means far less time standing at the stove. To start, brown meatloaf mix, add the sauce, and let it all simmer together briefly; then add a touch of cream for richness. Covering the lasagna with aluminum foil prevents it from drying out in the oven, but then removing the foil for the last few minutes of baking achieves the browned, cheesy top layer found on a full-size lasagna. If you cannot find meatloaf mix, substitute equal parts 80 percent lean ground beef and sweet Italian sausage, casings removed. Do not substitute fat-free ricotta here.

1 Heat oil in large saucepan over medium heat until shimmering. Stir in meatloaf mix and ¼ teaspoon salt and cook, breaking up meat with wooden spoon, until it is no longer pink, about 2 minutes.

2 Stir in tomato sauce. Bring to simmer and cook until flavors meld, about 2 minutes. Stir in cream. Season with salt and pepper to taste. Turn off heat.

— TAKE A 10-MINUTE BREAK —

3 Preheat oven to 400 degrees. Combine ricotta, ½ cup Parmesan, basil, egg, remaining ⅛ teaspoon salt, and pepper in bowl.

4 Spread ½ cup meat sauce over bottom of 9 by 5-inch loaf pan, avoiding large chunks of meat. Place 1 noodle in pan and spread one-third of ricotta mixture over top. Sprinkle evenly with ¼ cup mozzarella and spoon ½ cup sauce evenly over top.

5 Repeat layering process of noodle, ricotta mixture, mozzarella, and sauce twice more. Place remaining noodle on top, cover with remaining 1 cup sauce, and sprinkle with remaining ¼ cup mozzarella and remaining 2 tablespoons Parmesan.

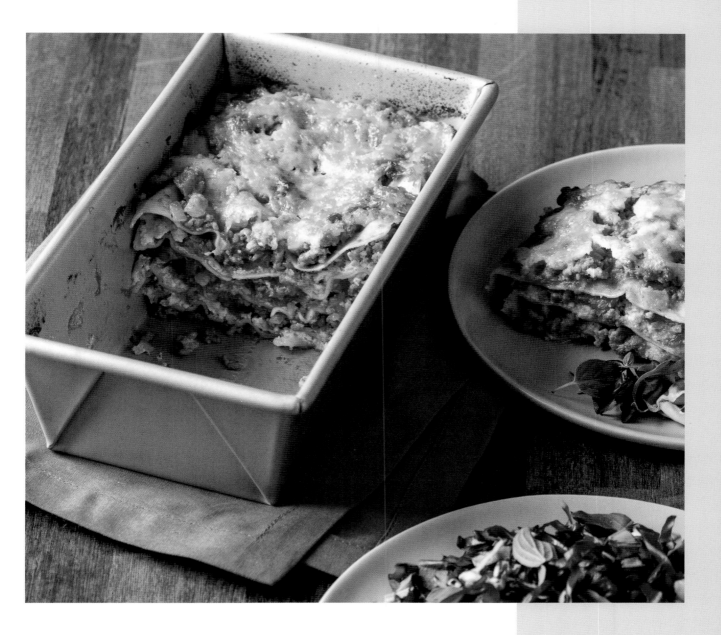

6 Cover dish tightly with aluminum foil sprayed with vegetable oil spray. Bake, on middle rack, until sauce bubbles lightly around edges, about 30 minutes.

— **TAKE A 30-MINUTE BREAK** —

7 Remove foil and continue to bake until lasagna is hot throughout and cheese is browned in spots, about 10 minutes.

— **TAKE A 10-MINUTE BREAK** —

8 Let cool for 15 minutes before serving.

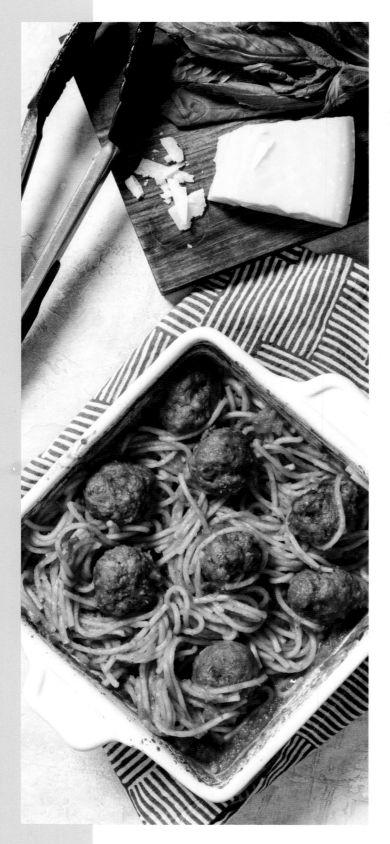
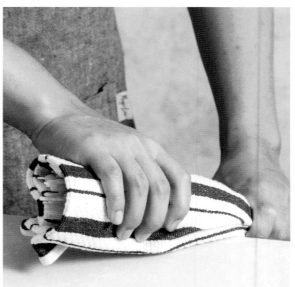
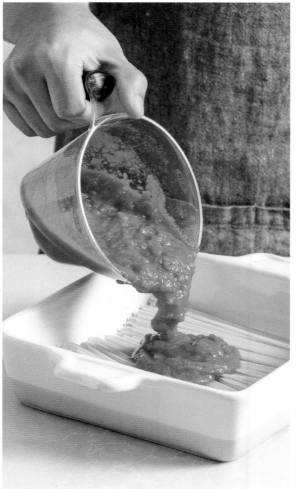

Baked Spaghetti and Meatballs

SERVES 2 — SUPER EASY

Why This Recipe Works An entirely hands-off dinner of spaghetti and meatballs sounds like a dream: no long wait for the water to boil, no tedious browning of the meatballs, no time-consuming sauce. For a supersimple one-pot spaghetti and meatballs, this version pares it down to the basics to deliver the nostalgic, satisfying meal of childhood. An easy combination of ground beef, store-bought pesto, and panko bread crumbs yields meatballs with plenty of flavor. To cook the pasta right in the sauce, the first step is to spread spaghetti in a casserole dish and cover it with jarred marinara sauce that is thinned with water to ensure that there is enough moisture to properly cook the strands. Then simply nestle the meatballs into the sauce and let everything bake, covered, in a very hot oven for 30 minutes. These conditions simulate boiling on the stovetop, enabling our pasta to cook in the sauce and absorb the flavors surrounding it. Once the pasta is al dente, uncover the baking dish, give the pasta a stir, and let the meatballs brown and the sauce thicken for the last few minutes of baking.

6	ounces spaghetti
1½	cups jarred marinara sauce
1	cup water, plus extra as needed
⅓	cup panko bread crumbs
3	tablespoons milk
8	ounces 85 percent lean ground beef
2	tablespoons store-bought basil pesto
½	teaspoon table salt
⅛	teaspoon pepper
1	tablespoon chopped fresh basil

1   Preheat oven to 475 degrees. Spray 8-inch square baking dish with vegetable oil spray. Loosely wrap pasta in dish towel, then press bundle against corner of counter to break noodles into 6-inch lengths. Spread pasta in prepared dish. Pour marinara sauce and water over pasta and toss gently with tongs to coat.

2   Using fork, mash panko and milk in large bowl until smooth paste forms. Add beef, pesto, salt, and pepper and knead mixture with your hands until well combined. Pinch off and roll mixture into 1½-inch meatballs (you should have about 8 meatballs). Place meatballs on top of pasta in dish. Cover dish tightly with aluminum foil and bake, on middle rack, for 30 minutes.

—   TAKE A 30-MINUTE BREAK   —

3   Remove dish from oven and stir pasta thoroughly, scraping sides and bottom of dish. Return uncovered dish to oven and continue to bake until pasta is tender and sauce is thickened, about 6 minutes.

4   Remove dish from oven. Toss to coat pasta and meatballs with sauce, adjusting sauce consistency with extra hot water as needed. Let cool for 10 minutes. Season with salt and pepper to taste. Sprinkle with basil and serve.

PREP AHEAD
You can form the meatballs up to 1 day ahead and refrigerate.

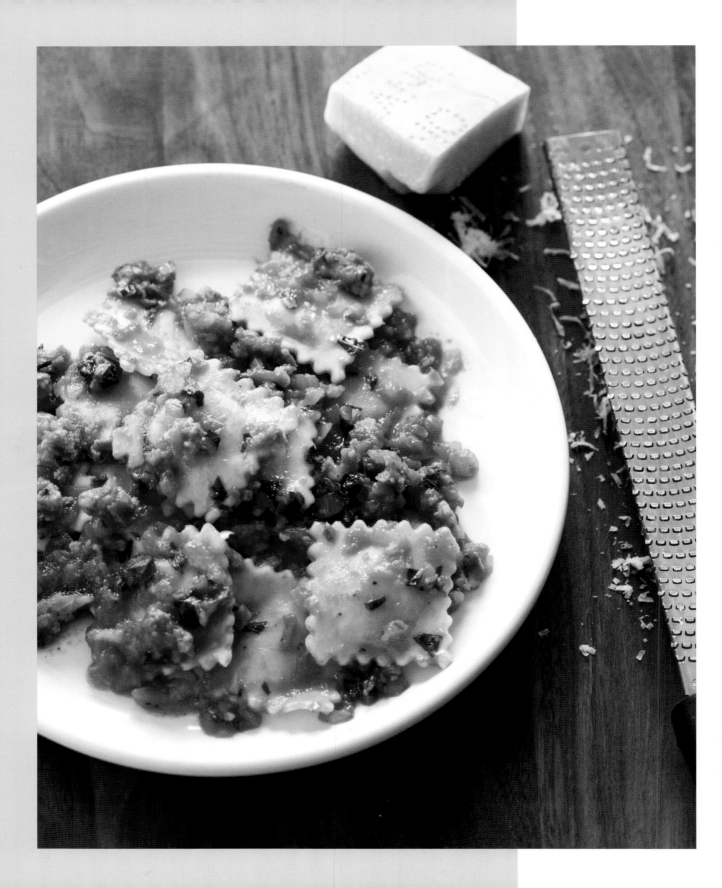

Skillet Ravioli with Meat Sauce

SERVES 2

Why This Recipe Works A staple on every Italian restaurant menu, cheese-stuffed ravioli covered in meaty tomato sauce is the ultimate comfort food. For an effortless take on this dish, fresh store-bought ravioli cooks right in the sauce. This not only eliminates extra pans but also allows the ravioli to soak up even more flavor. Crumbled fresh Italian sausage stands in for the usual ground beef, adding welcome herbal and aromatic notes on top of meaty flavor. A little minced porcini enhances the sauce's savory depth in short order, and a small can of diced tomatoes plus a little water provide the base of the sauce as well as the liquid for simmering the pasta. Because the ravioli cooks right in the sauce, use fresh ravioli; do not substitute frozen ravioli.

1   Heat oil in 12-inch skillet over medium heat until shimmering. Add onion and cook until softened and lightly browned, about 6 minutes. Stir in garlic and porcini and cook until fragrant, about 1 minute.

2   Add sausage and cook, breaking up meat with wooden spoon, for 1 minute. Turn off heat.

—   TAKE A 15-MINUTE BREAK   —

3   Add tomatoes and pepper to skillet, bring to simmer over medium heat, and cook until sauce is slightly thickened, about 10 minutes.

—   TAKE A 10-MINUTE BREAK   —

4   Add water and pasta to skillet, bring to vigorous simmer over medium heat, and cook, stirring often, until pasta is tender and sauce is thickened, about 8 minutes; if sauce becomes too thick, add extra water as needed. Off heat, stir in basil and season with salt and pepper to taste. Serve with Parmesan.

Ingredients

- 1 tablespoon extra-virgin olive oil
- 1 small onion, chopped fine
- 2 garlic cloves, minced
- ⅛ ounce dried porcini mushrooms, rinsed and minced
- 8 ounces sweet Italian sausage, casings removed
- 1 (14.5-ounce) can crushed tomatoes (1½ cups)
- ⅛ teaspoon pepper
- 1½ cups water, plus extra as needed
- 1 (9-ounce) package fresh cheese ravioli
- 2 tablespoons chopped fresh basil
- Grated Parmesan cheese

PREP AHEAD
You can chop the onion and mince the porcini up to 1 day ahead and refrigerate separately.

Skillet Ziti with Sausage and Peppers

SERVES 4

1 pound sweet Italian sausage, casings removed

6 garlic cloves, minced

¼ teaspoon red pepper flakes

1 (28-ounce) can crushed tomatoes

8 ounces (2½ cups) ziti

1½ cups water

1 red bell pepper, stemmed, seeded, and cut into ½-inch pieces

½ teaspoon table salt

1 ounce grated Parmesan cheese (½ cup)

⅓ cup heavy cream

¼ cup chopped fresh basil

6 ounces shredded mozzarella cheese (1½ cups)

Why This Recipe Works Baked ziti with sausage and bell peppers is an Italian American classic, and here it's made faster using a hybrid stovetop-to-oven approach—without sacrificing any of its bold flavor. Although this recipe has a few steps, there are breaks built in so you can pace yourself if you need to. For pronounced meatiness, render crumbled sweet Italian sausage in a skillet and then add canned crushed tomatoes and simmer to rid the tomatoes of their raw flavor and concentrate their sweetness. Add water to the skillet along with the ziti and cook the pasta right in its sauce until it's just tender. To finish, stir in cream and Parmesan, sprinkle the whole thing with shredded mozzarella, and transfer the skillet to the oven to finish cooking the pasta and brown the topping. You will need a 12-inch nonstick ovensafe skillet with a tight-fitting lid for this recipe.

1   Preheat oven to 450 degrees. Cook sausage in 12-inch ovensafe nonstick skillet over medium-high heat, breaking up meat with wooden spoon, until lightly browned, about 4 minutes. Stir in garlic and pepper flakes and cook until fragrant, about 30 seconds. Stir in tomatoes and simmer gently until tomatoes no longer taste raw, about 10 minutes.

—   TAKE A 10-MINUTE BREAK   —

2   Add ziti, water, bell pepper, and salt to skillet; cover; and bring to vigorous simmer over medium-high heat. Reduce heat to medium and cook, covered, stirring often, until pasta is nearly tender, about 16 minutes.

3   Off heat, stir in Parmesan, cream, and basil and season with salt and pepper to taste. Sprinkle mozzarella evenly over top. Transfer skillet to oven and bake, on middle rack, until cheese is melted and browned, about 10 minutes.

—   TAKE A 12-MINUTE BREAK   —

4   Let ziti rest for 10 minutes before serving.

PREP AHEAD
You can cut up the pepper up to 1 day ahead and refrigerate.

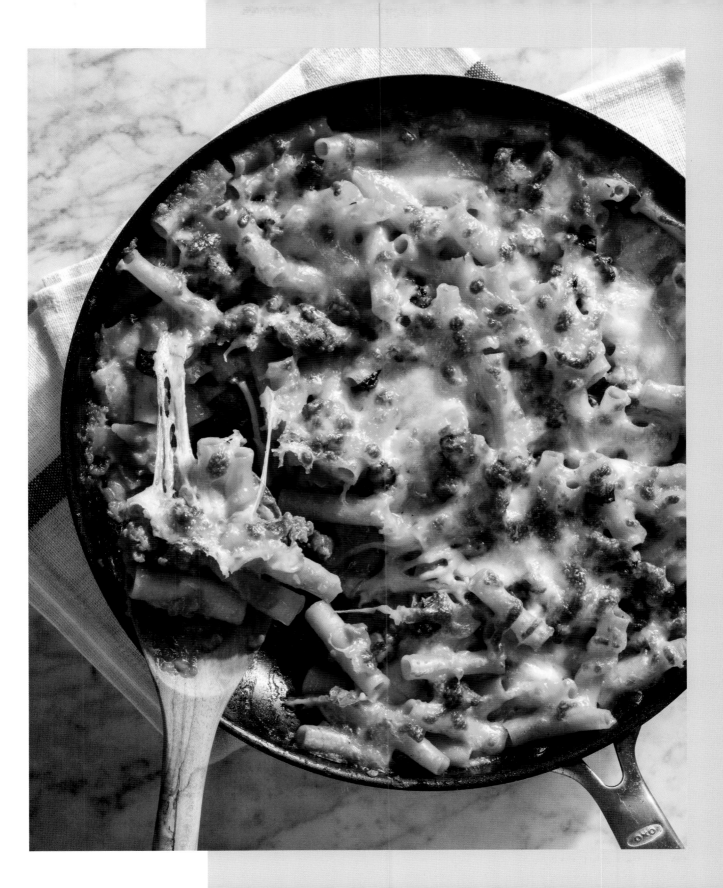

Cheesy Tex-Mex Chili Mac

SERVES 4 — SUPER EASY

1 tablespoon vegetable oil

1 onion, chopped fine

1 tablespoon chili powder

1 tablespoon ground cumin

½ teaspoon table salt

3 garlic cloves, minced

1 tablespoon packed brown sugar

1 pound 90 percent lean
ground beef

2 cups water

1 (15-ounce) can tomato sauce

8 ounces (2 cups) elbow macaroni
or small shells

1 cup frozen corn, thawed

1 (4.5-ounce) can chopped
green chiles, drained

2 tablespoons minced
fresh cilantro

8 ounces shredded Mexican
cheese blend (2 cups), divided

Why This Recipe Works I don't know anyone who doesn't love the combo of beef chili, macaroni, and cheese; the combo, and all its many permutations, is the definition of comfort food in my book. This easy-to-prep and easy-to-cook version will have you making it once again if you've lost sight of its charms. Many recipes are a sorry mix of canned chili and jarred salsa stirred into packaged macaroni and cheese. This quick skillet version combines the best spicy beef chili, real cheese, and perfectly cooked macaroni. Starting with the chili, a mix of onion and garlic along with chili powder and cumin jump-start the flavor base before the addition of lean ground beef. Then a can of tomato sauce (and some water) provides enough liquid to cook the macaroni. Brown sugar helps tame the acidity of the tomato sauce, and stirring in canned green chiles, sweet corn, and cilantro at the end ensures heartiness and flavor. Finally, a shredded Mexican cheese blend helps bind the mixture together and enriches the dish with cheesy flavor. For more spice, add ½ teaspoon red pepper flakes along with the chili powder.

1   Heat oil in 12-inch nonstick skillet over medium heat until shimmering. Add onion, chili powder, cumin, and salt and cook, stirring often, until onion is softened, about 6 minutes. Stir in garlic and brown sugar and cook until fragrant, about 30 seconds. Stir in beef, breaking up meat with wooden spoon, and cook until lightly browned and no longer pink, about 4 minutes. Turn off heat and cover skillet.

— TAKE A 15-MINUTE BREAK —

2   Add water, tomato sauce, and macaroni to skillet; cover; and cook over medium-high heat at vigorous simmer, stirring often, until macaroni is nearly tender, about 11 minutes.

3   Off heat, stir in corn, green chiles, cilantro, and 1 cup cheese. Season with salt and pepper to taste. Sprinkle remaining 1 cup cheese over top, cover, and let stand off heat until cheese melts, about 3 minutes. Serve.

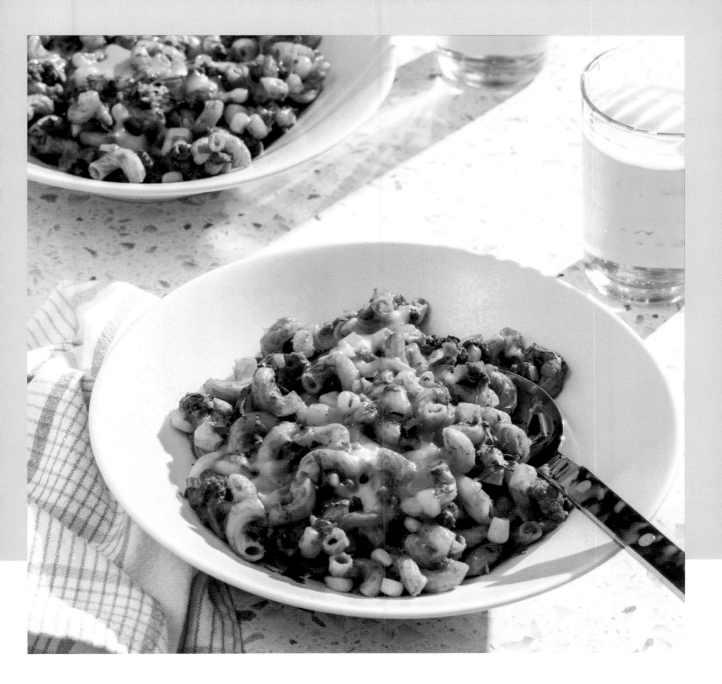

PREP AHEAD

You can chop the onion up to 1 day ahead and refrigerate. You can make the chili mac through step 2 up to 1 day ahead and refrigerate; reheat in a 12-inch skillet over medium heat, then add the corn, green chiles, and cilantro and top with cheese, following the instructions in step 3.

TAKE IT UP A NOTCH

Serve with sour cream, chopped red onion, and chopped avocado.

Simple Stovetop Macaroni and Cheese

SERVES 4

1½ cups water

1 cup milk

8 ounces (2 cups) elbow macaroni

4 ounces shredded American cheese (1 cup)

½ teaspoon Dijon mustard

Pinch cayenne pepper

4 ounces shredded extra-sharp cheddar cheese (1 cup)

⅓ cup panko bread crumbs

1 tablespoon extra-virgin olive oil

⅛ teaspoon table salt

⅛ teaspoon pepper

2 tablespoons grated Parmesan cheese

Why This Recipe Works If you held a secret vote among my family members, I suspect that all of us (myself included) would vote macaroni and cheese as one of our top three favorite dishes of all time. Most from-scratch macaroni and cheese recipes require making a béchamel sauce, which means watching the pan closely until the sauce just emulsifies (and before it scorches your pan). And then you have to boil the macaroni in a separate big pot before adding it and the cheese to the sauce in increments. That adds up to a lot of standing time, which of course works against anyone with back pain. Here, using science and a emulsifying trick, the process of creating a rich and comforting stovetop macaroni and cheese is reinvented. An innovative macaroni and cheese recipe that called for adding sodium citrate was the inspiration for the trick: Sodium citrate is an emulsifying salt added to cheese to keep it smooth when heated. So the sauce here is based on American cheese, which contains a similar ingredient, instead of a béchamel. Because American cheese has plenty of emulsifier but not a lot of flavor, extra-sharp cheddar is added to boost the cheesy flavor, along with a bit of mustard and cayenne pepper. Cooking the macaroni in a smaller-than-usual amount of water (along with some milk), means there is no draining required; the liquid left after the pasta is hydrated is just enough to form the base of the sauce. Cheesy toasted panko bread crumbs provide the crunch factor and eliminate the need for baking. Because the macaroni is cooked in a measured amount of liquid, don't use different shapes or sizes of pasta. Use a 4-ounce block of American cheese from the deli counter rather than presliced cheese.

1 Bring water and milk to boil in medium saucepan over high heat. Stir in macaroni and reduce heat to medium-low. Cook, stirring frequently, until macaroni is soft (slightly past al dente), about 7 minutes. Add American cheese, mustard, and cayenne and cook, stirring constantly, until cheese is completely melted, about 1 minute. Off heat, stir in cheddar until evenly distributed but not melted. Cover saucepan and let stand for 5 minutes.

2 Meanwhile, combine panko, oil, salt, and pepper in 8-inch nonstick skillet until panko is evenly moistened. Cook over medium heat, stirring frequently, until evenly browned, about 3 minutes. Off heat, sprinkle Parmesan over panko mixture and stir to combine. Transfer panko mixture to small bowl.

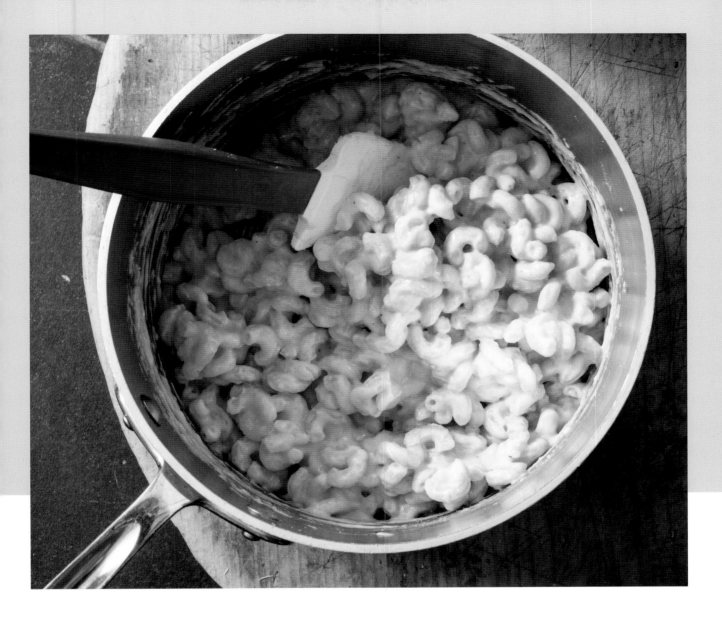

3 Stir macaroni until sauce is smooth (sauce may look loose but will thicken as it cools). Season with salt and pepper to taste. Transfer to warm serving dish and sprinkle panko mixture over top. Serve immediately.

PREP AHEAD
You can shred the American cheese up to 1 day ahead and refrigerate. You can make the panko mixture up to 1 day ahead and refrigerate.

VARIATION

Grown-Up Stovetop Macaroni and Cheese
Increase water to 1¾ cups. Substitute ¾ cup shredded Gruyère cheese and 2 tablespoons crumbled blue cheese for cheddar.

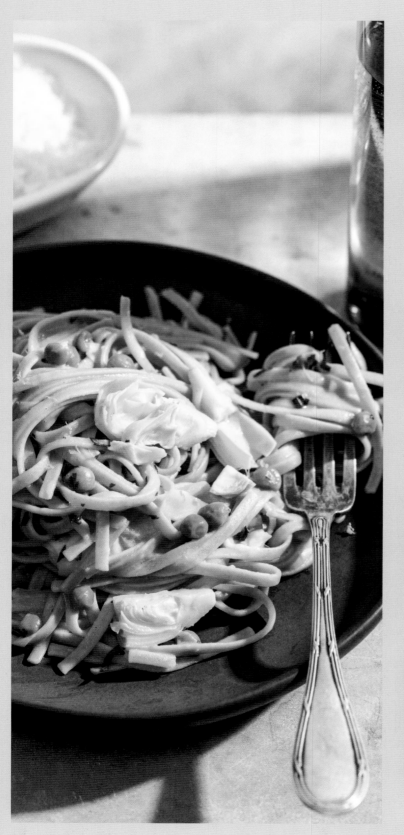

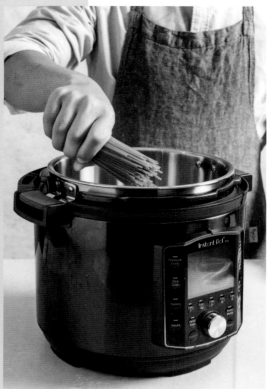

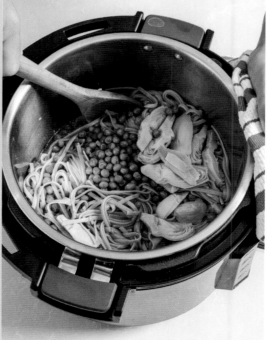

Instant Pot Creamy Spring Vegetable Linguine

SERVES 4 TO 6 — SUPER EASY

Why This Recipe Works This uncomplicated pasta dish was a revelation to me: perfect al dente noodles in a silky sauce, with a vibrant mix of vegetables and flavors—but without multiple pots, boiling water, or messy draining. Linguine is the best shape to use here, as the thicker strands retain their bite in the ultrahigh heat of the Instant Pot. After cooking the pasta at pressure, you simply stir in convenient frozen baby artichokes and frozen peas. By using exactly the right amount of water, there is no need to drain the pasta; instead, all of the starch that the linguine releases makes it a cinch to emulsify grated Pecorino and the residual cooking liquid into a luscious sauce. To finish, lemon zest and fresh tarragon enliven this springy, light dish. You can substitute traditional linguine for the whole-wheat linguine; however, do not substitute other pasta shapes. Note that it will take the Instant Pot about 10 minutes to come up to pressure and start the cook cycle.

1   Loosely wrap half of pasta in dish towel, then press bundle against corner of counter to break noodles into 6-inch lengths; repeat with remaining pasta.

2   Add pasta, water, oil, and salt to electric pressure cooker, making sure pasta is completely submerged. Lock lid into place and close pressure-release valve. Select high pressure-cook function and cook for 4 minutes.

—   TAKE A 14-MINUTE BREAK   —

3   Turn off electric pressure cooker and quick-release pressure. Carefully remove lid, allowing steam to escape away from you.

4   Stir artichokes and peas into pasta. Partially cover pot and let sit until pasta is tender, vegetables are heated through, and sauce is thickened, about 7 minutes. Stir in Pecorino and pepper until cheese is melted and fully combined. Stir in lemon zest and tarragon and season with salt and pepper to taste. Serve, passing extra Pecorino separately.

1   pound 100 percent whole-wheat linguine

5   cups water

1   tablespoon extra-virgin olive oil

1½   teaspoons table salt

1   cup frozen artichoke hearts, thawed

1   cup frozen peas, thawed

4   ounces grated Pecorino Romano cheese (2 cups), plus extra for serving

½   teaspoon pepper

2   teaspoons grated lemon zest

2   tablespoons chopped fresh tarragon

TAKE IT UP A NOTCH
Dollop spoonfuls of high-quality, whole-milk ricotta, such as from Calabro, on top of the pasta when serving.

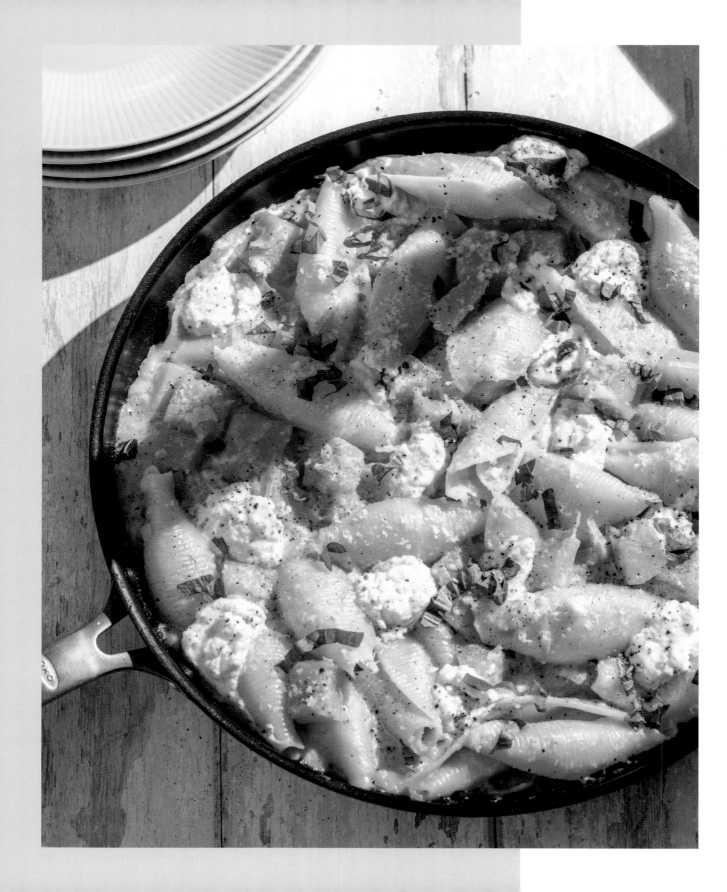

Unstuffed Shells with Butternut Squash and Leeks

SERVES 4

Why This Recipe Works Comforting dishes like this are so welcome, but only if they are easy on the back. Stuffed shells have their appeal, but boiling and then stuffing hot and slippery individual shells can be an ordeal. In this easy unstuffed version, jumbo pasta shells cook directly in a creamy sauce of butternut squash and leeks for a hearty vegetarian meal. Cooking the squash and leeks briefly before adding the pasta and liquid gives them more flavor and ensures that the pasta and squash finish cooking at the same time. Instead of stuffing the shells with cheese, simply sprinkle some Parmesan on top and dollop a lemony ricotta topping over everything. The skillet will be very full when you add the shells in step 3 but will become more manageable as the liquid evaporates. You will need a 12-inch nonstick skillet with a tight-fitting lid for this recipe.

1   Combine ricotta, ½ cup Parmesan, lemon zest, ¼ teaspoon salt, and pepper in bowl; cover and refrigerate until needed.

2   Heat oil in 12-inch nonstick skillet over medium heat until shimmering. Add squash, leeks, and remaining ½ teaspoon salt and cook until leeks are softened, about 5 minutes. Stir in garlic and cayenne and cook until fragrant, about 30 seconds. Stir in wine and cook until almost completely evaporated, about 1 minute. Turn off heat and cover skillet.

— TAKE A 15-MINUTE BREAK —

3   Add water and cream to skillet, then add pasta and bring to vigorous simmer over medium-high heat. Reduce heat to medium, cover, and cook, stirring gently and often, until pasta is tender and liquid has thickened, about 15 minutes.

4   Season with salt and pepper to taste. Sprinkle remaining ½ cup Parmesan over top, then dollop evenly with ricotta mixture. Sprinkle with basil and serve.

PREP AHEAD
You can cut the leeks up to 1 day ahead and refrigerate. You can make the ricotta topping up to 1 day ahead and refrigerate.

8   ounces (1 cup) whole-milk ricotta cheese

2   ounces grated Parmesan cheese (1 cup), divided

1   teaspoon grated lemon zest

¾   teaspoon table salt, divided

¼   teaspoon pepper

1   tablespoon extra-virgin olive oil

1½   pounds cubed butternut squash (5 cups)

1   pound leeks, white and light green parts only, halved lengthwise, sliced thin, and washed thoroughly

2   garlic cloves, minced

    Pinch cayenne pepper

¼   cup dry white wine

4   cups water

1   cup heavy cream

12   ounces jumbo pasta shells

2   tablespoons chopped fresh basil

Veggie Sheet Pan Pizza

SERVES 2

2 tablespoons plus 1 teaspoon extra-virgin olive oil, divided

8 ounces pizza dough, room temperature

4 ounces white mushrooms, trimmed and sliced thin

½ red or green bell pepper, sliced thin

½ small onion, chopped

4 ounces shredded whole-milk mozzarella cheese (1 cup)

¼ cup grated Parmesan cheese, divided

½ cup jarred marinara sauce

1 tablespoon chopped fresh basil

Why This Recipe Works I love homemade pizza and I make it from scratch quite often, but I know my patients would never have the stamina for the work involved. Using a pizza stone and bending down with a pizza peel to get a pizza into and out of the oven can be a bit challenging for anyone. This recipe will convince you that yes, you can make good pizza for two at home using just a small rimmed baking sheet, store-bought dough and sauce, and your toaster oven (or regular oven). To avoid excess moisture, which can cause soggy pizza, a two-tiered approach is in order: First, give the vegetable topping a head start in the microwave to drive off excess moisture. Second, parbake the bare crust with a layer of Parmesan to create a barrier and prevent any liquid from saturating the dough. Then top with the vegetables and briefly bake to produce a perfectly customizable, tasty pizza. Let the dough sit out at room temperature while preparing the other ingredients; otherwise, it will be difficult to stretch. You will need a small rimmed baking sheet with a cooking surface measuring at least 11 by 8 inches for this recipe, but a larger one will work as well (although it will not fit in a toaster oven). The recipe was developed using a light rimmed baking sheet; if using a dark one, start checking for doneness 5 minutes earlier than advised in step 4.

1   Coat small rimmed baking sheet with 2 tablespoons oil. Press and roll dough into 11 by 8-inch rectangle on lightly floured counter. (If dough springs back during rolling, let rest for 10 minutes before rolling again.) Transfer dough to prepared sheet and re-stretch dough into 11 by 8-inch rectangle. Brush dough evenly with remaining 1 teaspoon oil and cover with plastic wrap. Set in warm spot until slightly risen, about 20 minutes. Preheat oven to 450 degrees.

— TAKE A 20-MINUTE BREAK —

2   Microwave mushrooms, bell pepper, and onion in covered bowl, stirring occasionally, until softened and mushrooms release their liquid, about 4 minutes. Drain vegetables well and return to clean, dry bowl; let cool slightly. Add mozzarella and toss to combine.

3   Remove plastic from dough and, using your fingers, make indentations all over dough, pressing dough into corners. Sprinkle dough with 2 tablespoons Parmesan. Bake until dough has puffed slightly, about 6 minutes.

PREP AHEAD
You can prep the mushrooms, peppers, and onion up to 1 day ahead and refrigerate separately.

MAKE IT EVEN EASIER
Buy sliced mushrooms and peppers.

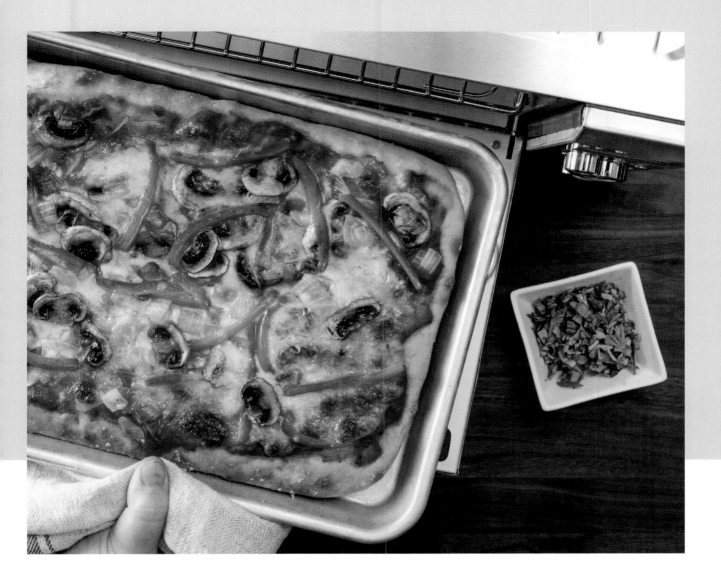

4   Remove sheet from oven. Spread sauce over crust, leaving ½-inch border. Sprinkle vegetable-mozzarella mixture evenly over sauce. Bake, on lowest rack, until cheese is melted and crust is golden brown on bottom, about 12 minutes.

— TAKE A 12-MINUTE BREAK —

5   Remove pizza from pan and transfer to wire rack; let rest for 5 minutes. Sprinkle with basil and remaining 2 tablespoons Parmesan. Cut into 8 equal pieces and serve.

VARIATIONS

Three-Cheese Sheet Pan Pizza

Omit mushrooms, bell pepper, and onion. Decrease mozzarella to 2 ounces. Toss ½ cup crumbled blue cheese with mozzarella and sprinkle cheese mixture over sauce before baking.

Meaty Sheet Pan Pizza

Omit mushrooms, bell pepper, and onion. Sprinkle mozzarella over sauce, then arrange 4 ounces hot or sweet Italian sausage, casings removed, pinched into dime-size pieces, and 1 ounce thinly sliced pepperoni, halved, on top.

Hearty
Soups
& Stews

* Try these recipes first if today is not one of your better days and you need a soul-refilling meal with high return on your energy investment.

Sun-Dried Tomato and White Bean Soup

SERVES 2 — SUPER EASY

1 (15-ounce) can small white beans

1¼ cups vegetable or chicken broth, plus extra as needed

3 tablespoons oil-packed sun-dried tomatoes, chopped coarse

2 tablespoons grated Parmesan cheese, plus extra for serving

1 tablespoon shredded fresh basil

Why This Recipe Works I think of this as a more grown-up version of classic tomato soup, and the perfect complement to a grilled cheese sandwich (for dipping). The complex taste of this fragrant soup belies its simplicity and the fact that it can be made in flash. An unexpected ingredient, canned white beans in their flavorful liquid, provides a velvety backdrop and subtle earthiness. Rather than using canned tomatoes, which can taste tinny if not cooked for an adequate amount of time, you just need to briefly simmer the beans and sweet and tangy sun-dried tomatoes—so potent (and pantry-friendly) that a mere 3 tablespoons is plenty. Parmesan cheese and shredded fresh basil provide rich and aromatic finishes. Creamy white beans bring buttery nuttiness, making this "from-a-can" soup an elegant lunchtime treat.

1   Bring beans and their liquid, broth, and tomatoes to simmer in medium saucepan and cook over medium-low heat, stirring occasionally, until beans begin to break down, about 6 minutes.

2   Off heat, add Parmesan and blend soup with immersion blender until smooth, about 3 minutes. Adjust consistency with extra hot broth as needed. Season with salt and pepper to taste and sprinkle with basil. Serve with extra Parmesan.

PREP AHEAD
You can refrigerate the soup for up to 3 days.

TAKE IT UP A NOTCH
Serve with a Grilled Cheese Sandwich
Heat a 12-inch skillet over medium-low heat. Sprinkle ¾ cup shredded mild cheddar cheese over two slices high-quality white sandwich bread. Top each with another bread slice, pressing down gently to set. Brush the sandwich tops with a tablespoon melted butter. Place each sandwich, buttered side down, in the skillet and brush the remaining side of each sandwich completely with another tablespoon melted butter. Cook until crisp and deep golden brown, 5 to 10 minutes per side, flipping the sandwiches back to the first side to reheat and crisp, about 15 seconds. Serve immediately. Makes 2 sandwiches.

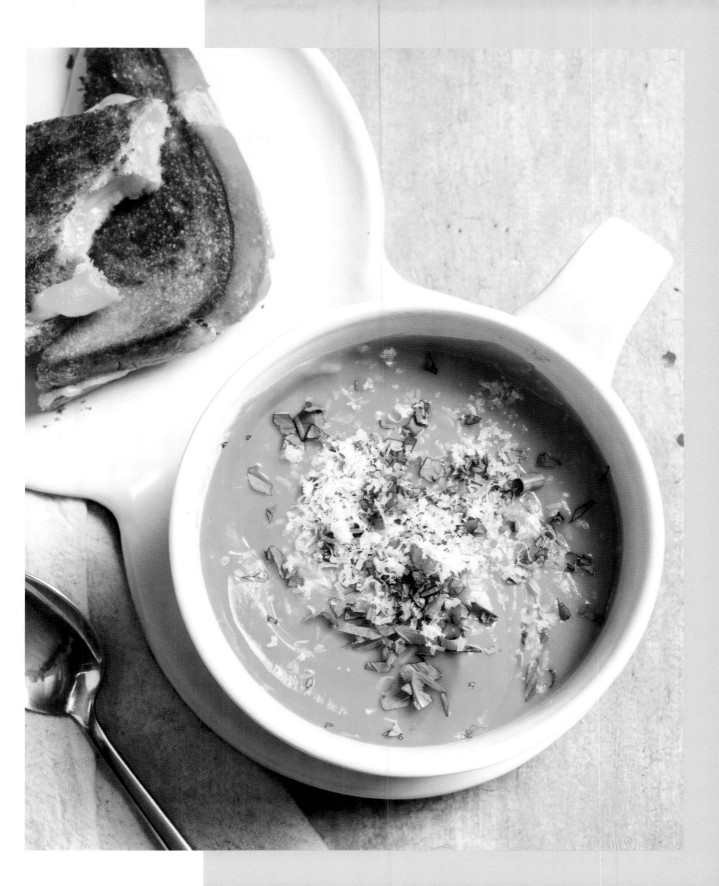

Creamy Chickpea and Roasted Garlic Soup

SERVES 2 — SUPER EASY

4 garlic cloves, unpeeled

1 (15-ounce) can chickpeas

1¼ cups vegetable or chicken broth, plus extra as needed

1 tablespoon minced fresh parsley, tarragon, or chives

1 tablespoon lemon juice

Why This Recipe Works If you have ever wanted to feel like a food magician, look no further than this gastronomic alchemy–inspired soup. Through the power of garlic, a can of chickpeas is transformed into a creamy, satisfying soup in mere minutes. To develop deep, nuanced flavor from such simple ingredients, start by quick-roasting four skin-on garlic cloves in a dry saucepan until they turn a beautiful golden color and become intensely fragrant. Roasting the garlic this way yields mellow, mildly sweet garlic that mimics the flavor of oven-roasted garlic in a fraction of the time. Next, peel the garlic and return it to the saucepan with some broth and a full can of chickpeas and their liquid and then blend the soup until it is smooth and velvety. A splash of lemon juice and some fresh parsley are more than just finishing elements here—they wake up the flavors by adding bright freshness and cutting through the rich, silky soup.

1   Toast garlic in medium saucepan over medium heat, stirring occasionally, until fragrant and skins are just beginning to brown, about 5 minutes. Remove garlic from saucepan and let cool slightly. Once cool enough to handle, peel garlic then return to now-empty saucepan along with chickpeas and their liquid and the broth. Bring to simmer and cook over medium-low heat, stirring occasionally, until chickpeas begin to break down, about 6 minutes.

2   Off heat, blend soup with immersion blender until smooth, about 3 minutes. Adjust consistency with extra hot broth as needed. Stir in parsley and lemon juice and season with salt and pepper to taste. Serve.

PREP AHEAD
You can refrigerate the soup for up to 3 days.

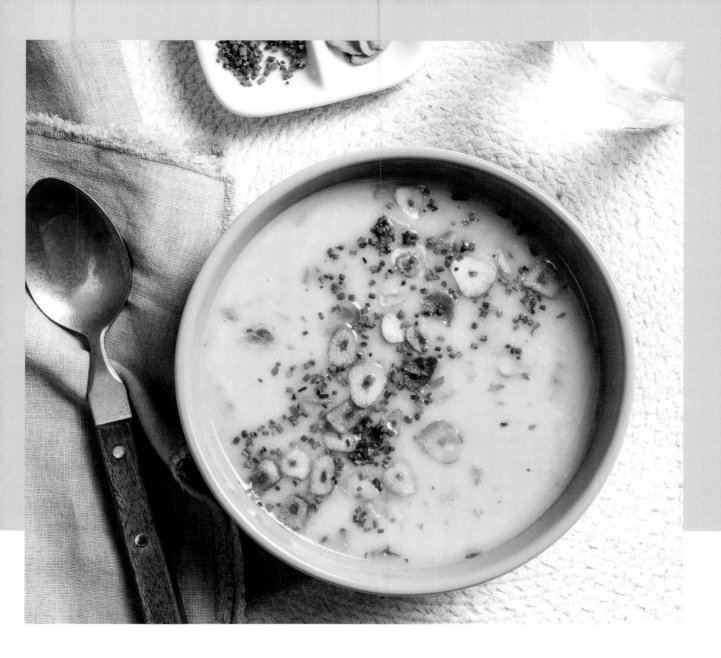

TAKE IT UP A NOTCH

Top with Crispy Garlic

Combine ¼ cup sliced garlic and ¼ cup vegetable oil in medium bowl. Microwave for 4 minutes. Stir and microwave for 1 minute. Repeat stirring and microwaving in 1-minute increments until garlic begins to brown (3 to 5 minutes). Repeat stirring and microwaving in 30-second increments until garlic is deep golden brown (30 seconds to 2 minutes). Using slotted spoon, transfer garlic to paper towel–lined plate. Sprinkle with ½ teaspoon confectioners' sugar (to offset any bitterness) and season with salt to taste. Use immediately. Leftover garlic oil can be stored in refrigerator for up to 1 week. Makes ¼ cup.

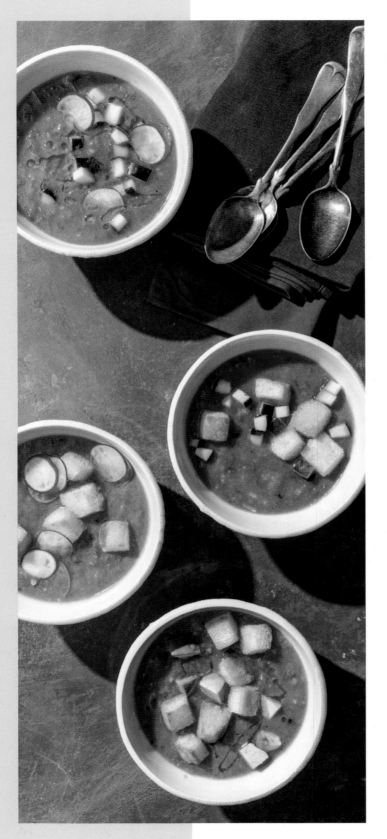
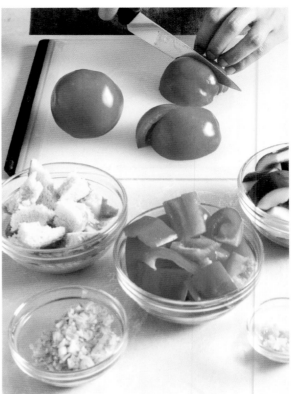
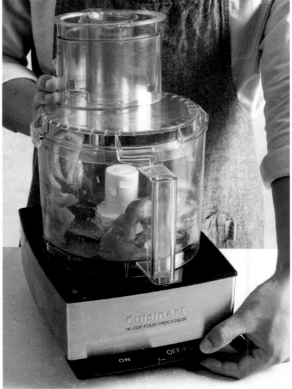

Easy Food-Processor Gazpacho

SERVES 4 TO 6

Why This Recipe Works I remember the first time I had gazpacho: What a revelation it was that a cold, tomatoey soup could be so delicious. Now I make this refreshing, summery soup often, especially after a trip to the farmers' market when I've come home with a bounty of fresh, ripe tomatoes. Traditional recipes for gazpacho call for chopping everything by hand into tiny pieces—a tedious job at best and too much standing time and knife work for anyone struggling with back pain, or a generalized lack of patience, or both! Here, you simply need to cut the vegetables into chunks and let the food processor finish up much of the process by pulsing all the vegetables into just the right size. Then simply transfer the vegetables to a bowl and stir in tomato juice, sherry vinegar, and a touch of hot sauce. To give the soup some body, puree 2 cups of the mixture with one slice of white bread and ¼ cup of oil. Garnish with finely chopped bell pepper and cucumber, if desired. Note that this recipe must be made and chilled at least 4 hours ahead.

1 Pulse tomatoes in food processor until broken into ½- to ¼-inch pieces, about 12 pulses; transfer to large bowl. Pulse bell pepper and cucumber in now-empty processor until broken down into ½- to ¼-inch pieces, about 8 pulses; add to bowl with tomatoes. Stir tomato juice, vinegar, hot sauce, salt, and pepper into the tomato mixture.

2 Process bread and 2 cups tomato mixture in now-empty processor until smooth, about 1 minute. With processor running, slowly drizzle in oil until incorporated. Return pureed tomato mixture to bowl with remaining tomato mixture and stir in shallot and garlic. Cover and refrigerate gazpacho for at least 4 hours.

12 ounces vine-ripened tomatoes, quartered

1 red bell pepper, stemmed, seeded, and cut into 1-inch pieces

1 cucumber, halved lengthwise, seeded, and cut into 1-inch pieces

2½ cups tomato juice

2½ tablespoons sherry vinegar

1 teaspoon hot sauce

1 teaspoon table salt

½ teaspoon pepper

1 slice hearty white sandwich bread, torn into pieces

¼ cup extra-virgin olive oil, plus extra for serving

1 shallot, minced

1 garlic clove, minced

PREP AHEAD
You can refrigerate the soup for up to 2 days.

TAKE IT UP A NOTCH
Try garnishing the soup with a mix of chopped radishes, cucumbers, and avocado. Another option is to top it with Homemade Garlic Croutons (page 67).

Cauliflower Soup

SERVES 4 TO 6

3 tablespoons unsalted butter

1 leek, white and light green parts only, halved lengthwise, sliced thin, and washed thoroughly

1 small onion, halved and sliced thin

1½ teaspoons table salt

4½–5 cups water

1¾ pounds cauliflower florets, coarsely chopped, divided

3 tablespoons chopped fresh chives

Why This Recipe Works Whenever I see cauliflower soup on a restaurant's appetizer menu, I order it. I cannot resist its rich taste and creamy consistency. If I had known how easy it was to make, this soup would have been on regular rotation in my house long ago. It's also a healthy choice given cauliflower's natural ability to turn into a lush puree without the addition of cream. And if you use packaged cauliflower florets, its preparation couldn't be simpler. To ensure that cauliflower flavor remains at the forefront, the cauliflower is cooked in seasoned water (instead of broth), and the soup is bolstered with sautéed onion and leek. Prepping all the vegetables earlier in the day means you're in the kitchen for just over 30 minutes before dinner. The cauliflower is simmered in two stages to unlock the grassy flavor of just-cooked cauliflower as well as the sweeter, nuttier taste of longer-cooked florets. If you are cutting up a whole head of cauliflower (you will need about a 2-pound head), be sure to thoroughly trim the cauliflower's core of green leaves and leaf stems, which can be fibrous and contribute to a grainy texture in the soup.

1 Melt butter in large saucepan over medium-low heat. Add leek, onion, and salt and cook, stirring frequently, until softened but not browned, about 7 minutes.

2 Increase heat to medium-high, add 4½ cups water and half of cauliflower, and bring to simmer. Reduce heat to medium-low and simmer gently for 15 minutes.

— TAKE A 15-MINUTE BREAK —

3 Add remaining cauliflower to soup and continue to cook until cauliflower is tender and crumbles easily, about 17 minutes.

— TAKE A 17-MINUTE BREAK —

4 Off heat, blend soup with immersion blender until smooth, about 3 minutes. Return to simmer over medium heat, adjusting consistency with remaining water as needed: Soup should have thick, velvety texture but should be thin enough to settle with flat surface after being stirred. Season with salt to taste and serve, garnishing individual bowls with chives.

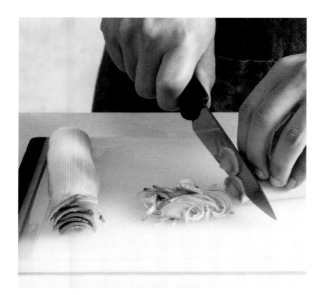

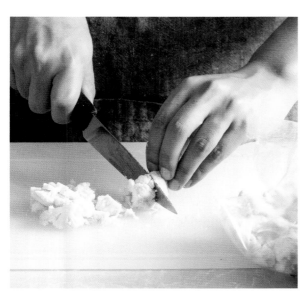

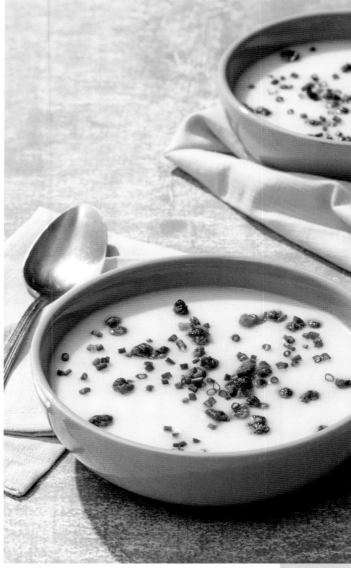

PREP AHEAD

You can slice and wash the leek, slice the onion, and chop the cauliflower up to 1 day ahead and refrigerate separately. You can refrigerate the soup for up to 2 days.

TAKE IT UP A NOTCH

Top with Crispy Capers

Microwave ¼ cup capers and ½ cup extra-virgin olive oil in bowl (capers should be mostly submerged) until capers are darkened in color and have shrunk, about 5 minutes, stirring halfway through. Using slotted spoon, transfer capers to paper towel–lined plate (they will continue to crisp as they cool). Makes ¼ cup.

Pasta e Piselli

SERVES 4 — SUPER EASY

- 2 tablespoons extra-virgin olive oil, plus extra for drizzling
- 1 onion, chopped fine
- 2 ounces pancetta, chopped fine
- ½ teaspoon table salt
- ½ teaspoon pepper
- 2½ cups chicken or vegetable broth
- 2½ cups water
- 7½ ounces (1½ cups) ditalini
- 1½ cups frozen petite peas, thawed
- ⅓ cup minced fresh parsley
- ¼ cup grated Pecorino Romano cheese, plus extra for serving
- 2 tablespoons minced fresh mint

Why This Recipe Works A cross between a soup and a brothy pasta, this rustic Italian dish is ultracomforting and easy to make, as it comes together all in one pot. The pasta is cooked in a broth flavored with sautéed onion and savory pancetta, simultaneously infusing the pasta with savoriness and thickening the rich, silky broth. Adding the peas next and immediately taking the pot off the heat preserves their tenderness and color. A sprinkle of Pecorino Romano contributes richness and tangy depth. Last-minute additions of minced herbs and extra-virgin olive oil punch up the aroma and flavors of the dish. If you'd prefer to substitute small pasta such as tubetti, ditali, elbow macaroni, or small shells for the ditalini, do so by weight, not by volume. Frozen petite peas (also labeled petit pois or baby sweet peas) work best in this recipe because they are sweeter and less starchy than fresh peas or regular frozen peas, but you can substitute regular frozen peas, if desired. Do not defrost the peas before using them. For a vegetarian version, omit the pancetta, substitute vegetable broth for the chicken broth, and add an extra 2 tablespoons grated cheese.

1   Heat oil in large saucepan over medium heat until shimmering. Add onion, pancetta, salt, and pepper and cook, stirring frequently, until onion is softened, about 8 minutes.

2   Add broth and water and bring to boil over high heat. Stir in pasta and cook, stirring frequently, until liquid returns to boil. Reduce heat to maintain simmer. Cover and cook until pasta is al dente, about 10 minutes.

—   TAKE A 10-MINUTE BREAK   —

3   Stir in peas and remove saucepan from heat. Stir in parsley, Pecorino, and mint and season with salt and pepper to taste. Serve, drizzling with extra oil and passing extra Pecorino separately.

PREP AHEAD
You can chop the onion and pancetta up to 1 day ahead and refrigerate separately.

MAKE IT EVEN EASIER
Buy diced pancetta.

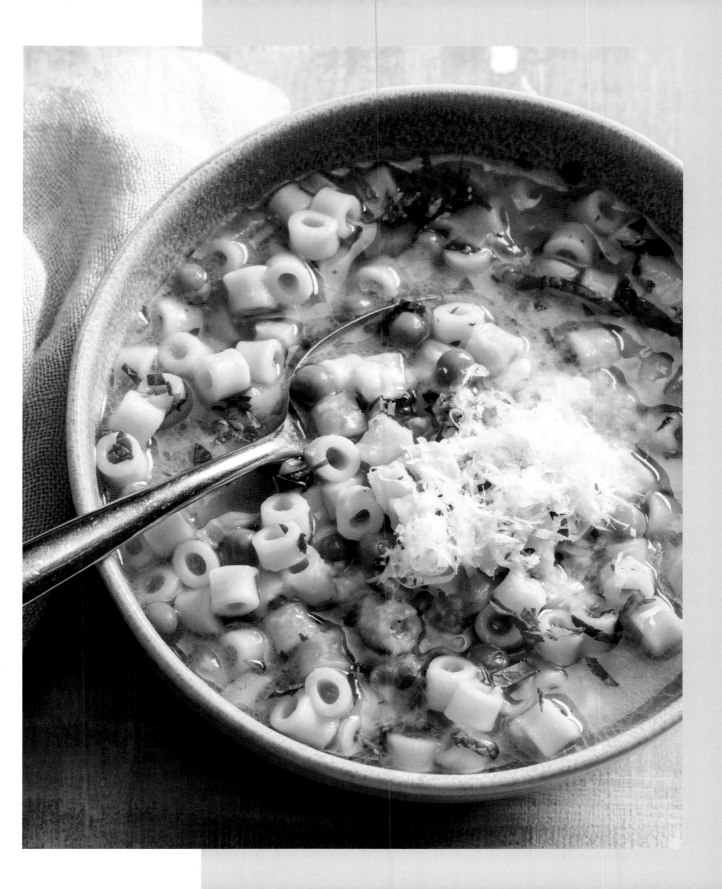

Tomato, Bulgur, and Red Pepper Soup

SERVES 6 TO 8

- 2 tablespoons extra-virgin olive oil
- 2 red bell peppers, stemmed, seeded, and chopped
- 1 onion, chopped
- ¾ teaspoon table salt
- ¼ teaspoon pepper
- 3 garlic cloves, minced
- 1 teaspoon dried mint, crumbled
- ½ teaspoon smoked paprika
- ⅛ teaspoon red pepper flakes
- 1 tablespoon tomato paste
- ½ cup dry white wine
- 1 (28-ounce) can diced fire-roasted tomatoes
- 4 cups vegetable or chicken broth
- 2 cups water
- ¾ cup medium-grind bulgur, rinsed
- ⅓ cup chopped fresh mint

Why This Recipe Works The biggest improvement in how I feel at the end of a meal has come as a result of incorporating more plant-based recipes into my diet, something I urge my patients to consider. Sometimes you need something that is hearty but that won't leave you feeling heavy and slowed down at the end of the meal—this soup is the perfect example of such a recipe. Inspired by Turkish red pepper soups, it relies on pantry ingredients, but the end result is a stunningly beautiful plant-based soup with layers of flavor. Many soups hailing from the region are often enriched with good-for-you grains that fill you up—and here, bulgur fits the bill. To start, soften red peppers and onion and then create a solid flavor backbone with garlic, tomato paste, white wine, dried mint, smoked paprika, and red pepper flakes. When stirred into the soup, the bulgur absorbs the surrounding flavors and gives off some of its starch, creating a silky texture. A sprinkle of fresh mint provides a final punch of flavor. When shopping, don't confuse bulgur with cracked wheat, which has a much longer cooking time and will not work in this recipe.

1 Heat oil in Dutch oven over medium heat until shimmering. Add bell peppers, onion, salt, and pepper and cook until vegetables are softened and lightly browned, about 7 minutes. Stir in garlic, dried mint, paprika, and pepper flakes and cook until fragrant, about 30 seconds. Stir in tomato paste and cook for 1 minute. Stir in wine, scraping up any browned bits, and bring to simmer until reduced by half, about 1 minute. Turn off heat.

— TAKE A 15-MINUTE BREAK —

2 Add tomatoes and their juice and cook over medium heat, stirring occasionally, until tomatoes soften and begin to break apart, about 12 minutes.

3 Stir in broth, water, and bulgur and bring to simmer. Reduce heat to low, cover, and simmer gently until bulgur is tender, about 20 minutes.

— TAKE A 20-MINUTE BREAK —

4 Season with salt and pepper to taste. Serve, sprinkling individual bowls with mint.

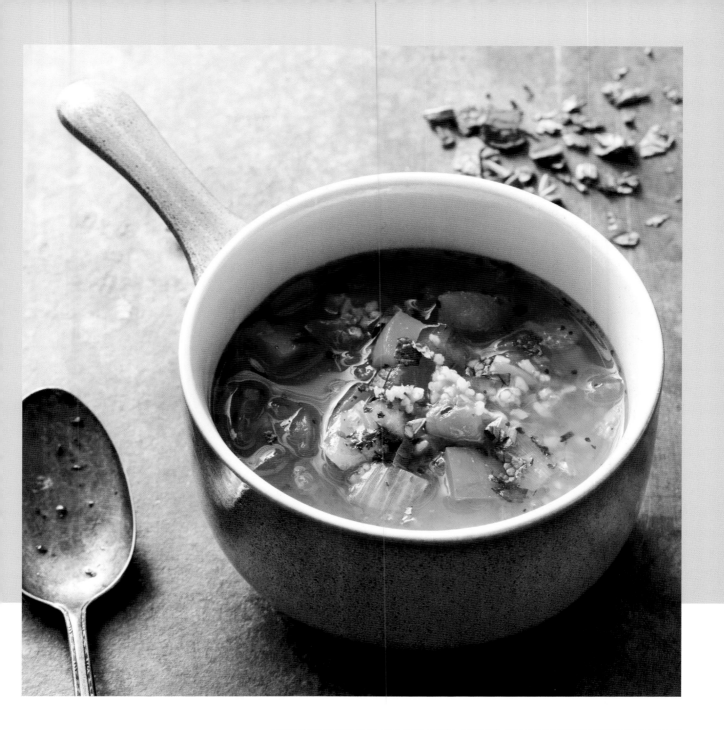

PREP AHEAD

You can chop the peppers and onion up to 1 day ahead and refrigerate
separately. You can refrigerate the soup for up to 2 days; add additional
broth or water to adjust consistency as needed.

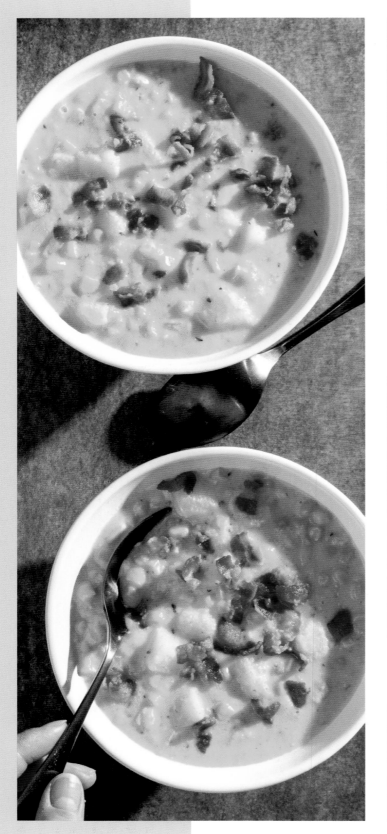
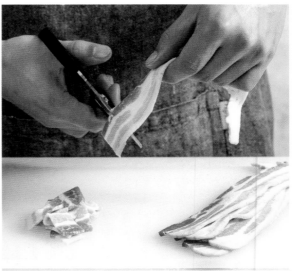
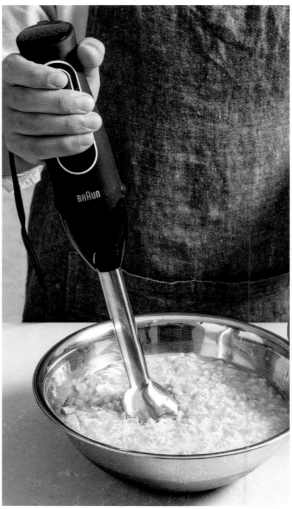

Easy Corn Chowder with Bacon

SERVES 4

Why This Recipe Works Growing up in the Midwest, I had ready access to fresh corn because it was available all summer at the roadside stands next to the farmers' fields along the drive from our home all the way to our local supermarket. And I love corn chowder; it's creamy, infused with the flavor of bacon (not to mention the topping of crispy bacon bits), and packed with potatoes. What could be more satisfying? That said, taking the corn off the cob is too much work when your back is on fire. This version uses frozen corn kernels, putting this rich chowder within reach of anyone at any time of the year. An immersion blender makes quick work of pureeing half the corn with chicken broth to imbue the chowder with a deep corn flavor. Cooking the onions and potatoes in the rendered bacon fat adds even more depth of flavor. Frozen corn can be quickly defrosted in a bowl in the microwave.

8 cups frozen corn kernels (about 2 pounds), thawed, divided

3 cups chicken broth, divided

6 slices bacon, chopped

1 onion, chopped fine

2 pounds russet potatoes, peeled and cut into ½-inch chunks

½ cup heavy cream

1 teaspoon minced fresh thyme

⅛ teaspoon cayenne pepper

1 Using immersion blender, puree 4 cups corn and 2 cups broth in medium bowl until smooth. Cook bacon in large saucepan over medium-high heat until crispy, about 5 minutes; transfer pieces to paper towel–lined plate, leaving fat in pan. Reduce heat to medium and cook onion and potatoes in bacon fat until onion is softened, about 5 minutes.

2 Whisk in pureed corn mixture, cream, thyme, cayenne, and remaining 1 cup broth and bring to simmer. Cook until potatoes are tender, about 15 minutes. Turn off heat.

— TAKE A 15-MINUTE BREAK —

3 Stir in remaining 4 cups corn and cook over medium heat until everything is heated through, about 5 minutes. Season with salt and pepper to taste. Sprinkle with crispy bacon and serve.

PREP AHEAD
You can chop the bacon, onion, and potatoes up to 1 day ahead (store potatoes in bowl covered with water) and refrigerate separately. You can refrigerate the chowder for up to 3 days.

Chicken Tortilla Soup

SERVES 4 TO 6

1 pound boneless, skinless chicken breasts, trimmed

¼ teaspoon table salt

¼ teaspoon pepper

1 tablespoon vegetable oil

1 onion, chopped fine

1 tablespoon minced canned chipotle chile in adobo sauce

2 garlic cloves, minced

2 teaspoons tomato paste

6 cups chicken broth

2 tablespoons lime juice

4 ounces tortilla chips, crushed into large pieces (4 cups), plus extra for serving

1 large tomato cut into ½-inch pieces, plus extra for serving

1 avocado, halved, pitted, and cut into ½-inch pieces, plus extra for serving

½ cup fresh cilantro leaves

PREP AHEAD

You can chop the onion and refrigerate and crush the tortilla chips up to 1 day ahead. You can refrigerate the soup (minus the garnishes) for up to 2 days.

Why This Recipe Works The all-time favorite soup at the Baum house is chicken tortilla soup. This streamlined version bypasses multiple steps, including toasting chiles and pureeing the aromatic base in a food processor as well as cutting up corn tortillas into strips and toasting them in the oven. This way, you don't have to sacrifice your back to enjoy it. To make this soup quickly without compromising any of its best qualities, the first step is to brown boneless, skinless chicken breasts right in the Dutch oven and then use the leftover fat to soften the onion. Chipotle in adobo sauce, garlic, and tomato paste are added next, and all contribute loads of bold flavors to the broth. Once the broth is built, the chicken goes back in to finish cooking. Coarsely crushed store-bought tortilla chips, creamy chunks of avocado, bright chopped tomato, and fresh cilantro leaves make for a panoply of flavors and textures. Because the saltiness of tortilla chips varies from brand to brand, sample the chips before seasoning the soup with additional salt.

1   Pat chicken dry with paper towels and sprinkle with salt and pepper. Heat oil in Dutch oven over medium-high heat until just smoking. Brown chicken lightly on both sides, about 5 minutes. Transfer to plate and cover with foil.

—   TAKE A 15-MINUTE BREAK   —

2   Add onion to fat left in pot and cook over medium heat until softened, about 5 minutes. Stir in chipotle, garlic, and tomato paste and cook until fragrant, about 30 seconds. Stir in broth, scraping up any browned bits.

3   Add browned chicken, cover, and simmer gently until it registers 160 degrees, about 10 minutes.

—   TAKE A 10-MINUTE BREAK   —

4   Transfer chicken to cutting board and let cool slightly. Using 2 forks, shred chicken into bite-size pieces.

5   Stir lime juice into soup and season with salt and pepper to taste. Divide shredded chicken, tortilla chips, tomato, and avocado among individual bowls. Ladle hot soup into bowls and sprinkle with cilantro. Serve, passing extra tortilla chips, tomato, and avocado separately.

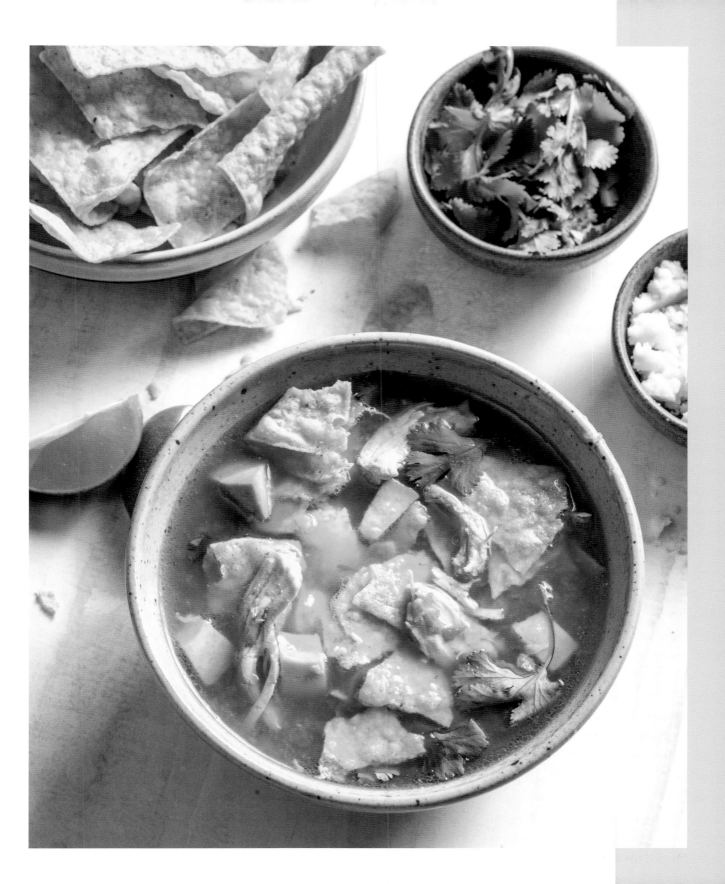

Almost-Instant Ginger Beef Ramen

SERVES 2 — SUPER EASY

4 ounces sirloin steak tips, trimmed and cut into 2-inch pieces

⅛ teaspoon table salt

⅛ teaspoon pepper

1 teaspoon vegetable oil

1½ cups chicken broth

2 teaspoons grated fresh ginger or ½ teaspoon ground ginger

½ teaspoon grated lime zest plus 1 teaspoon juice

1 (3-ounce) package ramen noodles, seasoning packet discarded

2 teaspoons soy sauce

1 scallion, sliced thin

Why This Recipe Works This isn't your dorm room ramen, though it's almost as easy to make. The recipe takes instant ramen to a new level, turning out a beefy, ginger-infused, soul-warming soup for two. To get all of the flavor of traditionally long-simmered ramen with the ease of the packaged instant versions, ditch the salty—but otherwise lackluster—flavor packet and keep the noodles. Gently browning pieces of sirloin steak tips in a medium saucepan, taking care not to burn the fond that develops as the meat browns—ensures that you keep all that flavor. While the meat rests, deglazing the flavorful, fond-coated saucepan with broth adds flavor, and the broth is further bolstered with a splash of soy sauce and healthy doses of aromatic ginger and floral lime zest. A single serving of widely available packaged ramen noodles cooks up quickly in this brew. Steak tips, also known as flap meat, can be sold as whole steaks, cubes, or strips. To ensure evenly sized pieces, it is best to cut up the steak tips yourself.

1 Pat beef dry with paper towels and sprinkle with salt and pepper. Heat oil in medium saucepan over medium heat until just smoking. Add beef and cook until well browned all over and registers 120 to 125 degrees (for medium-rare), about 5 minutes, reducing heat if saucepan begins to smoke. Transfer beef to plate, tent loosely with aluminum foil, and let rest for up to 15 minutes until ready to serve.

— TAKE A 15-MINUTE BREAK —

2 Add broth, ginger, and lime zest to now-empty saucepan; bring to a boil, scraping up any browned bits. Add noodles and cook, stirring often, until tender, about 3 minutes. Off heat, stir in lime juice, soy sauce, scallion, and any accumulated juices from beef. Season with salt and pepper to taste and transfer soup to serving bowls. Slice steak thin against grain and place on top of noodles. Serve.

PREP AHEAD

You can cut up the beef up to 1 day ahead and refrigerate. Broth (minus the ramen) and cooked beef can be refrigerated, separately, for up to 3 days. To serve, bring beef to room temperature, then bring broth to a boil, add the ramen, and finish the recipe.

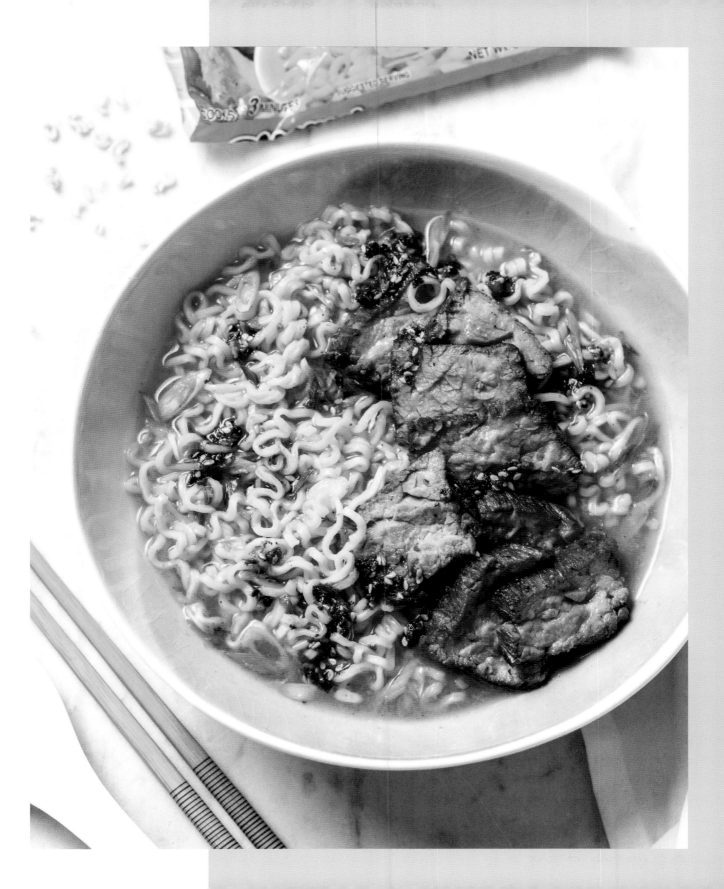

Beef and Barley Soup

SERVES 2 — SUPER EASY

8 ounces beef blade steak, trimmed and cut into ½-inch pieces

⅛ teaspoon table salt

Pinch pepper

2 teaspoons vegetable oil

6 ounces cremini mushrooms, trimmed and sliced thin

2 carrots, peeled and cut into ½-inch pieces

1 small onion, chopped fine

2 tablespoons tomato paste

3 garlic cloves, minced

2 teaspoons minced fresh thyme or ½ teaspoon dried

2 cups beef broth

2 cups chicken broth

4 teaspoons soy sauce

½ cup quick-cooking barley

2 tablespoons chopped fresh parsley

Why This Recipe Works This small-batch beef and barley soup uses quick-cooking blade steak instead of chuck roast and is made in a saucepan instead of the usual Dutch oven. Browning the meat in the saucepan provides plenty of savory fond. After browning the meat, it is easy to build a flavorful base with sautéed aromatics and vegetables. Tomato paste makes a big difference here, as it contributes umami flavor without the need of a long cooking time, while soy sauce boosts the savory depth even further. Since beef broth can add a tinny flavor, the key is to mix it with an equal amount of chicken broth. Letting the barley cook in the enhanced broth infuses the grains with flavor.

1 Pat beef dry with paper towels and sprinkle with salt and pepper. Heat oil in large saucepan over medium-high heat until just smoking. Brown beef on all sides, about 6 minutes; transfer to bowl.

2 Add mushrooms, carrots, and onion to fat left in saucepan and cook over medium heat until any mushroom juice has evaporated and vegetables begin to brown, about 7 minutes. Stir in tomato paste, garlic, and thyme and cook until fragrant, about 30 seconds.

3 Stir in beef broth, chicken broth, and soy sauce, scraping up any browned bits. Stir in browned beef and any accumulated juices, bring to simmer, and cook for 15 minutes.

— TAKE A 15-MINUTE BREAK —

4 Stir barley into the soup and simmer until barley and beef are tender, about 13 minutes.

— TAKE A 13-MINUTE BREAK —

5 Stir parsley into the soup and season with salt and pepper to taste. Serve.

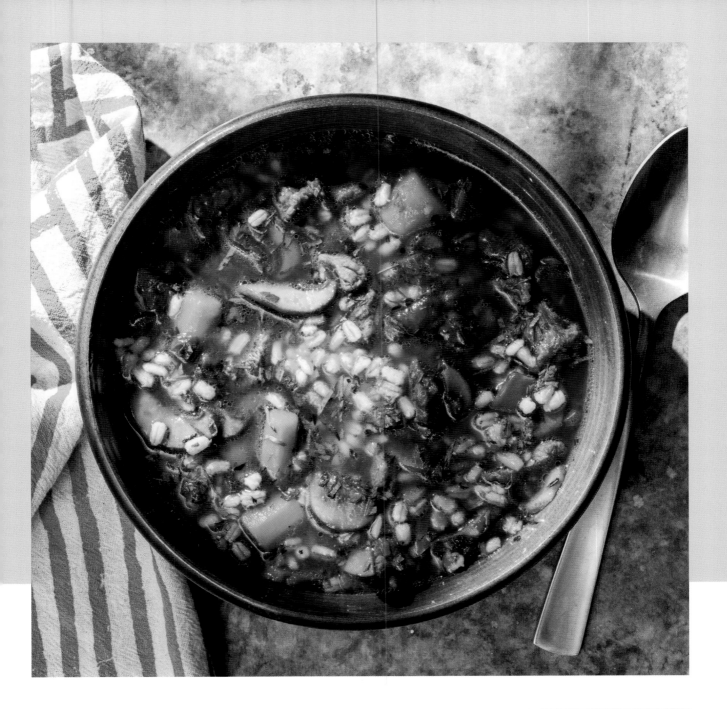

PREP AHEAD

You can cut up the meat, chop the onion and carrots, and slice the mushrooms up to 1 day ahead and refrigerate separately. You can refrigerate the soup for up to 3 days.

MAKE IT EVEN EASIER

Buy chopped carrots and sliced mushrooms.

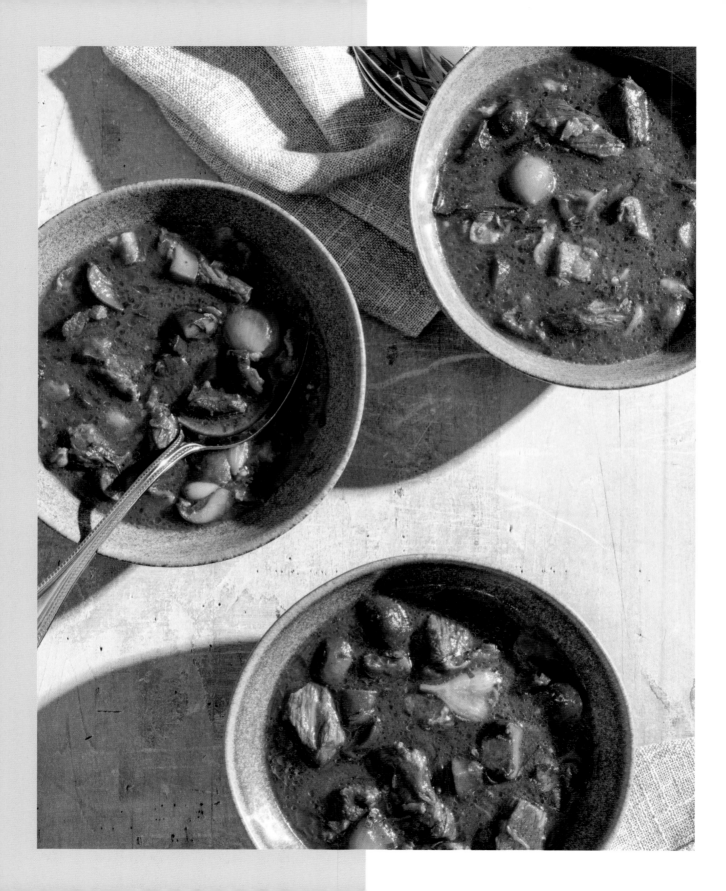

Easy Instant Pot Beef Stew with Mushrooms and Bacon

SERVES 4 — SUPER EASY

Why This Recipe Works What I love about this recipe is that, unlike most beef stews that require hours of simmering and a lot of heavy lifting, this one can be on the table with a modicum of prep work and after just 30 minutes of cooking under pressure. Thanks to the Instant Pot, a rich beef stew is within reach any night, especially if you do the prep work the night before. It starts with beefy boneless short ribs. To make this recipe even more streamlined, skip the time-consuming step of browning the beef and instead build flavor by sautéing bacon and using the rendered fat to cook tomato paste and thyme. Umami-rich mushrooms and soy sauce contribute savory depth. Flour thickens the stew, and frozen pearl onions lend this rich stew subtle sweetness with zero additional prep work. Note that it will take the Instant Pot about 10 minutes to come up to pressure and start the cook cycle.

1 Using highest sauté or browning function, cook bacon in electric pressure cooker until rendered and crispy, about 6 minutes. Using slotted spoon, transfer bacon to paper towel–lined plate; set aside.

2 Add tomato paste and thyme to fat left in pot and cook until fragrant, about 30 seconds. Stir in flour and cook for 1 minute. Slowly whisk in broth and soy sauce, scraping up any browned bits and smoothing out any lumps. Stir beef, mushrooms, and onions into pot.

3 Lock lid in place and close pressure release valve. Select high pressure cook function and cook for 30 minutes.

— TAKE A 40-MINUTE BREAK —

4 Turn off pressure cooker and quick-release pressure. Carefully remove lid, allowing steam to escape away from you.

5 Using wide, shallow spoon, skim excess fat from surface of stew. Adjust consistency with extra hot broth as needed. Stir in parsley and reserved bacon. Season with salt and pepper to taste, and serve.

4 slices bacon, chopped

¼ cup tomato paste

1 teaspoon minced fresh thyme or ¼ teaspoon dried

¼ cup all-purpose flour

1½ cups beef or chicken broth, plus extra as needed

2 tablespoons soy sauce

1½ pounds boneless beef short ribs, trimmed and cut into 1-inch pieces

1½ pounds cremini mushrooms, trimmed and quartered

1 cup frozen pearl onions, thawed

2 tablespoons minced fresh parsley

PREP AHEAD
You can chop the bacon, cut up the meat, and quarter the mushrooms up to 1 day ahead and refrigerate separately. You can refrigerate the stew for up to 3 days or freeze for up to 1 month.

MAKE IT EVEN EASIER
Ask the butcher at your market to cut up the meat for you.

Weeknight Beef Chili

SERVES 4

2 tablespoons chili powder

¾ teaspoon dried oregano

2 teaspoons ground cumin

1½ teaspoons ground coriander

⅛ teaspoon cayenne pepper

¾ teaspoon red pepper flakes

¼ teaspoon table salt

3 tablespoons vegetable oil

1 onion, chopped fine

1 red bell pepper, stemmed, seeded, and cut into ½-inch pieces

2 tablespoons tomato paste

4 garlic cloves, minced

1 pound 85 percent lean ground beef

1½ cups chicken broth

1 (15-ounce) can red kidney beans, rinsed

1 (15-ounce) can tomato sauce

Why This Recipe Works This is the chili to make when you need a restorative meal, but you can't handle the long cooking that other recipes require. There is no toasting of dried chiles, no cutting up a chuck roast—just a straightforward method that delivers a satisfyingly flavorful ground beef chili. It is also scaled down, since most recipes feed a crowd and require transferring a heavy Dutch oven from the stovetop to the oven, a back-straining task for sure. Instead of starting with a tomato base, you build a robust foundation by sweating onion and bell pepper and adding tomato paste, garlic, and chili powder reinforced with spices. Next up is the ground beef, which is simply cooked until no longer pink, followed by kidney beans. Then chicken broth is added, an unusual step, but one that provides enough liquid to simmer the chili without using canned tomatoes (which can take a while to lose their sharpness). Cooking the chili with the lid off for half the simmering time results in a rich, thick consistency, especially since this recipe uses a skillet, which allows for more evaporation than a Dutch oven. Stirring in a can of tomato sauce at the very end and then simmering for a few minutes allows the flavors to meld and provides just enough tomato flavor. Serve with your favorite chili toppings.

1   Combine chili powder, oregano, cumin, coriander, cayenne pepper, pepper flakes, and salt in bowl.

2   Heat oil in 12-inch skillet over medium heat until shimmering. Add onion and bell pepper and cook until softened, about 5 minutes. Stir in spice mixture, tomato paste, and garlic and cook until fragrant, about 1 minute.

3   Add ground beef and cook, breaking up meat with wooden spoon, until no longer pink, about 6 minutes. Stir in broth and beans, scraping up any browned bits, and bring to simmer. Reduce heat to gentle simmer, cover, and cook for 20 minutes.

— TAKE A 20-MINUTE BREAK —

4   Uncover skillet and continue to cook, stirring occasionally, until beef is tender and chili is thickened, about 20 minutes. (If chili begins to stick to bottom of skillet, stir in water as needed.) Stir in tomato sauce and cook until flavors meld, about 5 minutes. Season with salt and pepper to taste, and serve.

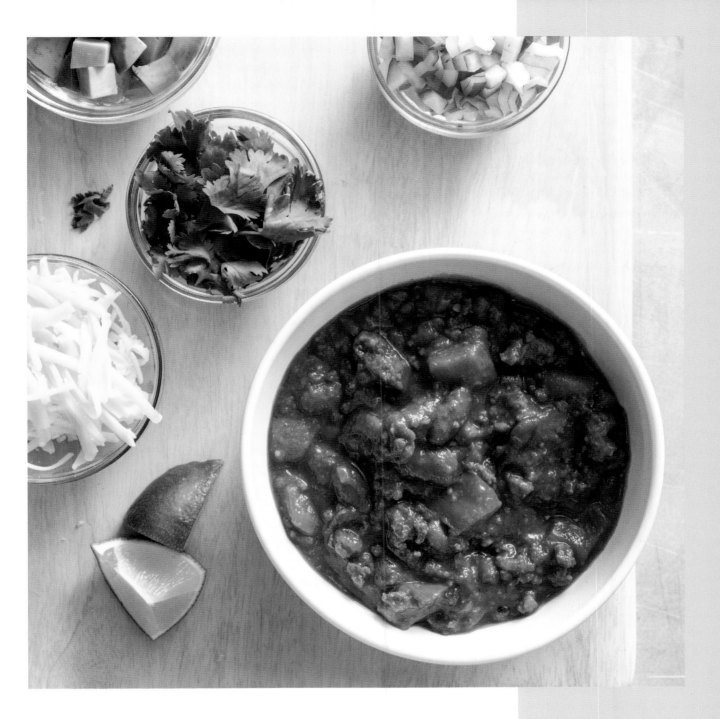

PREP AHEAD

You can make the spice blend, cut up the pepper, and chop the onion up to 1 day ahead and refrigerate separately. You can refrigerate the chili for up to 3 days or freeze for up to 1 month.

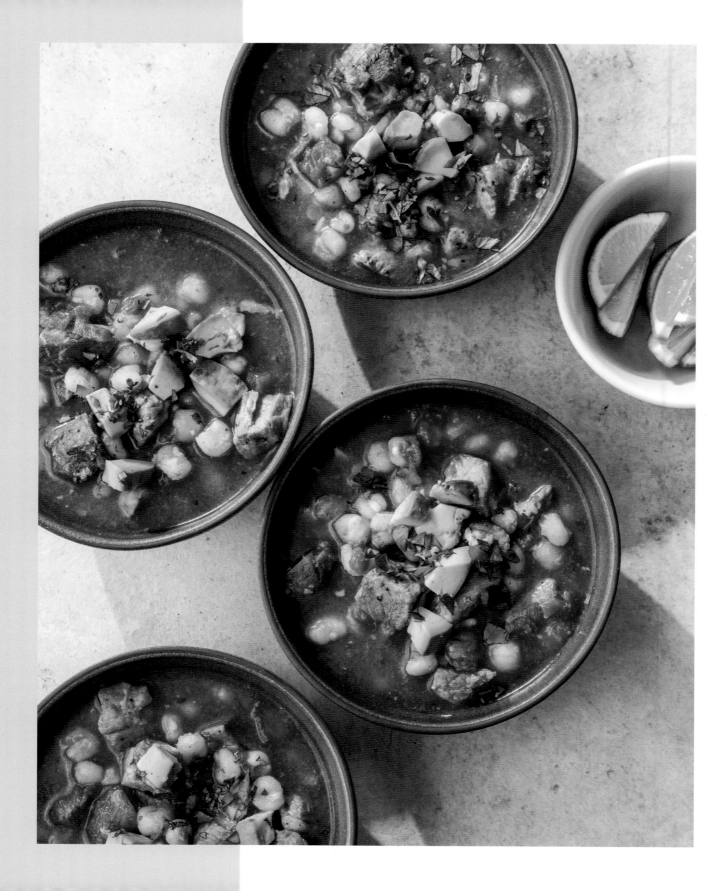

Slow-Cooker Pork Posole

SERVES 6 TO 8

Why This Recipe Works If I could only eat one thing for the rest of my life, posole just might be it: The meltingly tender pork, creamy hominy, and fragrant broth hit all the high notes for me. Here, the slow cooker does all the work, so you have almost a full day of walkaway time while the pork becomes fork tender and the broth incredibly rich tasting. There is a little up-front work on the stovetop before everything goes into the slow cooker, but it is well worth the effort. To achieve richness while also being mindful of effort, brown just half the pork before adding it to the slow cooker. Softening onion and blooming some garlic, chili powder, and oregano in the same skillet takes advantage of the dark fond left behind after browning the pork. Do not rinse the hominy after draining it; its starchiness gives the soup extra body. Serve posole with toppings such as diced avocado, sliced radishes, chopped cilantro, and lime wedges.

1   Sprinkle pork with 1 teaspoon salt and pepper. Heat oil in 12-inch nonstick skillet over medium-high heat until just smoking. Add half of pork and cook until browned on all sides, about 7 minutes. Transfer all pork (browned and raw) to slow cooker.

2   Add onion and remaining ½ teaspoon salt to now-empty skillet and cook over medium heat until softened and browned, about 5 minutes. Stir in garlic, chili powder, and oregano and cook until fragrant, about 1 minute. Transfer onion mixture to slow cooker. Stir in hominy, broth, and tomatoes and their juice. Cover and cook until pork is tender, 6 to 7 hours on high or 7 to 8 hours on low.

—   TAKE A BREAK   —

3   Using large spoon or ladle, skim fat from surface of stew. Season with salt and pepper to taste. Serve.

PREP AHEAD
You can cut up the pork and chop the onion up to 1 day ahead and refrigerate separately. You can refrigerate the posole for up to 2 days. I do not recommend freezing it.

MAKE IT EVEN EASIER
Ask the butcher at your market to cut up the pork for you.

2½	pounds boneless pork butt roast, trimmed and cut into 1-inch pieces
1½	teaspoons table salt, divided
½	teaspoon pepper
1	tablespoon vegetable oil
1	onion, chopped
5	garlic cloves, minced
1½	tablespoons chili powder
1	teaspoon dried oregano
3	(15-ounce) cans white or yellow hominy, drained
3	cups chicken broth
1	(14.5-ounce) can diced tomatoes

Skillet Meals

* Try these recipes first if today is not one of your better days and you need a soul-refilling meal with a high return on your energy investment.

Pan-Seared Chicken with Warm Bulgur Pilaf

SERVES 4

1½ cups medium-grind bulgur, rinsed

2¼ cups water

½ teaspoon table salt, divided

4 (6- to 8-ounce) boneless, skinless chicken breasts, trimmed

¼ teaspoon pepper

3 tablespoons vegetable oil, divided

10 ounces cherry tomatoes, halved

4 ounces feta cheese (1 cup), crumbled

¾ cup minced fresh parsley

½ cup pitted kalamata olives, halved

1 tablespoon lemon juice, plus lemon wedges for serving

Why This Recipe Works This Mediterranean-inspired meal pairs hearty and nutritious bulgur with simple pan-seared boneless, skinless chicken breasts. The bulgur is easy to cook, no draining required (and you can make it ahead), and the chicken takes less than 15 minutes to cook in a skillet. But what I love about this recipe is the combination of ingredients that brings the bulgur to life: cherry tomatoes, pungent feta cheese, a hefty dose of parsley, plus olives and lemon juice.

1 **For the bulgur** Bring 2¼ cups water, bulgur, and ¼ teaspoon salt to boil in large saucepan over medium-high heat. Reduce heat to low, cover, and simmer gently until bulgur is tender, about 17 minutes.

— TAKE A 17-MINUTE BREAK —

2 Remove pot from heat and let sit, covered, for 10 minutes.

— TAKE A 10-MINUTE BREAK —

3 **For the chicken** Pat chicken dry with paper towels and sprinkle with salt and pepper. Heat 1 tablespoon oil in 12-inch skillet over medium-high heat until just smoking. Cook chicken until golden brown and meat registers 160 degrees, about 7 minutes per side. Transfer to cutting board, tent with aluminum foil, and let rest for 5 minutes.

4 Fluff bulgur with fork, add tomatoes, feta, parsley, olives, lemon juice, and remaining 2 tablespoons oil and stir gently to combine. Season with salt and pepper to taste. Slice chicken breasts ¼ inch thick on bias. Serve with bulgur and lemon wedges.

PREP AHEAD

You can refrigerate cooked bulgur for up to 3 days; just rewarm before adding the remaining ingredients in step 4. You can halve the tomatoes and crumble the feta up to 1 day ahead and refrigerate separately.

MAKE IT EVEN EASIER

Buy crumbled feta.

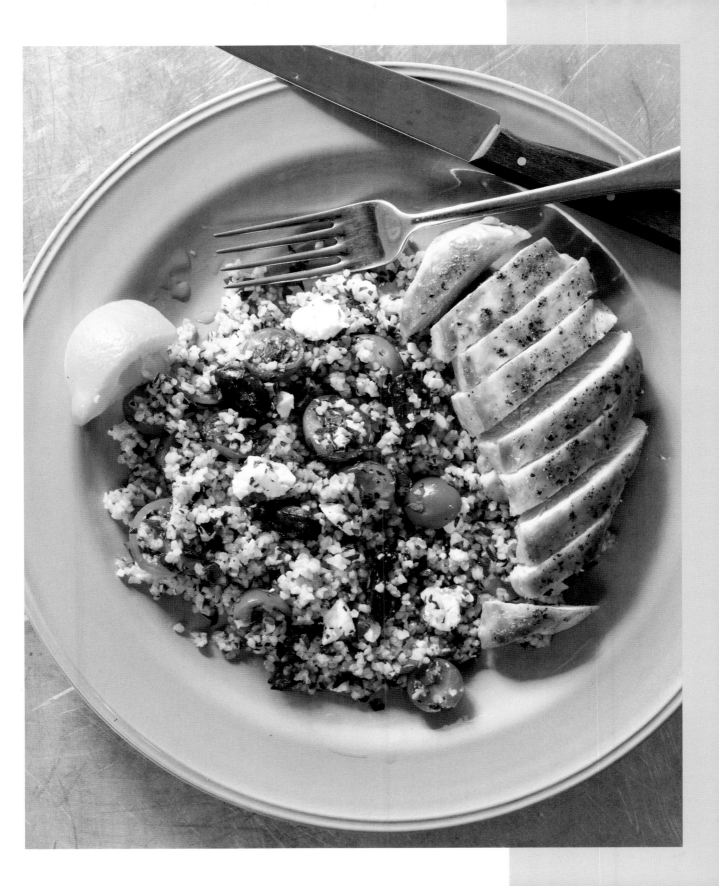

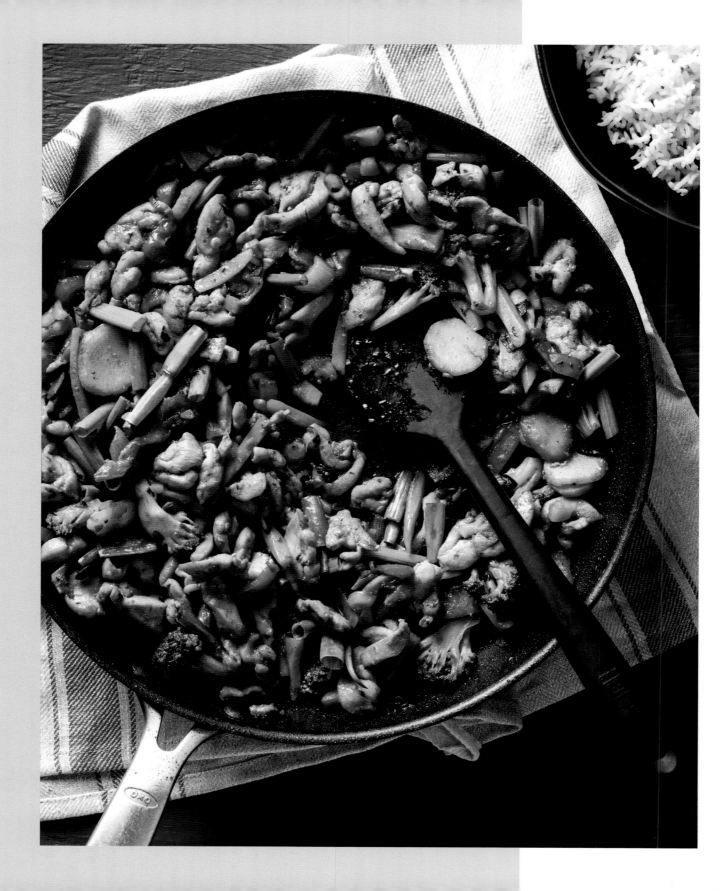

Stir-Fried Chicken and Vegetables with Black Bean Garlic Sauce

SERVES 4 — SUPER EASY

Why This Recipe Works Black bean garlic sauce, made from fermented black soybeans, garlic, and spices, is an umami-rich ingredient (with a long shelf life) that's full of salty, sweet, and slightly funky flavors. It's the shining star of this extraordinarily easy stir-fry. Thinned out with a bit of soy sauce and Shaoxing wine, it is the perfect marinade for the chicken as well as a finishing sauce. A little brown sugar in the mix gives the marinade and sauce some balancing sweetness. Scallion whites help build the aromatic base and a bag of frozen veggies (you can really use any you have on hand) plus the remaining scallion greens bring this simple stir-fry to life.

1   Whisk black bean garlic sauce, soy sauce, Shaoxing wine, and sugar in bowl. Measure 3 tablespoons sauce mixture into medium bowl, then stir in chicken and let sit for 10 minutes. Set aside remaining sauce mixture.

— TAKE A 10-MINUTE BREAK —

2   Heat 1½ teaspoons oil in 12-inch nonstick skillet over high heat until just smoking. Add half of chicken, breaking up any clumps, and cook until cooked through, about 4 minutes; transfer to bowl. Repeat with 1½ teaspoons oil and remaining chicken.

3   Heat 2 teaspoons oil in now-empty skillet over high heat until shimmering. Add stir-fry vegetables and cook for 30 seconds. Stir in water, then cover skillet, reduce heat to medium, and cook until vegetables are crisp-tender, about 2 minutes. Push vegetables to sides of skillet. Add scallion whites and remaining 1 teaspoon oil to center and cook, mashing scallion whites into skillet, until fragrant, about 1 minute; stir into vegetables.

4   Stir chicken, along with any accumulated juices, into skillet with vegetables. Whisk remaining sauce mixture to recombine, then add to skillet and cook, stirring constantly, until sauce is slightly thickened, about 1 minute. Stir in scallion greens and serve.

⅓ cup black bean garlic sauce

3 tablespoons soy sauce

2 tablespoons Shaoxing wine or dry sherry

4 teaspoons packed brown sugar

1½ pounds boneless, skinless chicken thighs, trimmed and sliced ¼ inch thick

2 tablespoons vegetable oil, divided

1 pound frozen stir-fry vegetable blend, thawed

2 tablespoons water

6 scallions, whites sliced thin, and greens cut into 1-inch pieces, separated

PREP AHEAD
You can trim and slice the chicken up to 1 day ahead and refrigerate.

Chicken Lo Mein with Bok Choy

SERVES 4 — SUPER EASY

- 1 pound boneless, skinless chicken breasts, trimmed and sliced crosswise ¼ inch thick

- ¼ cup soy sauce, divided

- 12 ounces fresh Chinese noodles or 8 ounces dried Chinese noodles

- 3 tablespoons vegetable oil, divided

- 1 pound baby bok choy, halved lengthwise and sliced crosswise ½ inch thick

- 1 tablespoon chili-garlic sauce

PREP AHEAD

You can trim and slice the chicken and prep the bok choy up to 1 day ahead and refrigerate separately. You can cook, drain, and rinse the Chinese noodles up to 2 hours ahead; toss with 2 teaspoons sesame oil and refrigerate until using.

TAKE IT UP A NOTCH

Use peeled and deveined shrimp instead of chicken; cook shrimp for 30 to 90 seconds per side.

Why This Recipe Works I guarantee that this stir-fry has the fewest ingredients of any you'll ever make. Soy sauce and chili-garlic sauce, a powerhouse ingredient that delivers a punch of both garlic and heat, are the only sauce ingredients. Fresh (or dried) Chinese noodles need mere minutes to cook. Because they are drained and rinsed, you can do this ahead of time—making this dinner very fast to execute but still deeply flavorful. The chicken breast slices cook all at once in a large skillet, no need to cook them in batches, while baby bok choy, which adds flavor and color, also only takes minutes to cook in the hot skillet. A platter full of these fragrant noodles, chicken, and bok choy is sure to please, and making it is easy on the back.

1   Toss chicken with 1 tablespoon soy sauce in bowl; set aside while cooking noodles. Bring 2 quarts water to boil in large saucepan. Add noodles and cook, stirring often, until tender. Drain noodles and rinse thoroughly with cold water; set aside.

— TAKE A 15-MINUTE BREAK —

2   Heat 1 tablespoon oil in 12-inch nonstick skillet over medium-high heat until just smoking. Add chicken and cook until no longer pink, about 3 minutes. Transfer chicken to large serving bowl. Add 1 tablespoon oil to now-empty skillet and heat over medium-high heat until just smoking. Add bok choy and cook until beginning to soften and char in spots, about 3 minutes. Transfer to bowl with chicken.

3   Add remaining 1 tablespoon oil to again-empty skillet and heat over medium-high heat until just smoking. Add noodles, remaining 3 tablespoons soy sauce, and chili-garlic sauce and toss to combine. Cook until noodles are warmed through, about 2 minutes. Transfer noodles to bowl with chicken and bok choy and toss to combine. Serve.

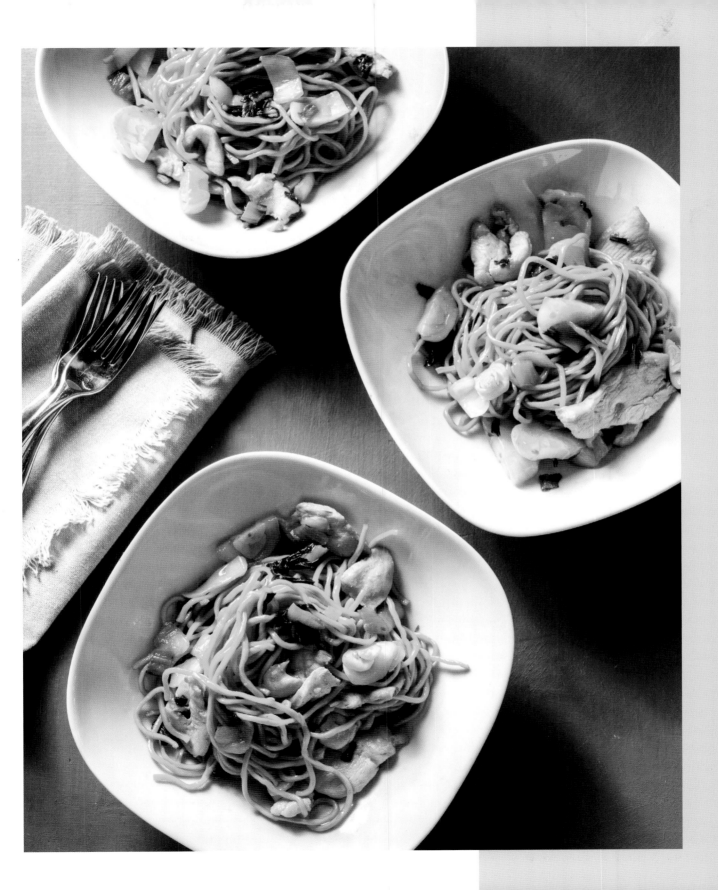

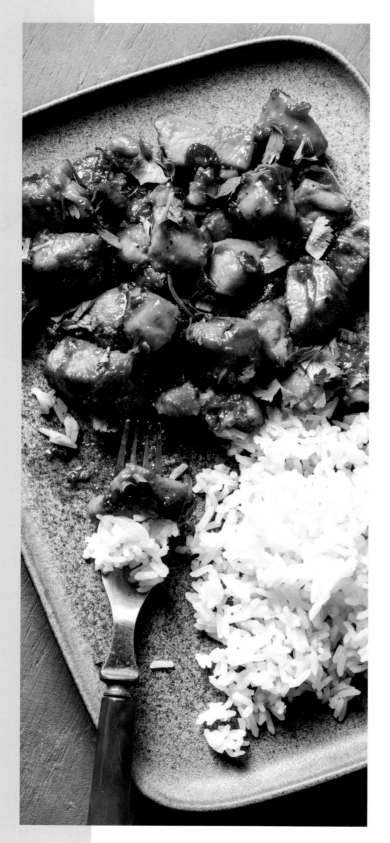
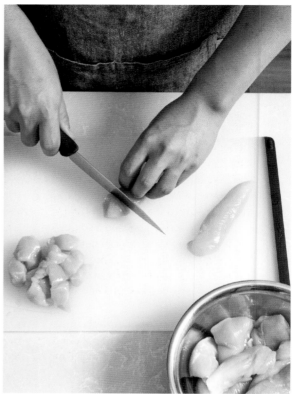
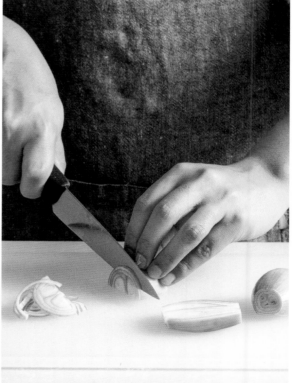

Caramelized Black Pepper Chicken

SERVES 4 — SUPER EASY

Why This Recipe Works This intensely flavored chicken is an exceptional Vietnamese pantry dish you can make in a flash. It is inspired by a recipe from Charles Phan, the chef-owner of the Slanted Door family of restaurants and his book of the same name. Here, it is streamlined by using brown sugar instead of making a caramel. Chunks of chicken and sliced shallots soak up the aromatic sauce packed with fresh ginger, fish sauce, rice vinegar and a whopping tablespoon of chili-garlic sauce. A full teaspoon of black pepper adds another layer of heat, so this dish is not for the faint of heart. The saltiness of fish sauce can vary; I recommend Red Boat 40°N fish sauce. This dish is highly seasoned, so serve it with plenty of steamed white rice, preferably jasmine.

1 Heat oil in 12-inch nonstick skillet over medium-high heat until shimmering. Add shallots and ginger and cook until softened, about 2 minutes. Stir in sugar, fish sauce, vinegar, chili-garlic sauce, and pepper and bring to simmer, stirring to dissolve sugar. Cook until very thick and syrupy, about 5 minutes.

2 Stir in chicken and cook, stirring occasionally, until cooked through, about 6 minutes (sauce will thin out as chicken exudes moisture). Sprinkle with cilantro and serve.

2 tablespoons vegetable oil

2 shallots, halved and sliced thin

1 teaspoon grated fresh ginger

⅓ cup packed dark brown sugar

3 tablespoons fish sauce

2 tablespoons unseasoned rice vinegar

1 tablespoon chili-garlic sauce

1 teaspoon coarsely ground pepper

1½ pounds boneless, skinless chicken breasts, trimmed and cut into ¾-inch pieces

¼ cup coarsely chopped fresh cilantro leaves and stems

PREP AHEAD
You can slice the shallots, grate the ginger, and trim and cut up the chicken up to 1 day ahead and refrigerate separately.

MAKE IT EVEN EASIER
Use chicken tenderloins instead of chicken breasts; they are easier to prep.

Chicken Curry with Tomatoes and Ginger

SERVES 4 — SUPER EASY

- 2 tablespoons vegetable oil
- 1 onion, chopped fine
- 1 teaspoon table salt
- 1 tablespoon yellow curry powder
- 4 garlic cloves, minced
- 1 teaspoon ground cardamom
- ¾ teaspoon ground ginger
- 1½ pounds boneless, skinless chicken thighs, trimmed and cut into 1-inch pieces
- ¾ cup chicken or vegetable broth
- 3 plum tomatoes, chopped coarse, divided
- ½ cup plain yogurt
- 2 tablespoons chopped fresh cilantro

Why This Recipe Works This lightning-fast skillet dish captures all the flavors of a fragrant curry with very little prep required (and you can do most of the prep work ahead). It is appealingly fresh and light and uses chopped fresh tomatoes instead of canned (added in two stages for flavor and brightness). And to pull it all together at the end, a bit of the fragrant and spice-infused broth in the skillet is mixed with yogurt and then swirled back into the skillet for creaminess without the cream that would dull the flavor of the spices.

1   Heat oil in 12-inch skillet over medium heat until shimmering. Add onion and salt and cook until softened, about 5 minutes. Add curry powder, garlic, cardamom, and ginger and cook until fragrant, about 30 seconds. Pat chicken dry with paper towels, then stir into spice mixture in skillet and cook until lightly browned, about 3 minutes. Turn off heat and cover skillet.

— TAKE A 15-MINUTE BREAK —

2   Return skillet to medium heat and add broth and half of tomatoes to skillet, scraping up any browned bits, and bring to boil. Reduce heat to medium-low and simmer until chicken is tender and sauce is slightly thickened and reduced by about half, about 9 minutes; remove skillet from heat.

3   In medium bowl, whisk yogurt until smooth. Whisking constantly, slowly ladle about 1 cup hot liquid from skillet into yogurt and whisk until combined, then stir yogurt mixture back into skillet until combined. Stir in cilantro and remaining tomatoes and season with salt and pepper to taste. Serve.

PREP AHEAD

You can chop the onion and tomatoes and trim and cut up the chicken up to 1 day ahead and refrigerate separately. You can make the curry up to 2 days ahead or freeze for up to 1 month.

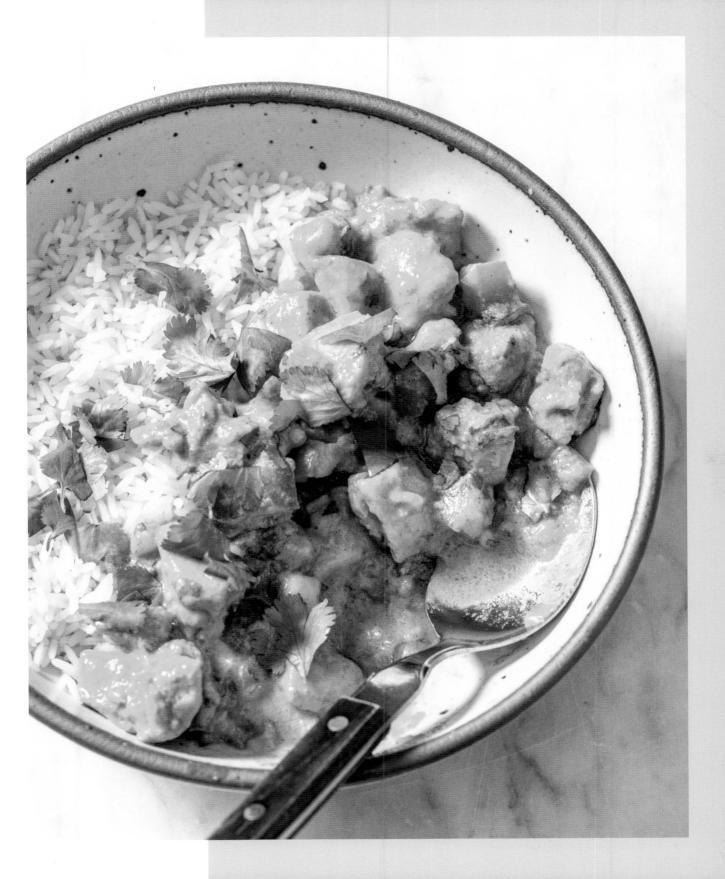

Chicken, Sun-Dried Tomato, and Goat Cheese Burgers

SERVES 4 — SUPER EASY

- 5 hamburger buns (1 bun torn into 1-inch pieces, 4 buns toasted, if desired)
- 2 tablespoons water
- 1 pound ground chicken
- 2 ounces goat cheese (½ cup), crumbled
- ⅓ cup oil-packed sun-dried tomatoes, chopped coarse, plus 1 tablespoon sun-dried tomato oil
- 1 shallot, minced
- 2 tablespoons chopped fresh basil
- ½ teaspoon table salt
- ¼ teaspoon pepper

Why This Recipe Works I like to have a few easy-to-assemble (and make-ahead) stovetop burger recipes in my repertoire for busy nights, but all too often simple burgers leave much to be desired in the flavor and satisfaction department. To jazz up chicken burgers, tangy goat cheese, minced shallot, fresh basil, and bright sun-dried tomatoes ensure that they are anything but dull. A panade made from mashing a torn hamburger bun with a little water allows the patties to hold their shape. Then, cooking them in a little of the oil from the sun-dried tomato jar helps them brown and also gives them a burst of flavor.

1   Using fork, mash bun pieces and water into paste in large bowl. Add chicken, goat cheese, tomatoes, shallot, basil, salt, and pepper and knead gently with your hands until combined. Divide mixture into 4 portions, form each into loose ball, then press gently into ¾-inch-thick patties. Refrigerate, covered, for 15 minutes.

— TAKE A 15-MINUTE BREAK —

2   Heat tomato oil in 12-inch nonstick skillet over medium-high heat until just smoking. Add patties and cook until lightly browned on first side, about 3 minutes. Flip patties and continue to cook until second side is lightly browned, about 3 minutes.

3   Reduce heat to low, partially cover, and continue to cook until meat registers 160 degrees, 8 to 10 minutes, flipping as needed. Place burgers on buns. Serve.

PREP AHEAD
You can crumble the goat cheese, chop the sun-dried tomatoes, and mince the shallot up to 1 day ahead and refrigerate separately. You can make the patties up to 1 day ahead and refrigerate until cooking.

MAKE IT EVEN EASIER
Buy jarred, chopped sun-dried tomatoes and crumbled goat cheese.

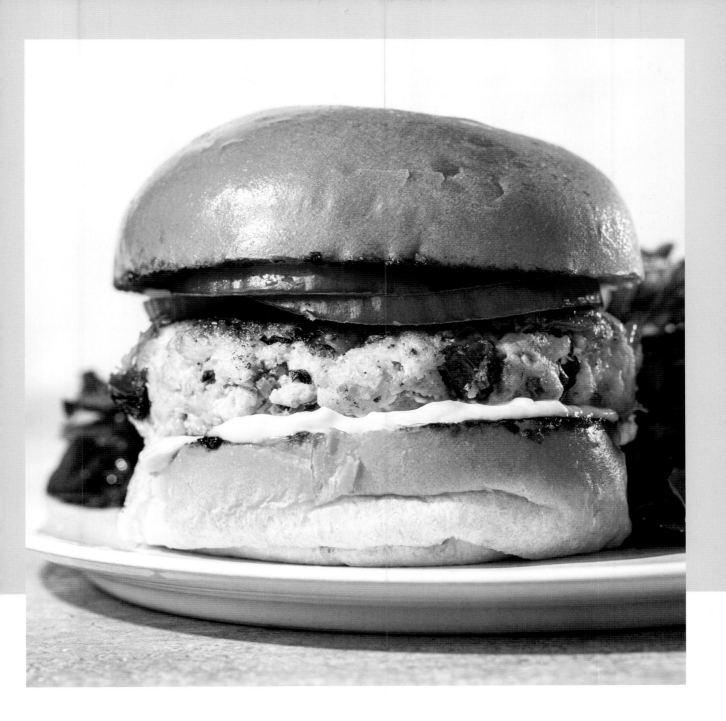

Serve with Sun-Dried Tomato and Caper Mayonnaise

Combine ½ cup mayonnaise, 2 tablespoons chopped oil-packed sun-dried tomatoes, and 2 teaspoons capers in small bowl. Season with salt and refrigerate for at least 30 minutes. The mayonnaise can be refrigerated for up to 3 days. Makes ½ cup.

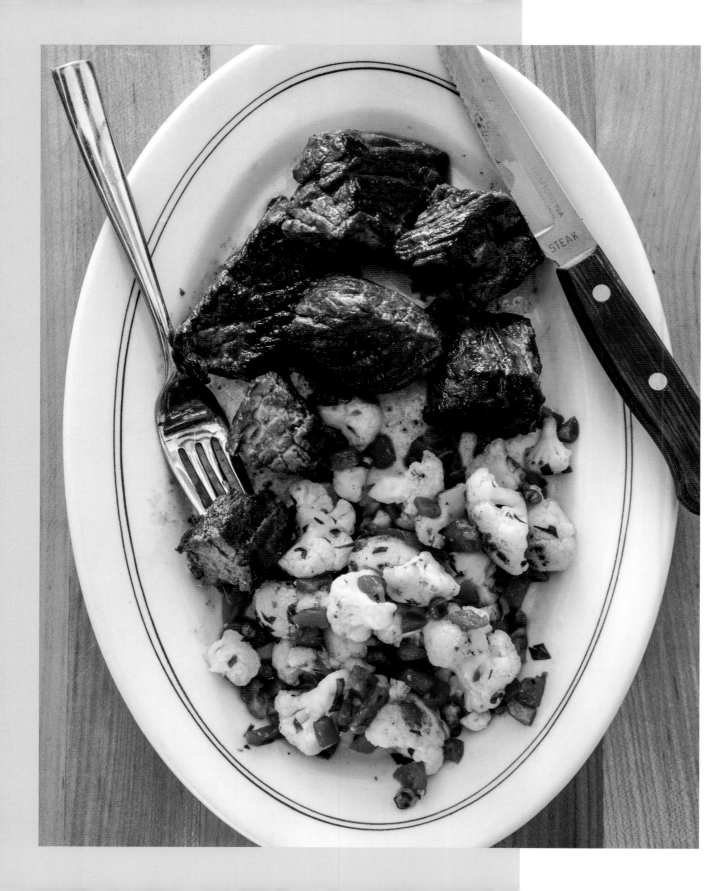

Steak Tips with Spicy Cauliflower

SERVES 2

Why This Recipe Works In the healthy back kitchen, steak tips are a star ingredient. They are easy to cut into pieces, deliver great beefy flavor, and cook in under 10 minutes. I like to pair them with an interesting side that can be cooked in the same skillet. Here, they accompany an exciting and unusual side that comes together with very little effort: cauliflower jazzed up with a pungent, no-cook relish of jarred roasted red peppers, hot cherry peppers, capers, and parsley. This keeps well in the fridge, so if you prep ahead, all you need to do to get dinner on the table is quickly sauté the cauliflower and then sear the steak tips. What could be better than dinner for two you can cook in 18 minutes with a break built in? Sirloin steak tips, also known as flap meat, can be sold as whole steaks, cubes, and strips. To ensure uniform pieces, it is best to purchase whole steaks and cut them yourself. You will need a 12-inch nonstick skillet with a tight-fitting lid for this recipe.

1   Combine 1½ tablespoons oil, red peppers, cherry peppers, parsley, capers, ⅛ teaspoon salt, and pinch pepper in medium bowl; set relish aside.

2   Heat 1½ teaspoons oil in 12-inch nonstick skillet over medium-high heat until shimmering. Add cauliflower, cover, and cook, stirring occasionally, until browned and tender, about 10 minutes. Add cauliflower to relish and toss to combine. Season with salt and pepper to taste and cover with foil.

—   **TAKE A 15-MINUTE BREAK**   —

3   Pat steak tips dry with paper towels and sprinkle with remaining ¼ teaspoon salt and remaining ⅛ teaspoon pepper. Heat remaining 1½ teaspoons oil in now-empty skillet over medium-high heat until just smoking. Add steak tips and cook until browned on all sides and meat registers 120 to 125 degrees (for medium-rare), about 8 minutes, flipping as needed. Serve steak tips with cauliflower.

2½   tablespoons extra-virgin olive oil, divided

¼   cup jarred roasted red peppers, patted dry and chopped

2   tablespoons finely chopped jarred hot cherry peppers

1   tablespoon chopped fresh parsley

1½   teaspoons capers, rinsed and minced

⅛   teaspoon plus ¼ teaspoon table salt, divided

Pinch plus ⅛ teaspoon pepper, divided

1½   pounds cauliflower florets, cut into 1-inch pieces

1   pound sirloin steak tips, trimmed and cut into 2-inch pieces

PREP AHEAD
You can make the red pepper mixture up to 1 day ahead and refrigerate; bring to room temperature before using. You can trim and cut the steak tips up to 1 day ahead and refrigerate.

MAKE IT EVEN EASIER
Buy jarred, chopped roasted red peppers and hot cherry peppers. Buy cauliflower florets.

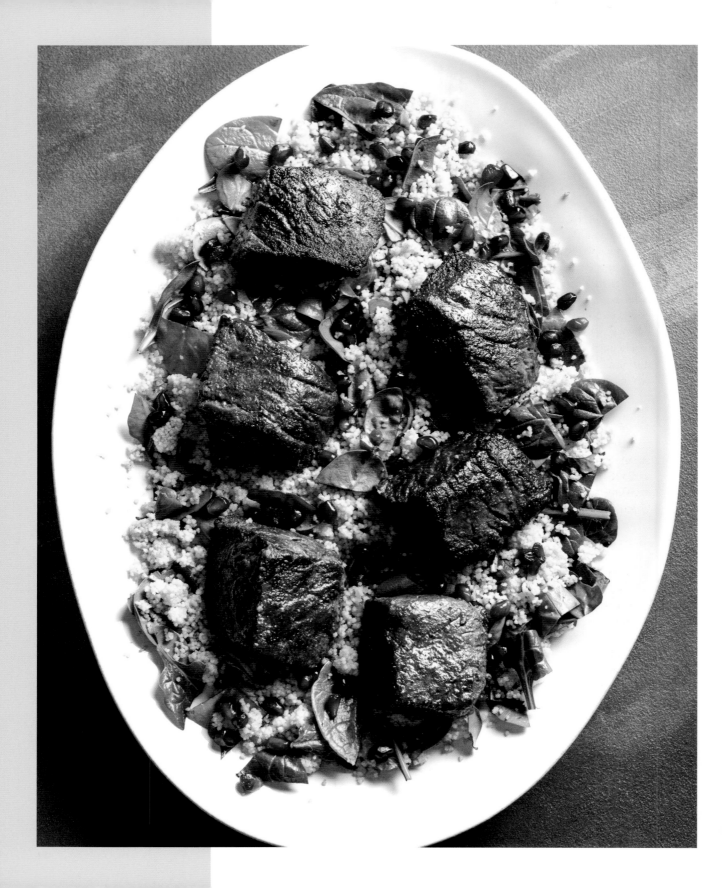

Steak Tips with Ras el Hanout and Couscous

SERVES 4

Why This Recipe Works The North African spice mix ras el hanout elevates humble steak tips with its mix of warm spices (black pepper, cumin, cinnamon, paprika, and turmeric) without the need to empty out your spice cabinet. Quickly sear steak tips and let rest and then add water to the fond-slicked skillet to make the couscous. This adds a noticeable depth of spice-infused flavor to the couscous in mere minutes. A little chopped baby spinach and bright pomegranate seeds mixed into the couscous elevates the flavor and belies the ease with which you can put it together. Sirloin steak tips, also known as flap meat, can be sold as whole steaks, cubes, and strips. To ensure uniform pieces, it is best to purchase whole steaks and cut them yourself. You will need a 12-inch nonstick skillet with a tight-fitting lid for this recipe.

1½ pounds sirloin steak tips, trimmed and cut into 2-inch pieces

2½ teaspoons ras el hanout, divided

1 teaspoon table salt, divided

¼ teaspoon pepper

2 tablespoons vegetable oil

1¼ cups water

¾ cup couscous

2 ounces (2 cups) baby spinach, chopped

¼ cup pomegranate seeds

1 Pat steak dry with paper towels and sprinkle with 2 teaspoons ras el hanout, ½ teaspoon salt, and pepper. Heat oil in 12-inch nonstick skillet over medium-high heat until just smoking. Add steak and cook until well browned all over and meat registers 120 to 125 degrees (for medium-rare), about 8 minutes, flipping as needed. Transfer to cutting board, tent loosely with aluminum foil, and let rest.

— TAKE A 15-MINUTE BREAK —

2 Add water, couscous, remaining ½ teaspoon salt, and remaining ½ teaspoon ras el hanout to now-empty skillet and bring to boil over medium-high heat. Remove from heat, cover, and let sit until couscous is tender, about 5 minutes.

3 Fluff couscous with fork, stir in spinach and pomegranate seeds, and season with salt and pepper to taste. Slice steak thin and serve with couscous.

PREP AHEAD
You can trim and cut the steak tips up to 1 day ahead and refrigerate.

MAKE IT EVEN EASIER
Ask the butcher at your local market to trim and cut up the steak tips.

Pan-Seared Strip Steaks with Crispy Potatoes

SERVES 2

¾ pound russet potatoes, unpeeled, cut lengthwise into 1-inch wedges

3 tablespoons vegetable oil, divided

⅛ plus ¼ teaspoon table salt, divided

Pinch plus ⅛ teaspoon pepper, divided

1 (1-pound) boneless strip steak, 1 to 1½ inches thick, trimmed and halved crosswise

¼ cup pesto

PREP AHEAD
You can trim and cut up the steaks up to 1 day ahead and refrigerate.

MAKE IT EVEN EASIER
Use frozen potato wedges (thawed) instead of the russet potatoes; you will not need to cook them as long in the skillet.

Why This Recipe Works What's better than a steak and potato dinner that you can easily whip up at home? This dinner for two is as good as one you can get at an expensive steak house, but it avoids a long dinner service. To make it speedy and easy to execute, simply parcook the potatoes in the microwave so you don't have to stand at the stove for long waiting for them to get crispy. After the meat is seared in a smoking hot skillet, let it rest on a platter while you cook the potatoes until they develop a gorgeous crust and soak up the meaty, savory fat left behind by the steak. A swoosh of store-bought pesto adds brightness to keep things from tipping into too-rich territory.

1 Combine potatoes, 1½ teaspoons oil, ⅛ teaspoon salt, and pinch pepper in bowl; cover and microwave until potatoes begin to soften, 7 to 10 minutes, stirring halfway through; drain well.

— TAKE A 15-MINUTE BREAK —

2 Pat steaks dry with paper towels and sprinkle with remaining ¼ teaspoon salt and remaining ⅛ teaspoon pepper. Heat 1½ teaspoons oil in 12-inch nonstick skillet over medium-high heat until just smoking. Add steak and cook, flipping every 2 minutes, until exteriors are well browned and meat registers 120 to 125 degrees (for medium-rare), about 11 minutes. Transfer to platter, tent loosely with aluminum foil, and let rest for 10 minutes.

— TAKE A 10-MINUTE BREAK —

3 Heat remaining 2 tablespoons oil in now-empty skillet over medium-high heat until shimmering. Add potatoes in single layer and cook until golden brown on both cut sides, about 5 minutes per side. Transfer potatoes to paper towel–lined plate and season with salt to taste.

4 Serve potatoes and steak with pesto.

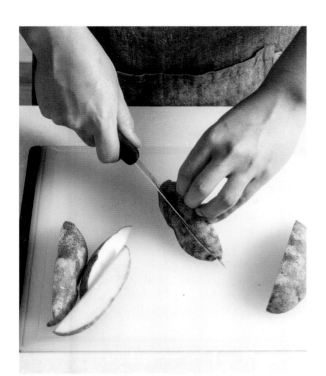

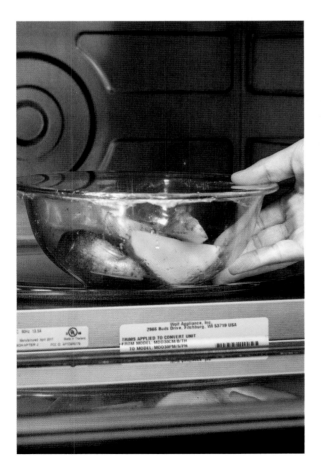

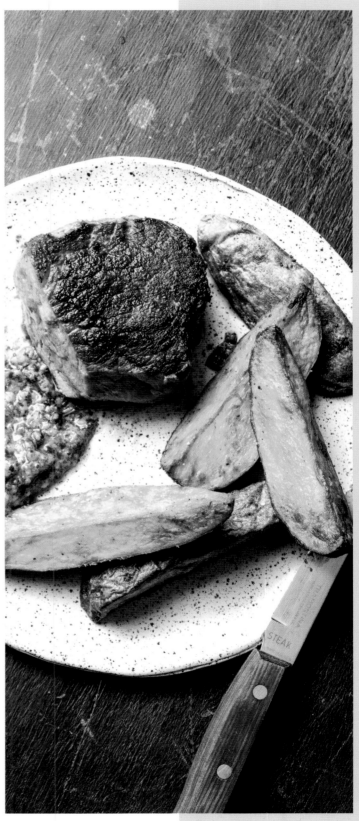

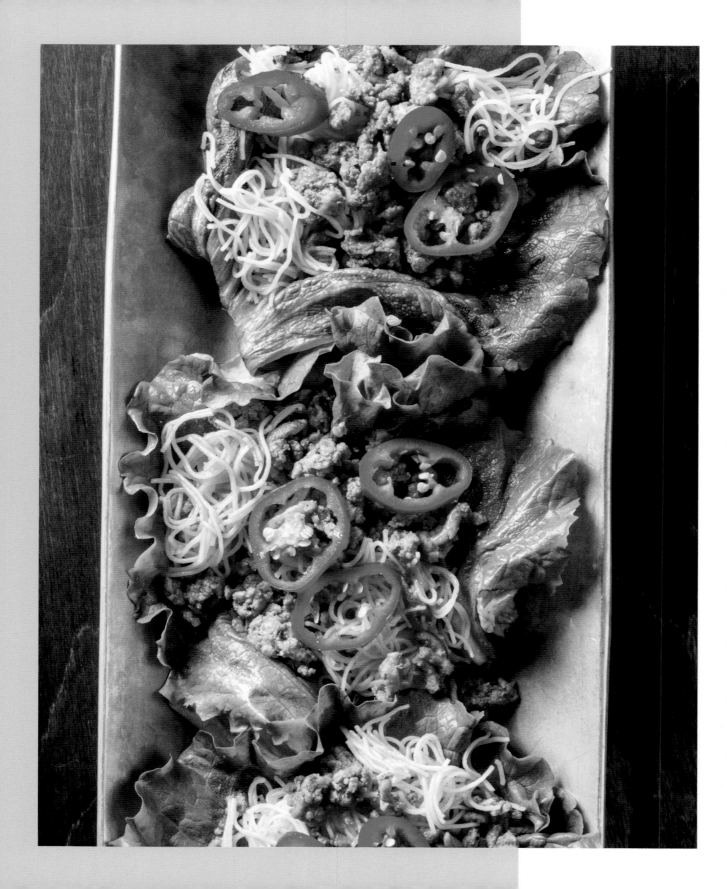

Red Curry Pork Lettuce Wraps

SERVES 4 — SUPER EASY

Why This Recipe Works This meal was a revelation to me because I thought lettuce wraps, which I'd never made before, were complicated. But this recipe is one of the easiest in this book. These wraps are super savory and come together in minutes thanks to Thai red curry paste, which provides concentrated flavors of galangal, shallots, lemongrass, and so much more. Ground pork, an underutilized ingredient, makes the perfect canvas for the delicious red curry flavor. Vermicelli noodles, which take just 5 minutes to become tender in boiling water, give these flavorful handheld wraps some heft.

8 ounces rice vermicelli

1 tablespoon vegetable oil

¼ cup Thai red curry paste

1½ pounds ground pork

1 head green leaf lettuce or Bibb lettuce, leaves separated

1 red bell pepper or jalapeño chile, stemmed, seeded, and sliced thin

1 Bring 2 quarts water to boil in large saucepan. Off heat, add noodles and let sit, stirring occasionally, until tender, about 5 minutes. Drain noodles, rinse with cold water, and drain again; set aside.

2 Meanwhile, heat oil in 12-inch nonstick skillet over medium heat until shimmering. Add curry paste and cook until fragrant and beginning to darken, about 2 minutes. Add pork and cook, breaking up meat with wooden spoon, until just beginning to brown, about 8 minutes. Season with salt and pepper to taste.

3 Using slotted spoon, serve pork in lettuce cups with noodles and bell pepper.

PREP AHEAD

You can cook, drain, and rinse the vermicelli noodles up to 2 hours ahead; toss with a teaspoon of sesame oil and refrigerate until using. You can separate the lettuce leaves and slice the pepper up to 1 day ahead and refrigerate separately.

Easy Salmon Burgers

SERVES 4 — SUPER EASY

1¼ pounds skinless salmon, cut into 1-inch pieces

2 tablespoons mayonnaise

2 scallions, sliced thin

1 tablespoon vegetable oil

½ teaspoon table salt

¼ teaspoon pepper

Why This Recipe Works I try to eat salmon at least once a week, and I recommend that my patients do the same. This recipe delivers easy, crave-worthy salmon burgers that you can serve on a bun and dress up with a sauce or sliced avocado and tomato or simply serve it on its own alongside a salad. The food processor makes easy work of chopping up the salmon (be sure to ask your fishmonger to remove the skin). Mayonnaise adds cohesiveness and moisture to the patties, while scallions bring color and texture. Refrigerating the formed patties for at least 15 minutes ensures that the burgers hold their shape when cooked. Like many burgers, these can be made in advance, giving you an easy dinner that can be on the table in less than 10 minutes.

1 Working in 3 batches, pulse salmon in food processor until chopped into ¼-inch pieces, about 2 pulses, transferring each batch to large bowl.

2 Add mayonnaise and scallions to chopped salmon and gently knead with your hands until well combined. Lightly moisten your hands, divide salmon mixture into 4 equal portions, then gently shape each portion into 1-inch-thick patty. Place patties on parchment paper–lined small rimmed baking sheet and refrigerate, covered, for 15 minutes.

— TAKE A 15-MINUTE BREAK —

3 Heat oil in 12-inch nonstick skillet over medium heat until shimmering. Season patties with salt and pepper. Cook patties, turning once, until browned, centers are still translucent when checked with tip of paring knife, and burgers register 125 degrees (for medium-rare), about 4 minutes per side. Serve.

PREP AHEAD

You can cut the salmon into pieces up to 1 day ahead and refrigerate. You can make the patties up to 1 day ahead and refrigerate.

TAKE IT UP A NOTCH
Serve with Chipotle Mayonnaise

Combine ½ cup mayonnaise, 1 tablespoon minced canned chipotle chile in adobo sauce, and 1 teaspoon grated lime zest plus 2 teaspoons juice in bowl. Mayonnaise can be refrigerated for up to 3 days. Makes ½ cup.

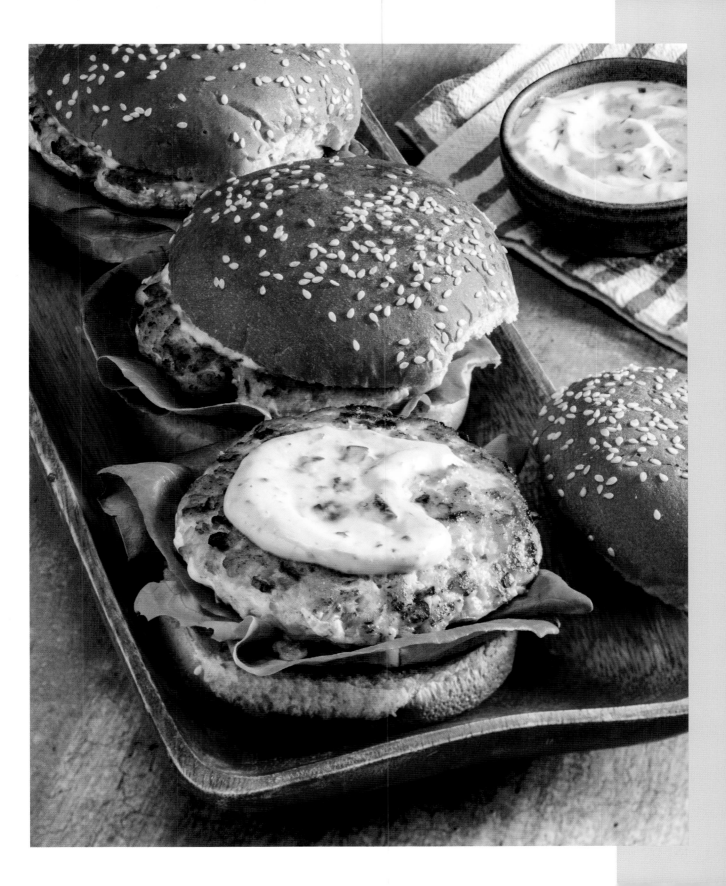

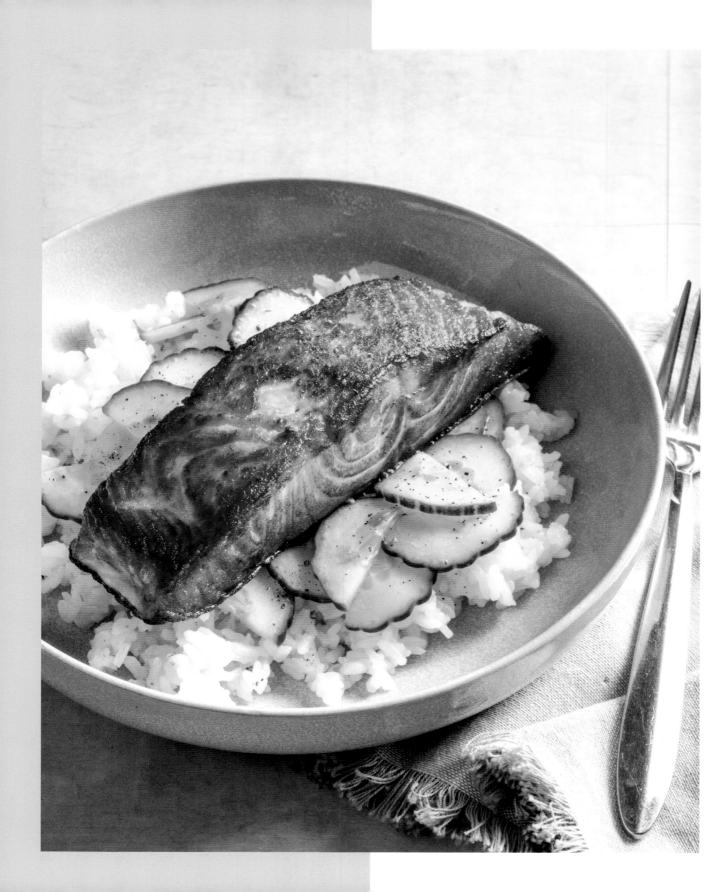

Salmon and Rice with Cucumber Salad

SERVES 2

Why This Recipe Works I will go out of my way to make seasoned sushi rice rather than regular white rice, and here use it as the base for an easy, fragrant salmon dinner for two. Making the sushi rice is simple with the right ratio of water to rice, and then the rice sits covered for 10 minutes before it is drizzled with seasoned rice vinegar. The salmon is cooked skin side up in a skillet, and turned once. And the special touch here to round out the meal is thinly sliced English cucumber tossed with more rice vinegar and a little toasted sesame oil.

1   Bring rice, water, and ¼ teaspoon salt to boil in small saucepan over high heat. Reduce heat to maintain bare simmer, cover, and cook until water is absorbed, about 20 minutes.

— **TAKE A 20-MINUTE BREAK** —

2   Remove pot from heat and let sit, covered, until rice is tender, about 10 minutes.

— **TAKE A 10-MINUTE BREAK** —

3   Drizzle rice with 1½ teaspoons vinegar, fluff with fork, and season with salt and pepper to taste. Cover to keep warm and set aside.

4   Pat salmon dry with paper towels and sprinkle with ¼ teaspoon salt and pepper. Heat vegetable oil in 10- or 12-inch nonstick skillet over medium-high heat until just smoking. Place salmon skin side up in skillet and cook until well browned and centers are still translucent when checked with tip of paring knife and register 125 degrees (for medium-rare), 4 to 6 minutes per side; remove from heat.

5   Toss cucumber with sesame oil, remaining 1½ tablespoons vinegar, and remaining ⅛ teaspoon salt in bowl, then season with salt and pepper to taste. Serve with salmon and rice.

½ cup sushi rice, rinsed

1 cup water

½ plus ⅛ teaspoon table salt, divided

2 tablespoons seasoned rice vinegar, divided

⅛ teaspoon pepper

2 (6- to 8-ounce) skin-on salmon fillets, 1 inch thick

½ teaspoon vegetable oil

½ English cucumber, halved lengthwise and sliced thin crosswise

1½ teaspoons toasted sesame oil

PREP AHEAD
You can slice the cucumber up to 1 day ahead and refrigerate.

MAKE IT EVEN EASIER
Make the sushi rice in a rice cooker; follow the seasoning instructions in step 3 after cooking rice.

Braised Halibut with Leeks and Mustard

SERVES 2

2 (6- to 8-ounce) skinless halibut fillets, ¾ to 1 inch thick

½ teaspoon table salt, divided

3 tablespoons unsalted butter

½ pound leeks, white and light green parts only, halved lengthwise, sliced thin, and washed thoroughly

½ teaspoon Dijon mustard

½ cup dry white wine

½ teaspoon lemon juice, plus lemon wedges for serving

1½ teaspoons minced fresh parsley

PREP AHEAD
You can slice the leeks up to 1 day ahead and refrigerate.

Why This Recipe Works When it comes to ways to cook fish, skillet braising has a lot going for it. As a moist-heat method, braising is gentle and thus forgiving, all but guaranteeing tender fish. Plus, it allows for a great one-pan meal: It's easy to add vegetables to the skillet to cook at the same time, and the cooking liquid becomes a sauce. Halibut is a great choice given its sweet, delicate flavor and its firm texture, which makes for easier handling. It pairs naturally with the classic French flavors of leeks, white wine, and Dijon mustard. Because the portions of the fillets submerged in liquid cook more quickly than the upper halves (which cook in steam), cook the fillets for a few minutes in the pan on just one side and then braise them, parcooked side up, to even out the cooking. For the liquid component, wine supplemented by the juices released by the fish and leeks during cooking deliver a bright and balanced sauce. Striped bass and swordfish are good substitutes for the halibut. To ensure that your fish cooks evenly, purchase fillets that are uniformly thick. You will need a 10-inch skillet with a tight-fitting lid for this recipe.

1 Pat halibut dry with paper towels and sprinkle with ¼ teaspoon salt. Melt butter in 10-inch skillet over low heat. Place halibut skinned side up in skillet, increase heat to medium, and cook, shaking skillet occasionally, until butter begins to brown (fish should not brown), 2 to 3 minutes. Turn off heat; Using spatula, carefully transfer halibut to large plate, raw side down.

— TAKE A 10-MINUTE BREAK —

2 Return skillet to medium heat and add leeks, mustard, and remaining ¼ teaspoon salt and cook, stirring frequently, until leeks begin to soften, about 3 minutes. Stir in wine and bring to gentle simmer. Place halibut, raw side down, on top of leeks. Cover skillet and cook, adjusting heat to maintain gentle simmer, until halibut flakes apart when gently prodded with paring knife and registers 130 degrees, 8 to 10 minutes. Remove skillet from heat and, using 2 spatulas, transfer halibut and leeks to serving platter or individual plates. Tent with aluminum foil.

3 Return skillet to high heat and simmer briskly until sauce is thickened, about 2 minutes. Off heat, stir in lemon juice and season with salt and pepper to taste. Spoon sauce over halibut and sprinkle with parsley. Serve immediately with lemon wedges.

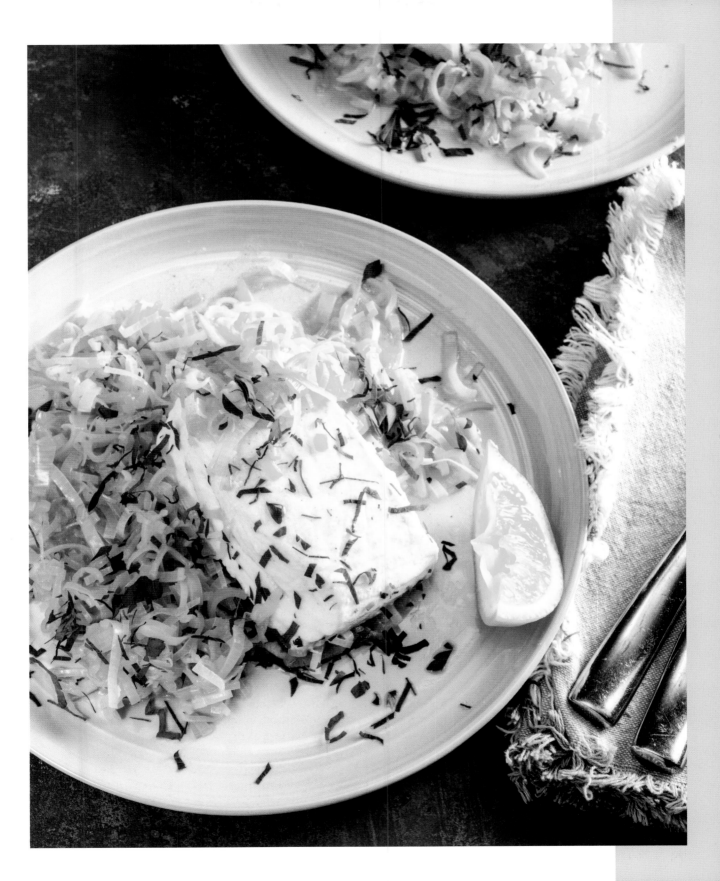

Red Curry Cod with Mushroom Rice

SERVES 4

1 tablespoon vegetable oil

1½ cups long-grain white rice

8 ounces white mushrooms, trimmed and sliced thin

1 (8-ounce) can bamboo shoots, rinsed

2 teaspoons grated fresh ginger

3 scallions, white and green parts separated and sliced thin

2¼ cups water

1 teaspoon table salt, divided

¾ cup canned coconut milk

3 tablespoons red curry paste

4 (6- to 8-ounce) skinless cod fillets, 1 to 1½ inches thick

¼ teaspoon pepper

Lime wedges

PREP AHEAD
You can trim and slice the mushrooms and grate the ginger up to 1 day ahead and refrigerate separately.

MAKE IT EVEN EASIER
Buy sliced mushrooms.

Why This Recipe Works Cod's mild flavor makes it the perfect fish to pair with the zesty, aromatic flavors of a simple red curry sauce. Though the dish could easily involve lots of prep and multiple pans, this stream-lined version layers the fish and a rice-and-vegetable side all in one skillet for a minimalist but boldly flavored meal. Enhancing the rice with meaty mushrooms and crunchy bamboo shoots by sautéing them all in a gingery scallion oil builds lots of flavor quickly. After simmering the rice for 10 minutes, place the fresh cod fillets on top, so the fish and rice finish at the same time. A simple coconut–red curry sauce infuses the fish with flavor while it cooks. The cod exudes juices as it simmers, flavoring the rice from above and marrying all the elements. Haddock and striped bass are good substitutes for the cod. Thin tail-end fillets can be folded to achieve proper thickness. You will need a 12-inch nonstick skillet with a tight-fitting lid for this recipe.

1   Heat oil in 12-inch nonstick skillet over medium heat until shimmering. Add rice, mushrooms, bamboo shoots, ginger, and scallion whites. Cook, stirring often, until edges of rice begin to turn translucent, about 2 minutes. Stir in water and ½ teaspoon salt and bring to boil. Reduce heat to medium-low, cover, and simmer for 10 minutes.

— TAKE A 10-MINUTE BREAK —

2   Whisk coconut milk and curry paste together in bowl. Pat cod dry with paper towels and sprinkle with remaining ½ teaspoon salt and pepper. Lay cod skinned side down on top of rice mixture and drizzle with one-third of coconut-curry sauce. Cover and cook until liquid is absorbed and cod flakes apart when gently prodded with paring knife and registers 130 degrees, 10 to 12 minutes. Remove from heat.

— TAKE A 10-MINUTE BREAK —

3   Microwave remaining coconut-curry sauce mixture until warm, about 1 minute. Sprinkle scallion greens over fish and rice mixture. Serve with remaining coconut-curry sauce and lime wedges.

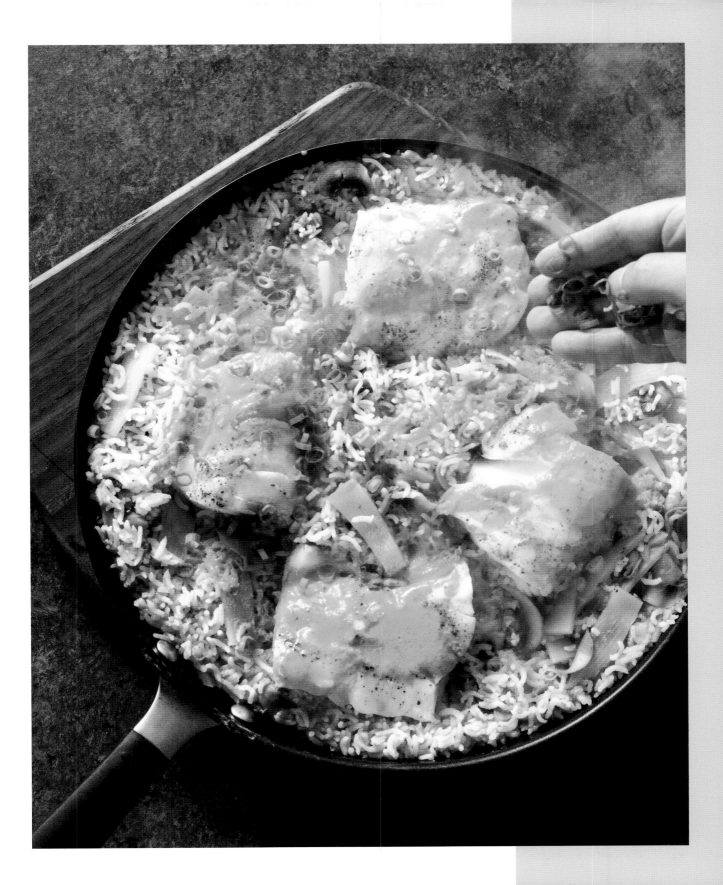

Spicy Shrimp and Ramen with Peanuts

SERVES 4

1 pound peeled and deveined extra-large shrimp (21 to 25 per pound)

¼ teaspoon table salt

⅛ teaspoon pepper

Pinch sugar

2 tablespoons vegetable oil, divided

1 red bell pepper, stemmed, seeded, and sliced thin

½ cup dry-roasted peanuts

3 garlic cloves, minced

1 tablespoon grated fresh ginger

1 teaspoon red pepper flakes

3½ cups chicken or vegetable broth

4 (3-ounce) packages ramen noodles, seasoning packets discarded

2 tablespoons hoisin sauce

1 tablespoon unseasoned rice vinegar

2 teaspoons toasted sesame oil

3 scallions, sliced thin on bias

Why This Recipe Works Shrimp meets instant ramen noodles in this dish with a spicy hoisin sauce so good no one will suspect how easy it is to make. After cooking the shrimp for less than 2 minutes, you can set them aside and take a break. Next up, sauté bell pepper slices and peanuts and then build a fragrant brothy base and add bricks of ramen noodles (sans the flavoring packets). As any college student will tell you, the ramen cooks in minutes. But that isn't the end of the story here, because a potent mix of hoisin sauce, seasoned rice vinegar, and toasted sesame oil is stirred into the noodles before the shrimp–bell pepper mixture is returned to the mix. The result is a dish that is the essence of noodle heaven. Do not substitute other types of noodles for the ramen noodles here. The sauce will seem brothy when finished, but the liquid will be absorbed quickly by the noodles when served.

1   Toss shrimp, salt, pepper, and sugar together in medium bowl. Heat 1 tablespoon vegetable oil in 12-inch nonstick skillet over high heat until just smoking. Add shrimp in single layer and cook without stirring until beginning to brown, about 1 minute. Stir shrimp and continue to cook until light pink and all but very centers are opaque, about 30 seconds. Transfer shrimp to bowl, cover to keep warm, and set aside.

— TAKE A 10-MINUTE BREAK —

2   Add remaining 1 tablespoon vegetable oil to now-empty skillet and heat over medium-high heat until shimmering. Add bell pepper and peanuts and cook until pepper is softened, about 2 minutes. Transfer to bowl with shrimp.

3   Add garlic, ginger, and pepper flakes to oil left in skillet and cook over medium-high heat until fragrant, about 30 seconds. Stir in broth. Break bricks of ramen into small chunks and add to skillet. Bring to simmer and cook, tossing ramen constantly with tongs to separate, until ramen is just tender but there is still liquid in pan, about 2 minutes.

4   Stir in hoisin, vinegar, and sesame oil and continue to simmer until sauce is thickened, about 1 minute. Return shrimp-pepper mixture to skillet and cook until warmed through, about 1 minute. Sprinkle with scallions and serve.

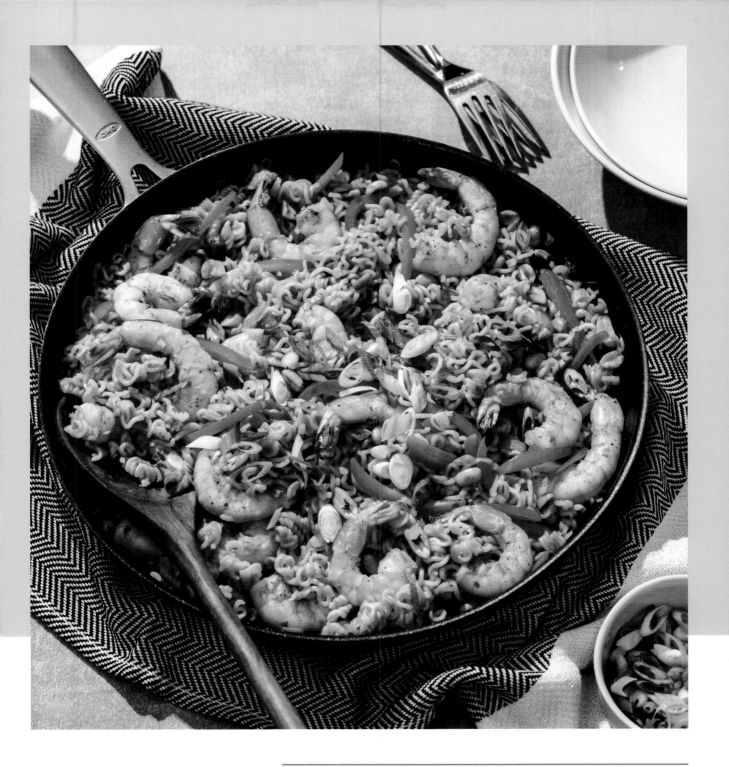

PREP AHEAD

You can slice the red pepper and scallions and grate the ginger up to 1 day
ahead and refrigerate separately.

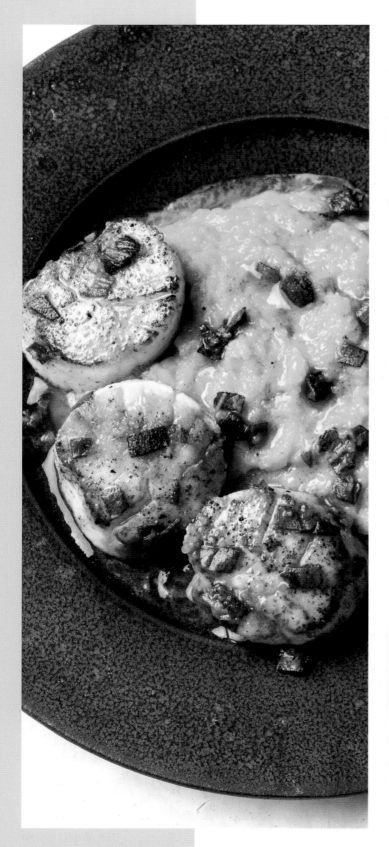

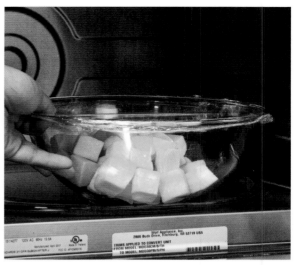

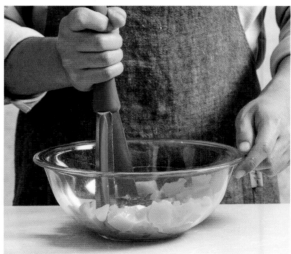

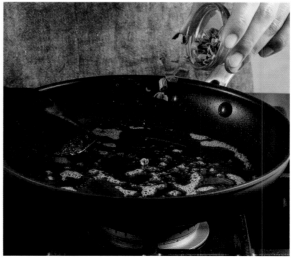

Seared Scallops with Sage Butter Sauce and Squash

SERVES 2

Why This Recipe Works Anytime I want to impress my wife, scallops are on the menu. And cooking scallops for two couldn't be easier, since you can sear them until they have an appealingly golden crust in just one batch. The dilemma I have is what to serve with them, because the usual starches don't seem to measure up. Here, an easy but luxurious-feeling side of buttery mashed butternut squash (effortlessly cooked in the microwave) pairs beautifully with the scallops. And for the perfect finishing touch, a buttery sage and lemon sauce drizzled over the scallops and squash will make you feel like you are eating in a fine restaurant.

- 1 pound large sea scallops, tendons removed
- 1 pound pre-cubed (1-inch) butternut squash pieces (2¾ cups)
- 4 tablespoons unsalted butter, divided
- ½ teaspoon table salt, divided
- ⅛ teaspoon pepper
- 1½ teaspoons chopped fresh sage
- 1½ teaspoons lemon juice

1 Place scallops on large plate lined with paper towels. Place layer of paper towels on top of scallops and press gently to blot liquid. Let scallops sit at room temperature for 10 minutes while towels absorb moisture.

— TAKE A 10-MINUTE BREAK —

2 Microwave squash in covered bowl until tender, about 10 minutes, stirring halfway through. Drain, if necessary, then add 1 tablespoon butter and ¼ teaspoon salt and mash with potato masher in large bowl until smooth and well combined. Cover and keep warm until ready to serve.

3 Sprinkle scallops with remaining ¼ teaspoon salt and pepper. Melt 1 tablespoon butter in 10-inch nonstick skillet over medium-high heat. Add scallops in single layer, flat side down, and cook until well browned, 1½ to 2 minutes. Flip scallops and cook until sides are firm and centers are opaque, 30 to 90 seconds (remove smaller scallops as they finish cooking). Transfer to plate and tent with aluminum foil.

4 Melt remaining 2 tablespoons butter in now-empty skillet over medium heat. Continue to cook, swirling skillet constantly, until butter begins to brown and has nutty aroma, about 1 minute. Add sage and cook until fragrant, about 1 minute. Off heat, stir in lemon juice. Drizzle sauce over scallops and squash puree and serve.

PREP AHEAD
You can cook and mash the butternut squash up to 1 day ahead; rewarm in the microwave before using.

Penne with Chicken, Mushrooms, and Gorgonzola

SERVES 2

8 ounces boneless, skinless chicken breasts, trimmed and sliced ¼ inch thick

⅛ plus ¼ teaspoon table salt, divided

⅛ teaspoon pepper

2 tablespoons extra-virgin olive oil, divided

4 ounces white mushrooms, trimmed and sliced

3 garlic cloves, minced

1 teaspoon minced fresh oregano or ¼ teaspoon dried

Pinch red pepper flakes

½ cup dry white wine

6 ounces (2 cups) penne

1½ cups chicken broth

1 cup water, plus extra as needed

1 ounce Gorgonzola cheese, crumbled (¼ cup), plus extra for serving

1 tablespoon unsalted butter

1 tablespoon minced fresh parsley

Why This Recipe Works The ingredient list for this hearty skillet dinner might look daunting, but it is actually not laborious, especially if you buy sliced mushrooms and chicken tenderloins (and simply slice them a bit thinner). And what's more, you can take a break after cooking the chicken, and then almost everything else, even the pasta, goes right into the skillet. A mix of white wine and broth infused with aromatics gives the pasta surprising richness and then just a little Gorgonzola and butter added at the end make the pasta feel special and ultrasatisfying. You will need a 10-inch nonstick skillet with a tight-fitting lid for this recipe.

1   Pat chicken dry with paper towels and sprinkle with ⅛ teaspoon salt and pepper. Heat 1 tablespoon oil in 10-inch nonstick skillet over medium-high heat until just smoking. Add chicken, breaking up any clumps, and cook, without stirring, until beginning to brown, about 1 minute. Stir chicken and continue to cook until just cooked through, about 2 minutes; transfer to bowl and cover.

— TAKE A 10-MINUTE BREAK —

2   Add remaining 1 tablespoon oil and mushrooms to now-empty skillet and cook over medium heat, stirring occasionally, until mushrooms have released their liquid and are golden brown, 5 minutes. Stir in garlic, oregano, and pepper flakes and cook until fragrant, about 30 seconds. Stir in wine, bring to simmer, and cook until nearly evaporated, about 2 minutes.

3   Stir in pasta, broth, water, and remaining ¼ teaspoon salt and bring to vigorous simmer. Reduce heat to medium, cover, and cook, stirring gently and often, until pasta is tender and sauce has thickened, about 12 minutes. (If sauce becomes too thick, add extra water as needed.)

4   Reduce heat to low and stir in chicken along with any accumulated juices, Gorgonzola, and butter. Cook, uncovered, stirring often, until pasta is well coated with sauce and chicken is warmed, about 3 minutes. Stir in parsley and season with salt and pepper to taste. Serve with extra Gorgonzola.

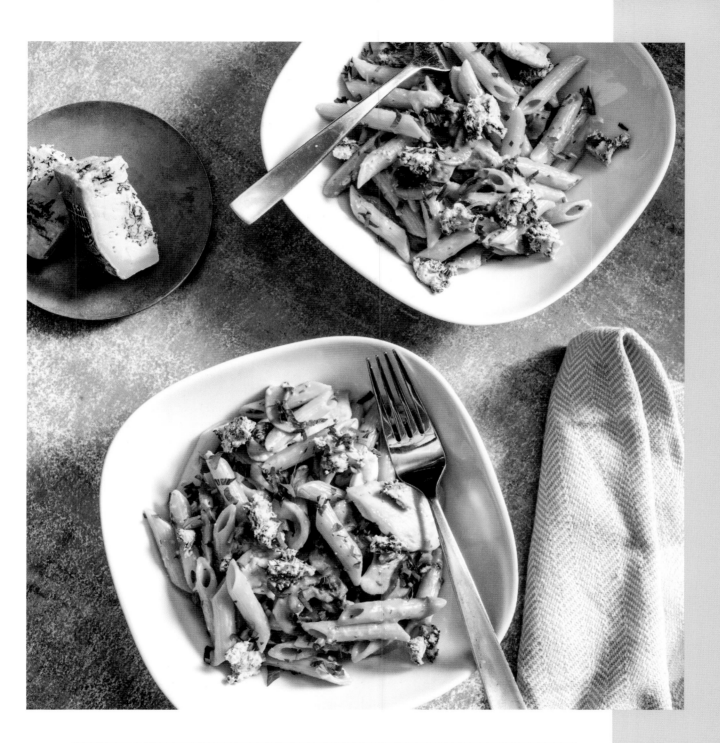

PREP AHEAD
You can trim and slice the chicken, slice the mushrooms, and crumble the Gorgonzola up to 1 day ahead and refrigerate separately.

MAKE IT EVEN EASIER
Buy sliced mushrooms and crumbled Gorgonzola or blue cheese. Buy chicken tenderloins, which are easier to slice.

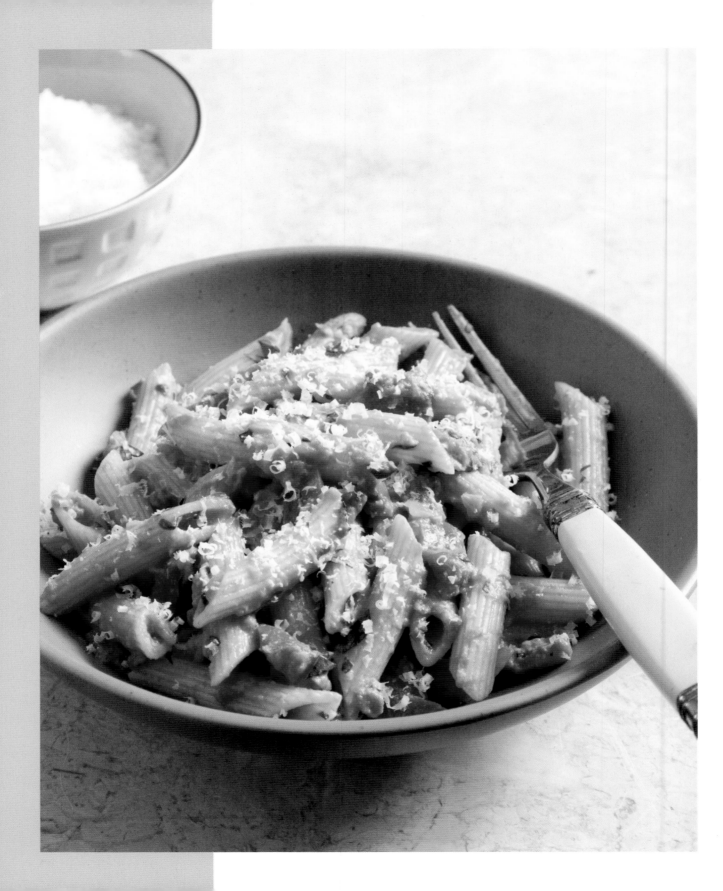

Skillet Penne alla Vodka

SERVES 4 TO 6

Why This Recipe Works Who doesn't love penne alla vodka? It's indulgent and screams comfort food. I don't eat it often, but when I do, I want the recipe to live up to my expectations and be worth the calories. This recipe does that and more. It's also a recipe I can recommend to back patients, because it bypasses the need to boil and drain a heavy pot of pasta filled with 4 quarts of water. It starts with a sweet, tangy, and spicy tomato sauce. Adding water and vodka to the pan provides enough liquid to cook the pasta. Once the pasta is done, heavy cream adds its signature richness, while basil and Parmesan are the finishing touches. If possible, use premium vodka; inexpensive brands will taste harsh in this sauce. Pepper vodka imparts a pleasant flavor and can be substituted for plain. Be sure to simmer the tomatoes gently in step 1 or the sauce will become too thick. You will need a 12-inch nonstick skillet with a tight-fitting lid for this recipe.

1 Heat oil in 12-inch nonstick skillet over medium heat until shimmering. Add onion, tomato paste, and salt and cook, stirring often, until softened, about 6 minutes. Stir in garlic and red pepper flakes and cook until fragrant, about 30 seconds. Stir in tomatoes. Reduce heat to medium-low and simmer gently, stirring occasionally, until tomatoes no longer taste raw, about 10 minutes. Turn off heat and cover skillet.

— TAKE A 15-MINUTE BREAK —

2 Return skillet to medium heat and cook tomato mixture until simmering. Stir in water and vodka, then add pasta. Cover, increase heat to medium-high, and cook, stirring often and adjusting heat to maintain gentle simmer, until pasta is tender, about 17 minutes.

3 Stir in cream and cook until hot, about 1 minute. Stir in basil and season with salt and pepper to taste. Serve, passing Parmesan separately.

PREP AHEAD
You can chop the onion up to 1 day ahead and refrigerate.

2 tablespoons extra-virgin olive oil

¼ cup finely chopped onion

1 tablespoon tomato paste

½ teaspoon table salt

2 garlic cloves, minced

¼–½ teaspoon red pepper flakes

3 (14.5-ounce) cans crushed tomatoes

2 cups water

⅓ cup vodka

1 pound penne

½ cup heavy cream

2 tablespoons minced fresh basil

Grated Parmesan cheese, for serving

Lemony Shrimp with Orzo, Feta, and Olives

SERVES 4

1 tablespoon grated lemon zest plus 1 tablespoon juice

½ teaspoon table salt

½ teaspoon pepper

1½ pounds peeled and deveined extra-large shrimp (21 to 25 per pound)

1 tablespoon extra-virgin olive oil, plus extra for drizzling

1 onion, chopped fine

2 garlic cloves, minced

2 cups orzo

4 cups chicken or vegetable broth

1 cup pitted Kalamata olives, chopped coarse

4 ounces feta cheese, crumbled (1 cup), divided

2 tablespoons chopped fresh parsley

Why This Recipe Works Fresh, tangy feta cheese and shrimp are a classic combination that is hard to beat—which is why you see it as an appetizer on just about every Greek diner menu. This easy weeknight skillet recipe turns the pairing into a satisfying dinner with the addition of olives and onion, plus creamy orzo. Tossing the shrimp with a lemon-salt mixture ensures that it is a far cry from bland. And cooking the orzo pilaf-style in a large skillet infuses it with onion and garlic flavors as it cooks in broth. After stirring in olives, some feta, and lemon juice, just nestle the shrimp on top so they cook gently in the covered skillet. For a bright finishing touch, a drizzle of extra-virgin olive oil and more feta take this meal over the top. You will need a 12-inch nonstick skillet with a tight-fitting lid for this recipe.

1 Mix lemon zest, salt, and pepper together. Pat shrimp dry with paper towels and toss with lemon-salt mixture to coat; set aside.

2 Heat oil in 12-inch nonstick skillet over medium-high heat until just smoking. Add onion and cook until softened, about 4 minutes. Stir in garlic and cook until fragrant, about 30 seconds. Stir in orzo and cook, stirring frequently, until orzo is coated with oil and lightly browned, about 4 minutes. Add broth, bring to boil, and cook, uncovered, until orzo is al dente, about 6 minutes. Stir in olives, ½ cup feta, and lemon juice. Season with salt and pepper to taste.

3 Reduce heat to medium-low, nestle shrimp into orzo, cover, and cook until shrimp are pink and cooked through, about 5 minutes. Sprinkle remaining ½ cup feta and chopped parsley over top and drizzle with extra oil. Serve.

PREP AHEAD

You can chop the onion and olives and crumble the feta cheese up to 1 day ahead and refrigerate separately.

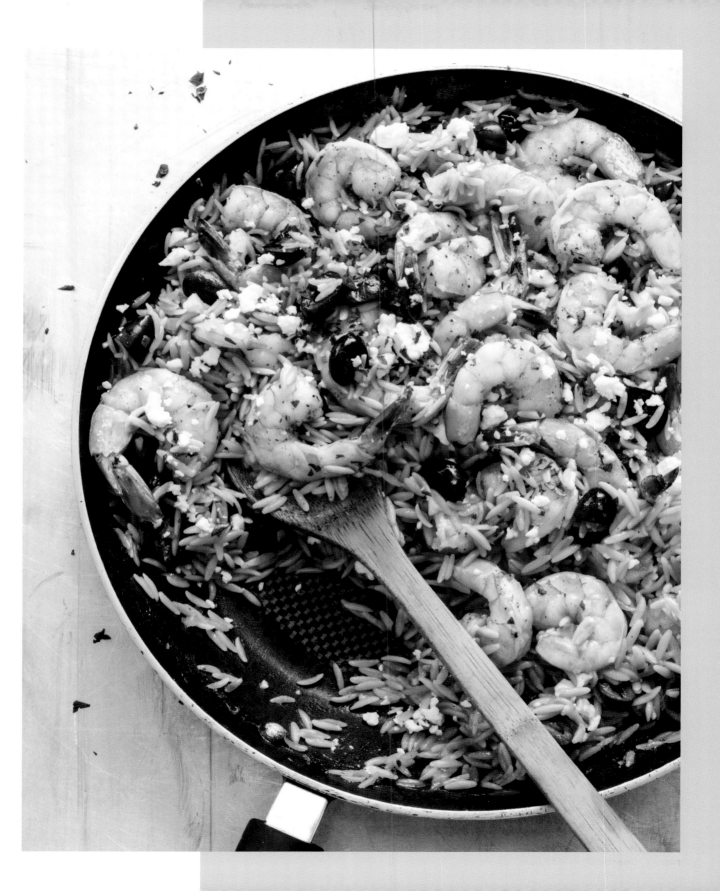

Fideos with Chickpeas

SERVES 4

8 ounces spaghettini or thin spaghetti, broken into 1- to 2-inch lengths

2 teaspoons plus 2 tablespoons extra-virgin olive oil, divided

1 onion, chopped fine

½ teaspoon table salt, divided

1 (14.5-ounce) can diced tomatoes, drained and chopped fine, juice reserved

3 garlic cloves, minced

1½ teaspoons smoked paprika

2¾ cups water

½ cup dry white wine

1 (15-ounce) can chickpeas, rinsed

½ teaspoon pepper

1 tablespoon chopped fresh parsley

Lemon wedges

Why This Recipe Works One of the biggest stars of traditional Spanish cooking is fideos, a richly flavored relative of paella that calls for breaking noodles into small lengths, toasting them until nut-brown and then cooking them in a garlicky, tomatoey stock with seafood and chorizo. Here, the bold tomato stock and toasted noodles work well with chickpeas, another common Spanish ingredient. For a sofrito, simply finely chop the onion (so it browns more quickly) and use chopped canned tomatoes. White wine and the juice from canned tomatoes, along with smoked paprika, ensure a stock with complex depth of flavor. You will need a 12-inch nonstick skillet with a tight-fitting lid for this recipe.

1 Toss pasta and 2 teaspoons oil in 12-inch nonstick skillet until pasta is evenly coated. Toast pasta over medium-high heat, stirring frequently, until it is browned and releases nutty aroma (pasta should be color of peanut butter), about 8 minutes; transfer to bowl.

— TAKE A 15-MINUTE BREAK —

2 Wipe out now-empty skillet, add remaining 2 tablespoons oil, and heat over medium-high heat until shimmering. Add onion and ¼ teaspoon salt and cook until onion is softened, about 5 minutes. Stir in tomatoes and cook until mixture is thick, dry, and slightly darkened in color, about 5 minutes.

3 Reduce heat to medium, stir in garlic and smoked paprika, and cook until fragrant, about 30 seconds. Stir in toasted pasta until thoroughly combined. Stir in water, wine, chickpeas, pepper, reserved tomato juice, and remaining ¼ teaspoon salt. Increase heat to medium-high and bring to simmer. Cook uncovered, stirring occasionally, until liquid is slightly thickened and pasta is just tender, about 9 minutes. Let cool for 5 minutes, then sprinkle with parsley; serve with lemon wedges.

PREP AHEAD

You can break the spaghetti and chop the onion and tomatoes (save the drained juice) up to 1 day ahead and refrigerate separately.

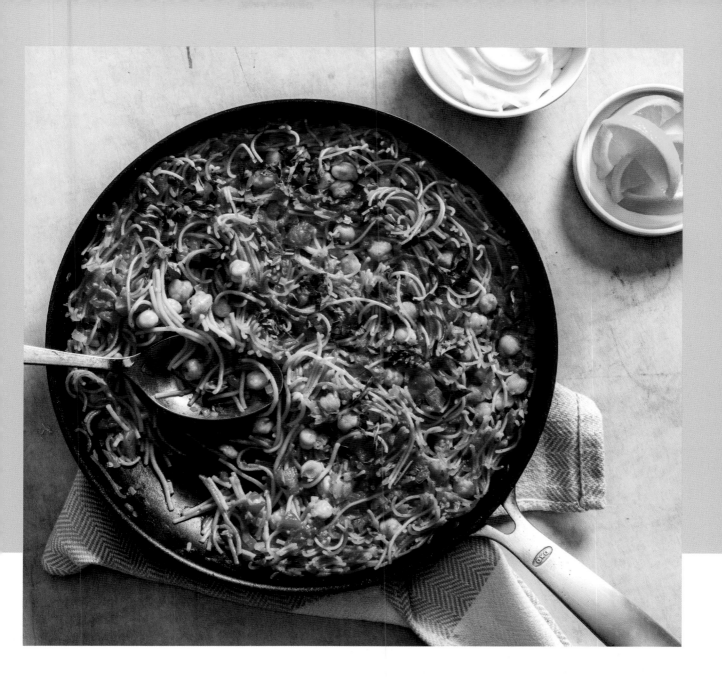

TAKE IT UP A NOTCH
Serve with Garlic Aioli

Process 2 large egg yolks, 2 teaspoons Dijon mustard, 2 teaspoons lemon juice, and 1 minced garlic clove in food processor until combined, about 10 seconds. With processor running, slowly drizzle in ¾ cup vegetable oil, about 1 minute. Transfer mixture to medium bowl and whisk in 1 tablespoon water, ½ teaspoon table salt, and ¼ teaspoon pepper. Whisking constantly, slowly drizzle in ¼ cup extra-virgin olive oil. Aioli can be refrigerated for up to 4 days. Makes about 1¼ cups.

Parmesan Polenta with Broccoli Rabe, Sun-Dried Tomatoes, and Pine Nuts

SERVES 4

Topping

- 3 tablespoons extra-virgin olive oil
- ½ cup oil-packed sun-dried tomatoes, chopped coarse
- 6 garlic cloves, minced
- ½ teaspoon red pepper flakes
- ½ teaspoon table salt
- 1 pound broccoli rabe, trimmed and cut into 1½-inch pieces
- ¼ cup vegetable or chicken broth
- 3 tablespoons pine nuts, toasted

Polenta

- 4 cups water
- 1 cup instant polenta
- ½ teaspoon table salt
- 2 ounces grated Parmesan cheese (1 cup), plus extra for serving
- 4 tablespoons unsalted butter

Why This Recipe Works Polenta is true comfort food, but normally making the polenta and a savory vegetarian topping is just too much work. Enter instant polenta and an easy method that uses only a skillet. For the topping, broccoli rabe, sun-dried tomatoes, garlic, and red pepper flakes are hearty enough to hold their own when paired with the polenta. After cooking the topping, which takes mere minutes, you simply wipe out the skillet and cook the instant polenta, which turns creamy and soft in just a few minutes. Parmesan cheese and butter add richness, and toasted pine nuts sprinkled on top offer a bit of crunch. Shopping for polenta can be confusing—instant polenta can look just like traditional polenta and is often identifiable only by the word "instant" in its title, which can be slightly hidden. Be sure to use instant polenta here; traditional polenta requires a slightly different cooking method. You will need a 12-inch nonstick skillet with a tight-fitting lid for this recipe.

1 For the topping Cook oil, tomatoes, garlic, pepper flakes, and salt in 12-inch nonstick skillet over medium-high heat until garlic is fragrant and slightly toasted, about 1½ minutes. Add broccoli rabe and broth, cover, and cook until broccoli rabe turns bright green, about 2 minutes. Uncover and continue to cook, stirring frequently, until most of broth has evaporated and broccoli rabe is just tender, about 2 minutes. Season with salt to taste. Transfer to bowl and cover to keep warm. Wipe skillet clean with paper towels.

— TAKE A 10-MINUTE BREAK —

2 For the polenta Bring water to boil in now-empty skillet. Gradually whisk in polenta and salt. Cook over medium heat, whisking constantly, until very thick, about 5 minutes. Off heat, stir in Parmesan and butter and season with salt and pepper to taste.

3 Portion polenta into 4 individual serving bowls, top with broccoli rabe mixture, and sprinkle with pine nuts. Serve with extra Parmesan.

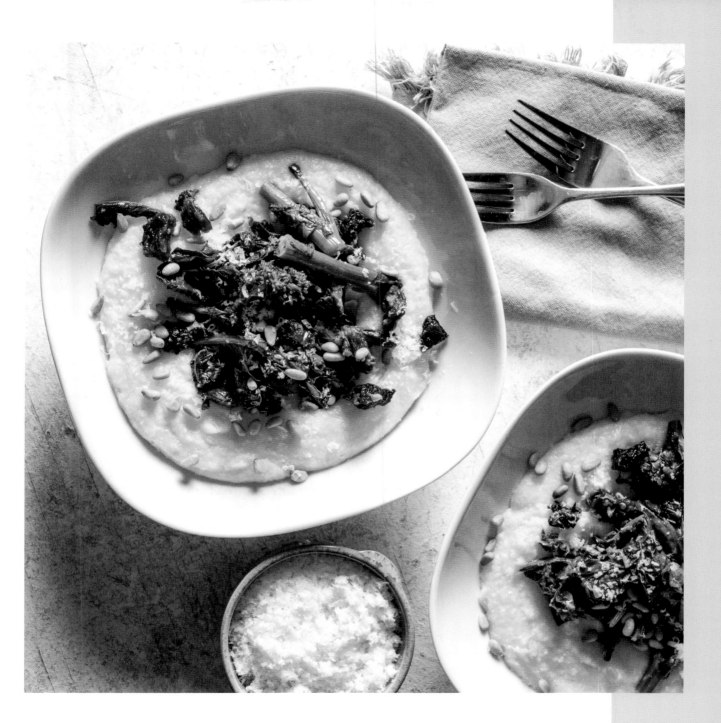

PREP AHEAD

You can chop the sun-dried tomatoes, trim and cut up the broccoli rabe, and toast the pine nuts up to 1 day ahead and refrigerate separately.

MAKE IT EVEN EASIER

Buy jarred, chopped sun-dried tomatoes. Toast the pine nuts in the microwave (see page 37).

Stir-Fried Eggplant in Garlic-Basil Sauce

SERVES 4 — SUPER EASY

Sauce

½ cup water

¼ cup fish sauce

2 tablespoons packed brown sugar

2 teaspoons grated lime zest plus 1 tablespoon juice

2 teaspoons cornstarch

⅛ teaspoon red pepper flakes

Vegetables

2 tablespoons plus 1 teaspoon vegetable oil

6 garlic cloves, minced

1 tablespoon grated fresh ginger

1 pound eggplant, cut into ¾-inch pieces

1 red bell pepper, stemmed, seeded, and cut into ¼-inch pieces

½ cup fresh basil leaves, torn into rough ½-inch pieces

2 scallions, sliced thin

Why This Recipe Works Once you've assembled the ingredients for this simple stir-fry, you are only 15 minutes away from a garlicky, basil-infused eggplant dish that is immensely satisfying. You can make this year-round, but it is especially delicious with eggplant, red bell pepper, and basil from your farmers' market at the height of summer. Leaving the skin on the eggplant keeps the prep work to a minimum and also adds extra color while increasing fiber. It is important to let the eggplant and bell pepper brown, as this gives them the deeper, caramelized flavor that adds richness. Mashing the garlic and ginger mixture into the center of the pan and cooking them until just fragrant makes it easier to infuse the entire dish with flavor once the sauce is added. A final sprinkle of torn basil leaves and sliced scallions adds color and a fragrant and fresh sweetness. Serve with rice.

1 For the sauce Whisk all ingredients together in bowl.

2 For the vegetables Combine 1 teaspoon oil, garlic, and ginger in bowl. Heat remaining 2 tablespoons oil in 12-inch nonstick skillet over high heat until shimmering. Add eggplant and bell pepper and cook, stirring often, until well browned and tender, about 9 minutes.

3 Clear center of skillet, add garlic mixture, and cook, mashing mixture into skillet, until fragrant, about 30 seconds. Stir garlic mixture into vegetables. Whisk sauce to recombine, then add to skillet. Cook, stirring constantly, until sauce is thickened, about 30 seconds. Off heat, stir in basil and scallions and serve.

PREP AHEAD

You can grate the ginger and cut up the pepper and scallions up to 1 day ahead and refrigerate separately. You can make the sauce up to 1 day ahead and refrigerate until using.

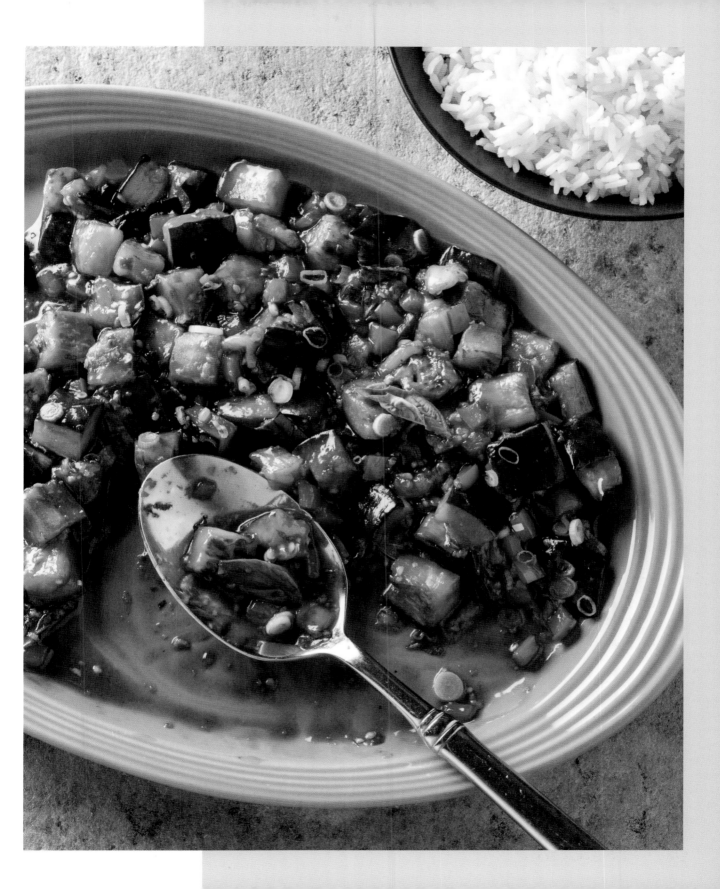

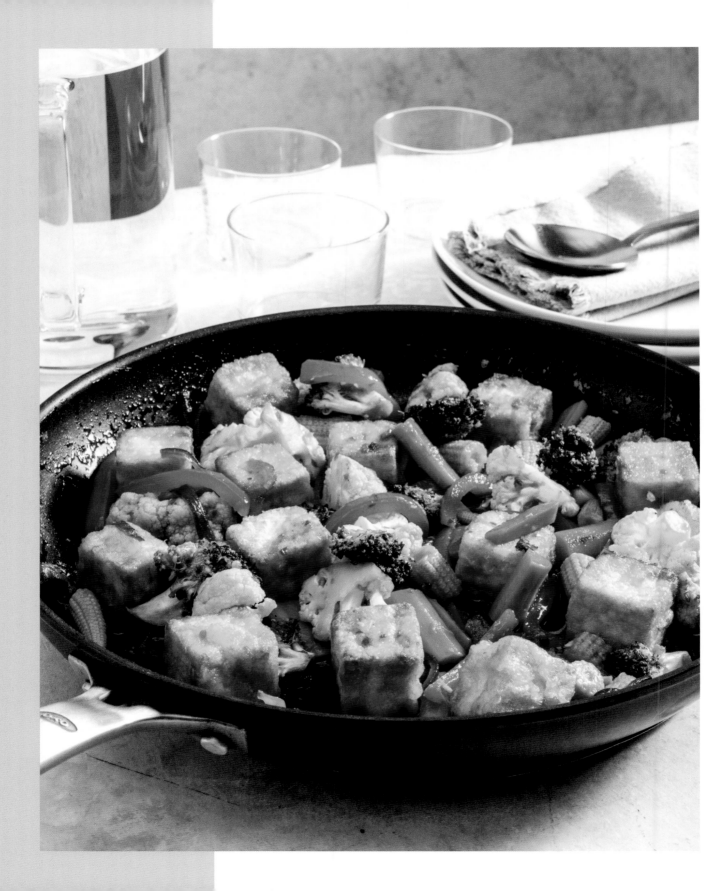

Salad Bar Stir-Fry with Tofu

SERVES 4 — SUPER EASY

Why This Recipe Works This is an endlessly variable stir-fry that puts crispy tofu at center stage. Memorize this method for making the tofu and the five-ingredient sauce and you'll have the formula for a lifetime of great, easy-to-execute stir-fries. To keep things nearly prep free, buy a combination of vegetables like broccoli, snow peas, and sliced bell peppers from your supermarket salad bar. This makes it possible to have array of vegetables with zero waste. I am in awe of this trick and wonder why I never thought of it before. Also, the method for dredging the tofu in cornstarch and then frying it in a hefty amount of vegetable oil creates a remarkable contrast between its crispy, browned exterior and appealingly soft and creamy interior. Do not use extra-firm tofu here, as it will not be as creamy. Be sure to dredge the tofu in cornstarch right before cooking, otherwise it will turn gummy.

14 ounces firm tofu, cut into
    1-inch cubes

¼ cup honey

3 tablespoons soy sauce

1 tablespoon chili-garlic sauce

1 tablespoon grated fresh ginger

½ cup cornstarch, divided

½ cup vegetable oil

1 pound salad bar vegetables,
    cut into bite-size pieces

1   Place tofu on paper towel–lined plate and let drain 15 minutes.

—   TAKE A 15-MINUTE BREAK   —

2   Whisk honey, soy sauce, chili-garlic sauce, ginger, and 1 teaspoon cornstarch in bowl.

3   Spread remaining cornstarch in shallow dish. Pat tofu dry with additional paper towels and dredge in cornstarch, shaking off excess. Heat oil in 12-inch nonstick skillet over medium heat until shimmering. Cook tofu, turning occasionally, until golden brown and crisp, about 7 minutes. Using slotted spoon, transfer tofu to plate lined with fresh paper towels.

4   Pour off all but 1 tablespoon oil from skillet. Add vegetables and cook until softened, about 5 minutes. Add tofu, then stir in honey mixture and cook until slightly thickened, about 2 minutes. Serve.

PREP AHEAD
You can cut up the tofu and the vegetables and grate the ginger up to 1 day ahead and refrigerate separately.

Xīhóngshì Chao Jīdàn

SERVES 4 — SUPER EASY

- 3 tablespoons vegetable oil, divided

- 4 scallions, white parts sliced thin, green parts cut into 1-inch lengths

- 3 garlic cloves, sliced thin

- 2 teaspoons grated fresh ginger

- 8 large eggs

- 2 tablespoons Shaoxing wine or dry sherry

- 1 teaspoon toasted sesame oil

- 1 teaspoon table salt, divided

- 1 (28-ounce) can whole peeled tomatoes, drained with juice reserved, cut into 1-inch pieces

- 2 teaspoons sugar

PREP AHEAD

You can prep the scallions, grate the ginger, and cut up the canned tomatoes (save the drained juice) up to 1 day ahead and refrigerate separately.

Why This Recipe Works This simple yet surprisingly complex dish, stir-fried tomatoes and eggs, deserves its reputation as one of China's most beloved comfort foods. It's included here because it can be made in a flash and because you likely have all the ingredients on hand. Xīhóngshì Chao Jīdàn didn't come onto the scene until the early 20th century, when Chinese cooks first began incorporating tomatoes into their cooking. But that hasn't stopped the combination of pillowy eggs enrobed in a savory-sweet tomato sauce from being one of the country's most beloved dishes. It's so popular, some Chinese food bloggers deem it the country's national dish. It's also an essential comfort food of Chinese immigrants and their families. In an ode to his mother's version, writer Francis Lam describes it in the *New York Times* as "the kind of dish that people say is the first thing they learned to cook, that fed them when they left home, that inspires sudden and irresistible cravings." Beating eggs with Shaoxing wine and sesame oil adds savory notes as well as tenderness—the liquid and oil dilute the egg proteins and keep them from bonding too closely and turning tough. Quickly cooking the eggs over medium-high heat promotes airier curds. Garlic, ginger, and scallions add savoriness to the tomato base, while canned tomatoes ensure year-round consistency. Simmering the tomatoes with a measured amount of sugar makes the base concentrated and rich before combining with the eggs. This dish is traditionally made in a wok; you can use a light-weight carbon steel wok instead of a skillet, if desired. Serve with rice.

1   Combine 1 tablespoon vegetable oil, scallion whites, garlic, and ginger in small bowl; set aside. Whisk eggs, Shaoxing wine, sesame oil, and ½ teaspoon salt together in separate bowl.

2   Heat remaining 2 tablespoons vegetable oil in 12-inch nonstick skillet over medium-high heat until shimmering. Add egg mixture. Using heatproof rubber spatula, slowly but constantly scrape along bottom and sides of pan until eggs just form cohesive mass, about 2 minutes (eggs will not be completely dry); transfer to clean bowl.

3   Add reserved garlic mixture to now-empty skillet and cook over medium heat, mashing mixture into pan, until fragrant, about 30 seconds. Add tomatoes and their juice, sugar, and remaining ½ teaspoon salt and simmer until almost completely dry, about 6 minutes. Stir in egg mixture and scallion greens and cook, breaking up any large curds, until heated through, about 1 minute. Serve.

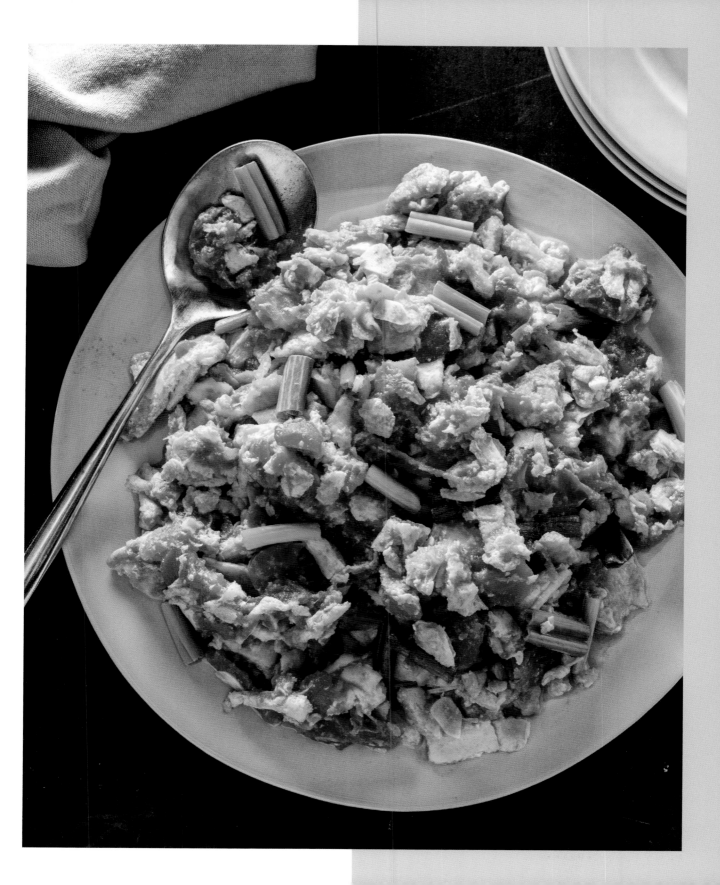

Simple Mains

That Won't Strain Your Back

* Try these recipes first if today is not one of your better days and you need a soul-refilling meal with high return on your energy investment.

Cooker Citrus-Braised Chicken Tacos

SERVES 6 — SUPER EASY

¼ cup thawed frozen orange juice concentrate

¼ cup tomato paste

1½ tablespoons Worcestershire sauce

4 garlic cloves, minced

1 tablespoon ground cumin

1 tablespoon dried oregano

2 teaspoons table salt

1 teaspoon pepper

1 teaspoon ground allspice

1 teaspoon ground cinnamon

3 pounds boneless, skinless chicken thighs, trimmed

1 onion, halved

3 (3-inch) strips orange zest

2 tablespoons distilled white vinegar or cider vinegar

18 (6-inch) corn tortillas, warmed or charred

Why This Recipe Works Tacos have a lot going for them in the healthy-back kitchen because they are easy, usually pretty healthy, and tailor-made to share around the table with friends and family. You can simply portion out the filling and liven up the table with all the fixings. Here, the slow cooker ensures that making the filling itself is hands-off. Boneless, skinless chicken thighs require no browning and stay moist during the long braise. To get complex, nuanced orange flavor without excess liquid in the slow cooker, orange juice concentrate (convenient, inexpensive, and packed with flavor) and orange zest (tangy and pleasantly bitter) are key. Added to the concentrate are umami-rich tomato paste and Worcestershire sauce, plus garlic, cumin, and oregano, creating a solid base of flavor. The addition of allspice and cinnamon provides a welcome kick of warm spice, and a little vinegar stirred in at the end invigorates the flavors. Spoon the chicken filling into warm tortillas and serve with sliced radishes, avocado chunks, cotija, fresh cilantro, hot sauce, and lime wedges. Use a vegetable peeler to remove the strips of zest from the orange. Orange juice concentrate is relatively soft even when it's frozen, so there's no need to defrost the whole container to get the ¼ cup you need.

1   Whisk orange juice concentrate, tomato paste, Worcestershire, garlic, cumin, oregano, salt, pepper, allspice, and cinnamon together in slow cooker.

2   Add chicken and toss to coat with orange juice concentrate mixture. Nestle onion and orange zest among chicken thighs. Cover and cook until chicken is tender, 3 to 4 hours on low.

— TAKE A 3- TO 4-HOUR BREAK —

3   Transfer chicken to cutting board and let cool slightly. Using 2 forks, shred into bite-size pieces. Meanwhile, turn slow cooker to high and cook until liquid is reduced, about 20 minutes.

4   Discard zest and onion. Stir in vinegar and return shredded chicken to slow cooker. Stir to combine with sauce. Season with salt and pepper to taste. Serve chicken on warmed or charred tortillas.

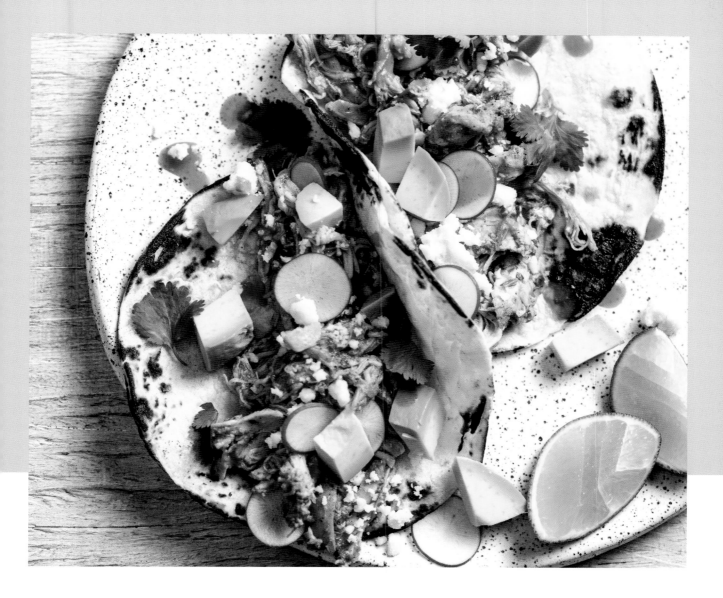

You can trim the chicken up to 1 day ahead and refrigerate.

TAKE IT UP A NOTCH

Serve with Avocado Crema

Process ½ avocado, ¼ cup chopped fresh cilantro, 3 tablespoons water, 1 tablespoon lime juice, and 1 tablespoon yogurt in food processor until smooth. Season with salt and pepper to taste. Crema can be refrigerated with plastic wrap pressed flush to surface for up to 2 days. Makes ½ cup.

TWO WAYS TO WARM TORTILLAS

Warming tortillas not only makes them more pliable but can also add flavorful toasty char, depending on the method. After warming, wrap the tortillas in foil or clean dish towels to keep them warm until serving.

Microwave Wrap up to 6 tortillas in damp, clean dish towel and microwave until warm, 30 to 45 seconds.

Skillet To char, toast tortilla in dry nonstick skillet over medium-high heat until softened and spotty brown, 20 to 30 seconds per side.

Slow-Cooker Sweet and Tangy Pulled Chicken Sandwiches

SERVES 4 — SUPER EASY

1 onion, chopped fine

¼ cup tomato paste

1 tablespoon chili powder

1 tablespoon vegetable oil

1 teaspoon paprika

½ teaspoon table salt

¼ teaspoon pepper

⅛ teaspoon cayenne pepper

¼ cup ketchup

2 tablespoons molasses

1½ pounds boneless, skinless chicken breasts

2 tablespoons cider vinegar

2 teaspoons Dijon mustard

4 hamburger buns

PREP AHEAD
You can chop the onion up to 1 day ahead and refrigerate. You can also make the pulled chicken 1 day ahead; rewarm before serving.

Why This Recipe Works If you are having friends over for lunch or a casual dinner, these pulled chicken sandwiches are a no-brainer, as the chicken requires only 15 minutes to be slow-cooker ready. Just spoon the chicken onto hamburger buns, put out store-bought potato salad, and you have a winning meal with hardly any work. A simple spice mixture and a quick-to-assemble homemade barbecue sauce turn slow-cooked boneless chicken breasts into tangy, silky, shredded chicken—perfect for piling onto buns. To start, microwave onions with tomato paste, chili powder, paprika, and cayenne to bloom the spices and soften the onions before they go into the slow cooker to be infused with layers of barbecue flavor. Add ketchup and molasses to finish the sauce and then simply season the chicken with salt and pepper before nestling the breasts in the sauce. In the slow cooker's low-and-slow moist heat, the chicken takes on the rich essence of the sauce. Stirring in 2 tablespoons of vinegar and a small amount of mustard at the end of cooking gives the sauce the perfect consistency and punch of bright flavor. You can double this recipe, but you will need to use a 7-quart slow cooker.

1   Combine onion, tomato paste, chili powder, oil, paprika, salt, pepper, and cayenne in bowl and microwave, stirring occasionally, until onion is softened, about 5 minutes; transfer to slow cooker.

2   Stir in ketchup and molasses. Sprinkle chicken with salt and pepper and add to slow cooker. Turn to coat, then nestle into sauce. Cover and cook until chicken registers 160 degrees, 2 to 3 hours on low.

— TAKE A 2- TO 3-HOUR BREAK —

3   Transfer chicken to cutting board and let cool slightly. Using 2 forks, shred into bite-size pieces. Stir vinegar and mustard into sauce left in slow cooker. (Adjust sauce consistency with hot water as needed.) Stir in shredded chicken and season with salt and pepper to taste. Portion chicken onto buns and serve with pickle chips, if desired.

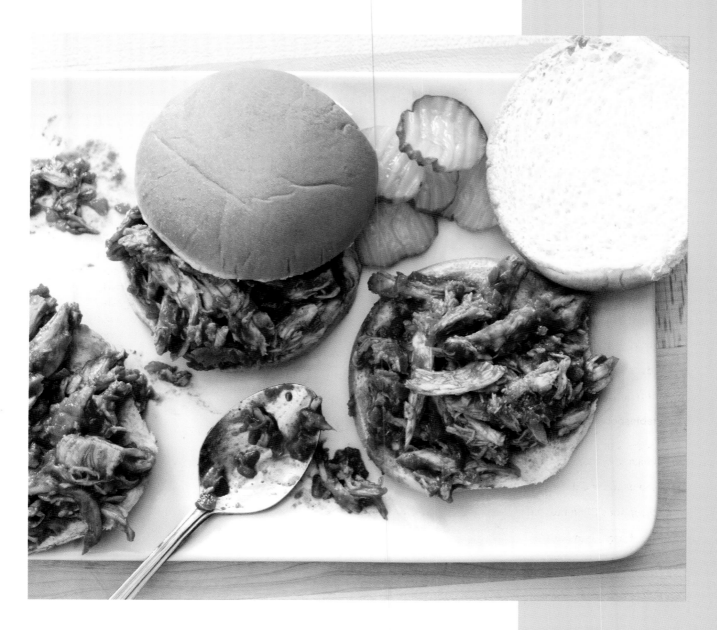

Quick Pickle Chips

Bring ¾ cup seasoned rice vinegar, ¼ cup water, 1 halved garlic clove, ¼ teaspoon ground turmeric, ⅛ teaspoon black peppercorns, and ⅛ teaspoon yellow mustard seeds to boil in medium saucepan over medium-high heat. Fill one 1-pint jar with hot tap water to warm. Drain jar, then pack with 8 ounces sliced pickling cucumbers and 2 dill sprigs. Using funnel and ladle, pour hot brine over cucumbers to cover. Let cool to room temperature, about 30 minutes. Cover and refrigerate until chilled and flavors meld, about 3 hours. Pickles can be refrigerated for up to 6 weeks. Makes about 2 cups.

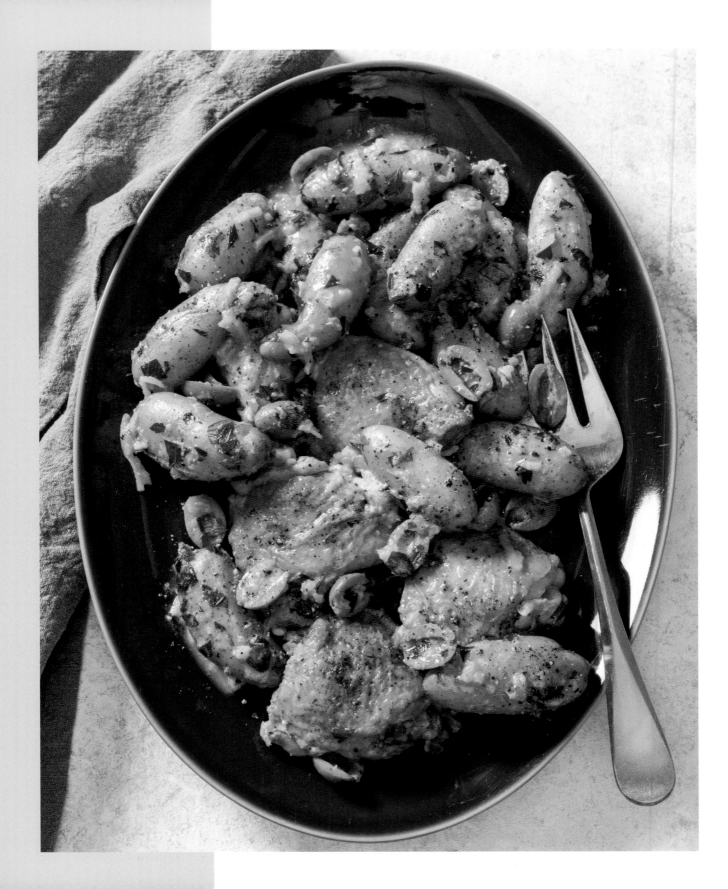

Instant Pot Lemony Chicken Thighs with Fingerling Potatoes and Lemon

SERVES 4 — SUPER EASY

Why This Recipe Works In this one-pot dinner, juicy chicken thighs and delicate fingerling potatoes absorb the bright aromas of a classic Provençal trio: garlic, lemon, and olives. To develop flavor, the first step is to brown the chicken thighs in olive oil and then set aside briefly. Next, toast smashed garlic cloves in the pot and add chicken broth and a whole sliced lemon to create a vibrant cooking liquid. Return the chicken to the pot, top with whole unpeeled fingerling potatoes, and cook it all under pressure. Finish off the potatoes with bright parsley and briny olives. Use potatoes that are approximately 1 inch in diameter. Slice the lemon as thinly as possible; this allows the slices to melt into the sauce. Note that it will take the Instant Pot about 10 minutes to come up to pressure and start the cook cycle.

1   Pat chicken dry with paper towels and sprinkle with salt and pepper. Using highest sauté function, heat oil in electric pressure cooker for 5 minutes (or until just smoking). Place chicken skin side down in pot and cook until well browned on one side, about 5 minutes; transfer to plate.

2   Add garlic to fat left in pot and cook, using highest sauté function, until golden and fragrant, about 2 minutes. Stir in broth and lemon, scraping up any browned bits. Return chicken to pot skin side up and add any accumulated juices. Arrange potatoes on top. Lock lid in place and close pressure release valve. Select high pressure cook function and cook for 9 minutes.

—   TAKE A 19-MINUTE BREAK   —

3   Turn off electric pressure cooker and quick-release pressure. Carefully remove lid, allowing steam to escape away from you. Transfer chicken to serving dish and discard skin, if desired. Stir olives and parsley into potatoes and season with salt and pepper to taste. Serve chicken with potatoes.

PREP AHEAD
You can trim the chicken and halve the olives up to 1 day ahead and refrigerate separately.

4   (5- to 7-ounce) bone-in chicken thighs, trimmed

½   teaspoon table salt

¼   teaspoon pepper

2   teaspoons extra-virgin olive oil

4   garlic cloves, peeled and smashed

½   cup chicken or vegetable broth

1   small lemon, sliced thin

1½   pounds fingerling potatoes, unpeeled

¼   cup pitted brine-cured green or black olives, halved

2   tablespoons coarsely chopped fresh parsley

Chicken and Chorizo Paella

SERVES 2

1½ cups water, divided

½ cup Valencia or arborio rice

⅛ plus ¼ teaspoon table salt, divided

4 teaspoons vegetable oil, divided

4 ounces chorizo sausage, halved lengthwise and sliced ¼ inch thick

8 ounces boneless, skinless chicken breast, trimmed and sliced ¼ inch thick

¼ teaspoon pepper

1 small onion, chopped fine

¾ cup canned diced tomatoes, drained with juice reserved

2 garlic cloves, minced

⅛ teaspoon saffron threads, crumbled

¼ cup large pitted green olives, quartered

¼ cup frozen peas

Why This Recipe Works Paella is something I make only when I'm entertaining, and honestly, it takes most of the day to organize and prep all the ingredients. That said, this ingenious recipe for two brings the flavors I love in paella to the table with a minimum of work. Using a combination of chorizo sausage and chicken, it's plenty hearty even without the traditional seafood. To ensure that the rice is evenly cooked, give it a head start in the microwave and finish it in the pan with the other ingredients. A rich sofrito of onion, garlic, and tomatoes gives the paella deep flavor, and bright peas and briny olives add color and dimension. Short-grain Valencia rice is best for this dish, but you can substitute arborio rice. Do not substitute long-grain rice. Look for large pitted green olives at the olive bar in the supermarket; pimento-stuffed olives can be substituted in a pinch. To make the chicken easier to slice, freeze it for 15 minutes. You will need a 10-inch skillet with a tight-fitting lid for this recipe.

1   Combine 1 cup water, rice, and ⅛ teaspoon salt in bowl. Cover and microwave until rice is softened and most of liquid is absorbed, about 7 minutes.

2   Heat 2 teaspoons oil in 10-inch nonstick skillet over medium-high heat until just smoking. Add chorizo and cook until lightly browned, about 2 minutes. Using slotted spoon, transfer chorizo to plate. Pat chicken dry with paper towels and sprinkle with pepper and remaining ¼ teaspoon salt. Add chicken to fat left in skillet, breaking up any clumps, and cook until lightly browned on all sides, about 4 minutes; transfer to plate with chorizo. Cover with foil to keep warm.

— TAKE A 15-MINUTE BREAK —

3   Heat remaining 2 teaspoons oil in now-empty skillet over medium heat until shimmering. Add onion and cook until softened, about 5 minutes. Stir in tomatoes and cook until beginning to soften and darken, about 4 minutes. Stir in garlic and saffron and cook until fragrant, about 30 seconds. Stir in remaining ½ cup water and reserved tomato juice, scraping up any browned bits. Stir in parcooked rice, breaking up any large clumps, and bring to simmer. Reduce heat to medium-low, cover, and simmer until rice is tender and liquid is absorbed, about 10 minutes.

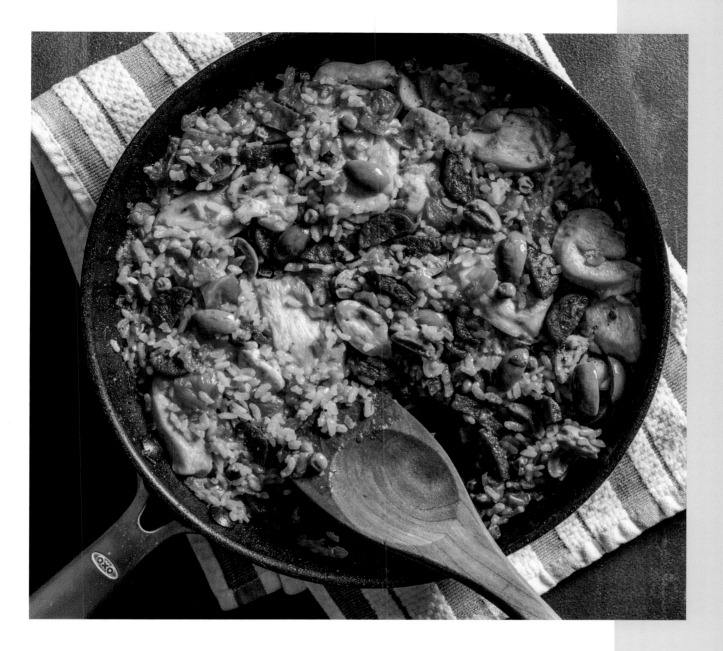

— TAKE A 10-MINUTE BREAK —

4　Stir in browned chorizo and chicken and any accumulated juices, olives, and peas and increase heat to medium-high. Cook, uncovered, until bottom layer of rice is golden and crisp, about 5 minutes, rotating skillet halfway through cooking to ensure even browning. Season with salt and pepper to taste, and serve.

PREP AHEAD

You can cut up the chorizo, chicken, onion, and olives up to 1 day ahead and refrigerate separately.

Instant Pot Chicken Sausage with White Beans and Spinach

SERVES 4 TO 6 — SUPER EASY

1 tablespoon extra-virgin olive oil, plus extra for drizzling

1½ pounds raw hot or sweet Italian chicken sausage

2 shallots, halved and sliced thin

3 garlic cloves, minced

½ cup dry white wine

½ cup chicken or vegetable broth

2 (15-ounce) cans cannellini beans, rinsed

12 ounces cherry tomatoes

1 sprig fresh rosemary

¼ teaspoon pepper

4 ounces (4 cups) baby spinach

2 ounces Parmesan cheese, shaved

PREP AHEAD

You can slice the shallots and shave the Parmesan up to 1 day ahead and refrigerate separately.

Why This Recipe Works This recipe is the perfect example of the benefits of the Instant Pot for anyone with back issues. The fact that you can make a delicious braise *and* a side in just 4 minutes of cooking under pressure with little prep is a game changer. Here, a simple combination of sausage, beans, and rosemary is transformed into a rich, warming ragout by the heat and pressure of the cooker. And the only ingredients requiring any knife work are shallots and garlic. Italian chicken sausage, which is full of spices (fennel and caraway) provides ample flavor to this hearty but not heavy dish. The combination of broth, wine, garlic, and rosemary delivers a flavorful liquid that seasons the beans beautifully as they cook. Once the sausages are cooked, just move them to a platter to rest and then stir some baby spinach into the beans before serving; this allows the spinach to wilt slightly, giving it a pleasing bite. Feel free to use any variety of uncooked chicken sausage that you think will work in the stew. Note that it will take the Instant Pot about 10 minutes to come up to pressure and start the cook cycle.

1 Using highest sauté function, heat oil in electric pressure cooker until just smoking. Add sausages and brown on all sides, about 7 minutes; transfer to plate. Turn off electric pressure cooker.

2 Add shallots and garlic to fat left in pot and cook, using residual heat, until shallots are softened, about 1 minute. Stir in wine, scraping up any browned bits. Stir in broth, beans, tomatoes, rosemary sprig, and pepper. Nestle sausages into bean mixture and add any accumulated juices.

3 Lock lid into place and close pressure-release valve. Select high pressure-cook function and cook for 4 minutes.

— TAKE A 14-MINUTE BREAK —

4 Turn off electric pressure cooker and quick-release pressure. Carefully remove lid, allowing steam to escape away from you. Transfer sausages to plate and let rest while finishing beans. Discard rosemary sprig. Stir spinach into bean mixture, 1 handful at a time, until wilted, about 1 minute. Season with salt and pepper to taste. Transfer beans to serving platter and top with sausages. Top with Parmesan and drizzle with extra oil. Serve.

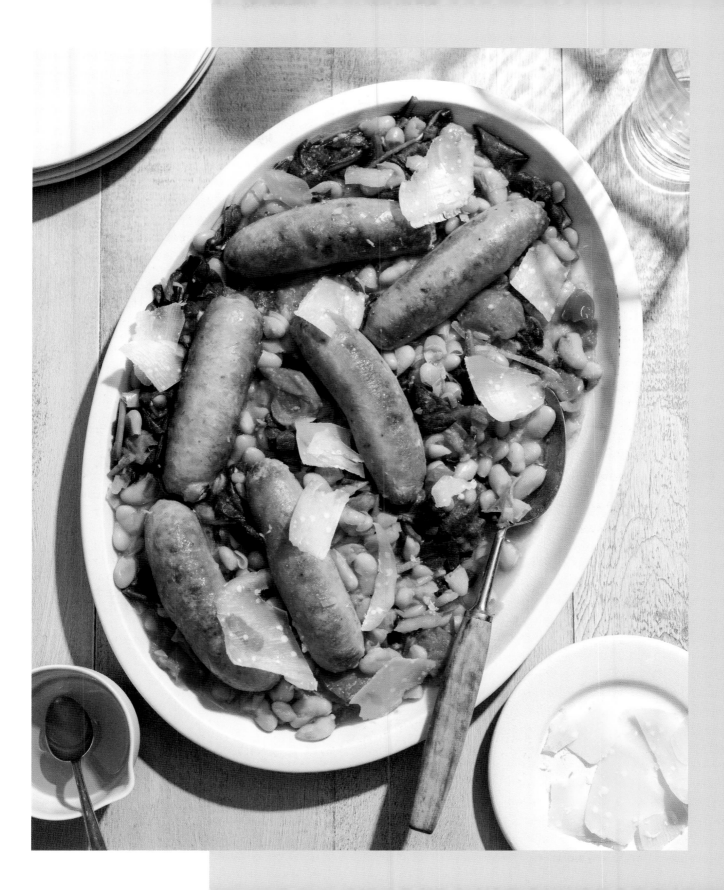

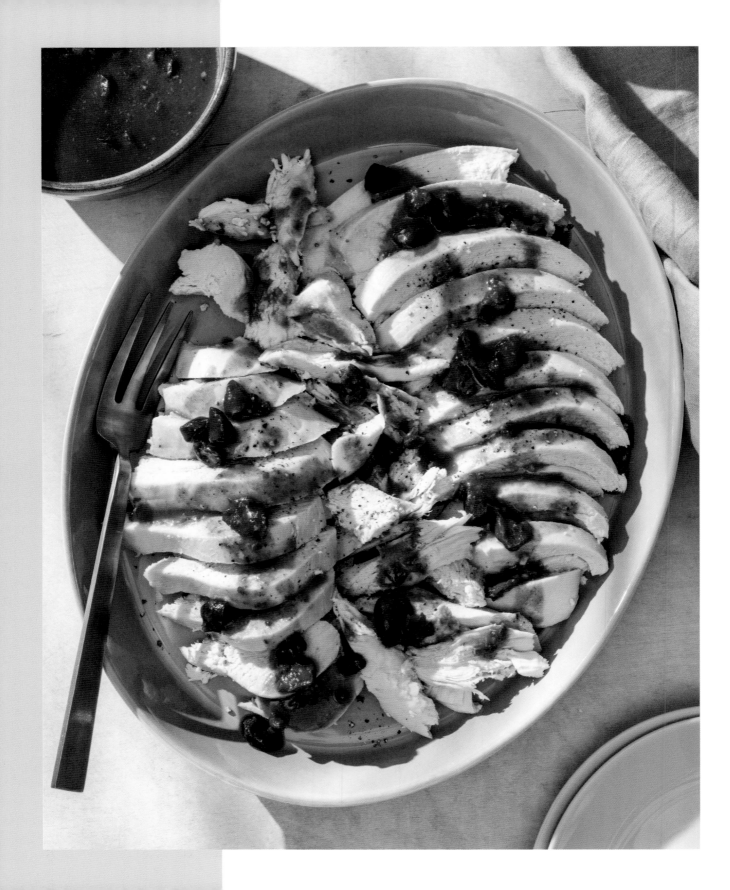

Slow-Cooker Turkey Breast with Cherry-Orange Sauce

SERVES 8 TO 10 — SUPER EASY

Why This Recipe Works Most of my patients have given up on hosting Thanksgiving or any big family meal requiring a centerpiece roast. But with this recipe, the slow cooker makes it entirely possible to cook a turkey breast and flavorful sauce without any heavy lifting. The bone-in turkey breast is nearly prep free, and the gentle heat of the slow cooker produces juicy and tender meat every time. For a fresh, simple accompaniment, cook the turkey in chopped frozen cherries combined with orange zest and a little thyme for aroma. By the time the turkey is fully cooked, the cherries are tender and the juices of the turkey, along with the aromatics, create the base for a flavorful sauce, lightly thickened with the addition of instant tapioca. While the turkey rests, just finish the sauce by whisking in apple butter for body and sweetness, butter for richness, and lemon juice for a hit of balancing acidity. Many supermarkets are now selling "hotel-cut" turkey breasts, which still have the wings and rib cage attached. If this is the only type of breast you can find, you will need to remove the wings and cut away the rib cage with kitchen shears before proceeding with the recipe. Check the turkey's temperature after 5 hours of cooking and continue to monitor until the breast registers 160 degrees. You will need a 5- to 7-quart oval slow cooker for this recipe.

12 ounces frozen sweet cherries, thawed and chopped

2 (2-inch) strips orange zest

1 teaspoon instant tapioca

½ teaspoon minced fresh thyme or ⅛ teaspoon dried

1¾ teaspoons table salt, divided

1 (6- to 7-pound) bone-in whole turkey breast, trimmed

¾ teaspoon pepper

½ cup apple butter

2 tablespoons unsalted butter

2 tablespoons lemon juice

1 Combine cherries, orange zest, tapioca, thyme, and ¼ teaspoon salt in slow cooker. Sprinkle turkey with remaining 1½ teaspoons salt and pepper and place skin side up in slow cooker. Cover and cook until breast registers 160 degrees, 5 to 6 hours on low.

— TAKE A 5- TO 6-HOUR BREAK —

2 Transfer turkey to carving board, tent loosely with aluminum foil, and let rest for 20 minutes.

— TAKE A 20-MINUTE BREAK —

3 Discard orange zest. Whisk apple butter, butter, and lemon juice into cherry mixture until combined. Season with salt and pepper to taste. Carve turkey and discard skin. Serve with sauce.

PREP AHEAD
You can trim and season the turkey, cover, and refrigerate for up to 2 days. You can chop the cherries and zest the orange up to 1 day ahead and refrigerate.

One-Pan Steak Fajitas

SERVES 2

2 small green and/or red bell peppers, stemmed, seeded, and cut into ½-inch-wide strips

1 red onion, halved and sliced ½ inch thick

2 garlic cloves, sliced thin

4 teaspoons vegetable oil, divided

½ teaspoon table salt, divided

½ teaspoon pepper, divided

2 teaspoons chili powder

1 teaspoon packed brown sugar

1 (12- to 16-ounce) flank steak, trimmed and cut with grain into 2½- to 3-inch wide strips

1½ teaspoons lime juice, plus lime wedges for serving

6–8 (6-inch) flour tortillas, warmed

PREP AHEAD
You can cut up the peppers and slice the onion up to 1 day ahead and refrigerate. You can trim and slice the flank steak up to 1 day ahead and refrigerate.

Why This Recipe Works Fajitas are a sizzling spectacle, but this recipe—more about flavor than theater—can be easily done in the oven on a small rimmed baking sheet, no searing required. Flank steak, chosen for its beefy flavor, tenderness, and availability, can get a boost from a dark-colored spice rub to mimic the color and flavor of searing: A mixture of chili powder, brown sugar, salt, and pepper works perfectly. Cooking peppers and onions spread out on a baking sheet ensures that the vegetables brown and don't steam. After 10 minutes, simply push them to one side to make room for the steak to roast to perfection while the vegetables finish cooking. While the meat rests, toss the tender peppers and onion with a spritz of lime juice to liven up the flavors. Feel free to use yellow or orange bell peppers for a more colorful presentation. Note that you can also make this recipe in a toaster oven. The recipe can be easily doubled; you will need either two small rimmed baking sheets or one large one. Serve with your favorite fajita toppings. For information on warming tortillas, see page 217.

1 Preheat oven to 450 degrees. Toss bell peppers, onion, and garlic with 1 tablespoon oil, ¼ teaspoon salt, and ¼ teaspoon pepper on small rimmed baking sheet, then spread into even layer. Roast, on lowest rack, until vegetables are starting to soften, about 10 minutes.

— TAKE A 10-MINUTE BREAK —

2 Remove baking sheet from oven and cover with foil. Combine chili powder, sugar, remaining ¼ teaspoon salt, and remaining ¼ teaspoon pepper in bowl. Pat steak dry with paper towels, rub with remaining 1 teaspoon oil, and sprinkle with spice mixture.

3 Remove foil from baking sheet and push vegetables to one side. Place steaks on now-empty side of baking sheet, spaced evenly apart. Roast until vegetables are spotty brown and meat registers 130 to 135 degrees (for medium), about 8 minutes.

4 Transfer steaks to cutting board, tent with aluminum foil, and let rest for 5 minutes. Toss vegetables with lime juice and any accumulated juices on sheet; transfer to serving platter. Slice steak pieces thin against grain and transfer to platter with vegetables. Serve steak and vegetables with tortillas and lime wedges.

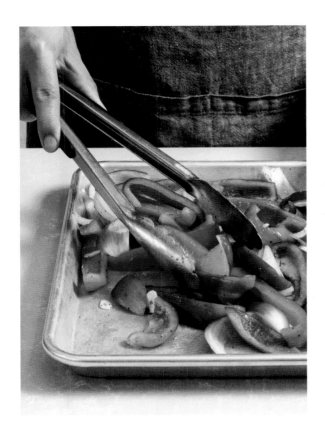

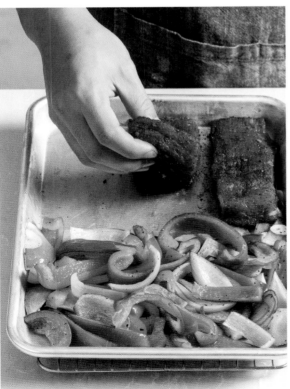

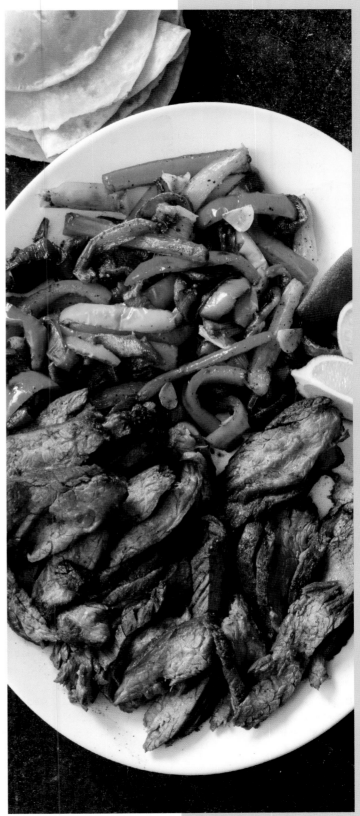

Spice-Roasted Steaks

SERVES 2

1 (12- to 16-ounce) boneless top sirloin, strip, or rib-eye steak, 1-inch thick, trimmed

1 teaspoon extra-virgin olive oil

4 teaspoons Steakhouse Spice Blend or Tex-Mex Spice Blend (recipes follow)

¼ teaspoon table salt

Why This Recipe Works Never overcook a steak again! If you forgo the grill and roast your steak in the oven, you not only eliminate a lot of standing time, you also avoid the too-common predicament of nailing a good sear on the grill only to cut into a well-done hockey puck. There are two hallmarks of a perfectly cooked medium-rare steak—a consistently pink, juicy interior and a dark brown, crusty exterior. Unfortunately, you need an even, gentle heat to achieve the former and an intense, direct heat for the latter. Alas, without a searing-hot direct heat, it just isn't possible to achieve a crust in the oven. Yet roasting produces steak with a perfectly medium-rare interior from edge to edge. The way to create a crust in the oven turns out to be a spice rub, which not only crisps up the exterior and adds color but also contributes delicious flavor. If you use a store-bought spice blend instead of homemade, you may need to reduce the amount of salt in the recipe. Note that you can also make this recipe in a toaster oven. The recipe can be easily doubled; you will need either two small rimmed baking sheets or one large baking sheet.

1 Preheat oven to 450 degrees. Cut steak crosswise to yield two 1-inch-thick steaks. Pat steaks dry with paper towels, rub evenly with oil, and sprinkle with spice blend and salt, pressing to adhere.

— TAKE A 15-MINUTE BREAK —

2 Arrange steaks on small rimmed baking sheet and roast, on lowest rack, until meat registers 120 to 125 degrees (for medium-rare), about 12 minutes, flipping steaks halfway through roasting. Transfer steaks to cutting board and let rest for 5 minutes. Slice steaks thin and serve.

PREP AHEAD
You can trim and cut the steak, rub it with the spice blend, and refrigerate it up to 1 day ahead.

MAKE IT EVEN EASIER
Use a store-bought spice blend instead of making your own.

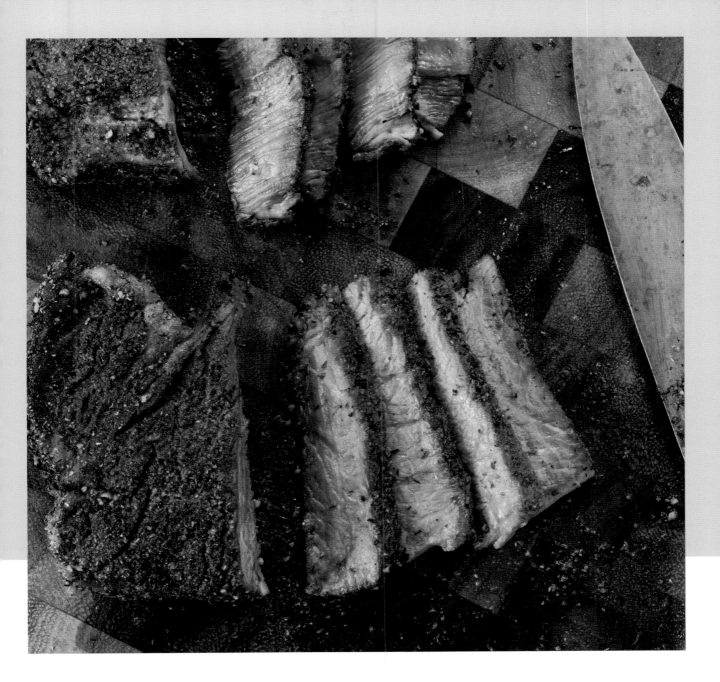

Steakhouse Spice Blend

Combine 4 teaspoons ground coriander, 2 teaspoons pepper, 1 teaspoon garlic powder, and 1 teaspoon dried dill weed or parsley together in bowl. Spice rub can be stored in airtight container for up to 3 months. Makes 8 teaspoons.

Tex-Mex Spice Blend

Combine 1 tablespoon paprika, 2 teaspoons ground coriander, 1½ teaspoons ground cumin and 1½ teaspoons garlic powder together in bowl. Spice rub can be stored in airtight container for up to 3 months. Makes 8 teaspoons.

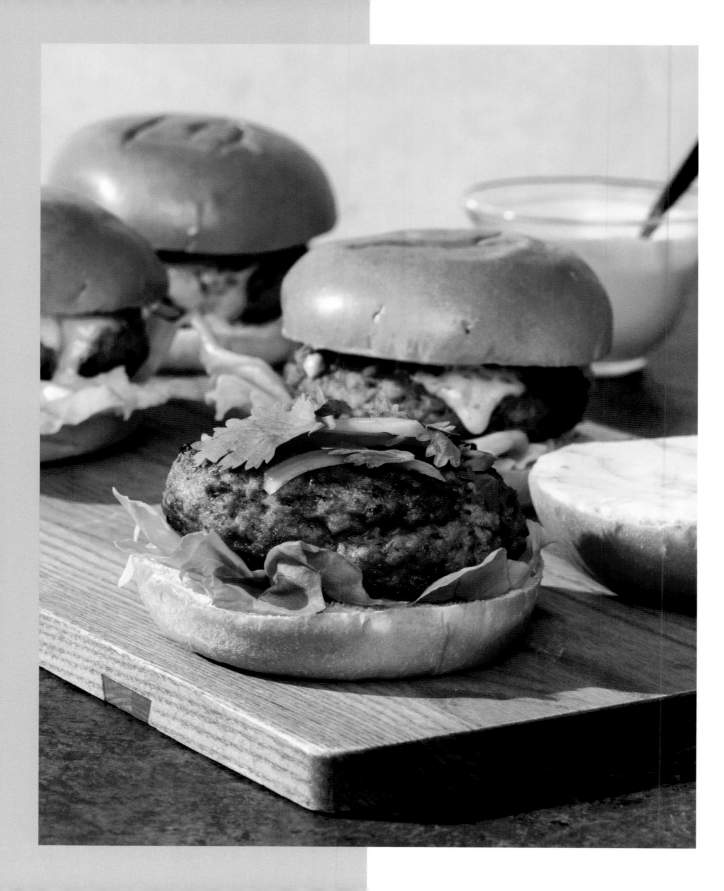

Pork Burgers with Lime and Sriracha

SERVES 4 — SUPER EASY

Why This Recipe Works When you want burger night to feel special but still be easy (and make-ahead), these superflavorful and unusual pork burgers fit the bill. They are umami-packed thanks to the combo of fish sauce and sriracha, while lime zest and a hefty dose of cilantro complete the flavor profile. Burgers made from ground pork can be dry and crumbly, so the addition of a panade (a mixture of bread and milk) keeps the burgers moist and cohesive.

1 Using fork, mash bun pieces and milk into paste in large bowl. Add cilantro, fish sauce, lime zest, sriracha, and pepper and mix to combine. Using your hands, add pork and mix until well combined.

2 Divide pork mixture into 4 equal balls, then flatten into ¾-inch-thick patties, about 4 inches wide. Cover and refrigerate for 20 minutes.

— TAKE A 20-MINUTE BREAK —

3 Heat oil in 12-inch nonstick skillet over medium-low heat until shimmering. Add patties and cook until well browned on first side, about 7 minutes. Flip patties and continue to cook until second sides are well browned and meat registers 150 degrees, about 8 minutes, flipping as needed to ensure even browning. Transfer patties to wire rack set in rimmed baking sheet and let rest for 5 minutes.

4 Transfer patties to buns and serve.

5 hamburger buns, 1 bun torn into 1-inch pieces, 4 buns toasted, if desired

3 tablespoons milk

3 tablespoons minced fresh cilantro

1 teaspoon fish sauce

1 teaspoon grated lime zest

2 teaspoons sriracha

1 teaspoon pepper

1½ pounds 80 to 85 percent lean ground pork

1 tablespoon vegetable oil

PREP AHEAD
You can form the patties up to 1 day ahead and refrigerate until cooking.

TAKE IT UP A NOTCH
Serve with Sriracha Mayonnaise
Whisk ½ teaspoon grated lime zest and 1 tablespoon juice, ¼ cup mayonnaise, and 2 teaspoons sriracha together in small bowl and refrigerate until serving. Mayonnaise can be made up to 1 day ahead and refrigerated. Makes about 6 tablespoons.

Salmon Tacos with Cilantro-Lime Slaw

SERVES 4 — SUPER EASY

- 3 cups (8¼ ounces) coleslaw mix
- 1 small red onion, halved and sliced thin
- ½ cup fresh cilantro leaves, divided
- 2 tablespoons lime juice, divided
- 1½ teaspoons table salt, divided
- ¾ teaspoon pepper, divided
- ¼ cup sour cream
- 1 teaspoon chili powder
- 2 (8-ounce) skin-on salmon fillets, 1 to 1½ inches thick
- 1 tablespoon vegetable oil
- 8 (6-inch) corn tortillas, warmed

Why This Recipe Works I don't think you can have too many recipes using salmon, which is why there are a variety of them in this book. There is something exciting about salmon tacos because they are a little bit out of the ordinary, but far easier to make than white-fish tacos, which require breading and frying and too much time standing at the stove. These salmon tacos are a game changer, delivering crisp seasoned salmon, a zesty slaw using coleslaw mix, and a sour cream–based topping. A rub of chili powder, salt, and pepper makes for flavorful salmon, and cooking the fillets skin-on ensures that they hold together in the skillet and stay moist. For information on warming tortillas, see page 217. If using wild salmon, cook the fillets until they register 120 degrees.

1   Combine coleslaw mix, onion, ¼ cup cilantro, 5 teaspoons lime juice, ½ teaspoon salt, and ¼ teaspoon pepper in bowl. Whisk sour cream, remaining 1 teaspoon lime juice, ¼ teaspoon salt, and ¼ teaspoon pepper together in separate bowl. Refrigerate slaw and sauce.

— **TAKE A 15-MINUTE BREAK** —

2   Combine chili powder, remaining ¾ teaspoon salt, and remaining ¼ teaspoon pepper; season salmon with spice mixture.

3   Heat oil in 12-inch nonstick skillet over medium heat until shimmering. Cook salmon, skin side up, until well browned, 6 to 8 minutes. Flip and continue to cook until salmon registers 125 degrees (for medium-rare), 6 to 8 minutes. Transfer salmon to plate and let cool slightly, about 2 minutes. Using 2 forks, flake fish into 1-inch pieces; discard skin. Divide fish evenly among tortillas. Top with coleslaw mixture, sour cream mixture, and remaining ¼ cup cilantro. Serve.

MAKE IT EVEN EASIER
Use store-bought coleslaw instead of making your own.

PREP AHEAD
You can make the slaw and the sour cream sauce up to 1 day ahead and refrigerate separately.

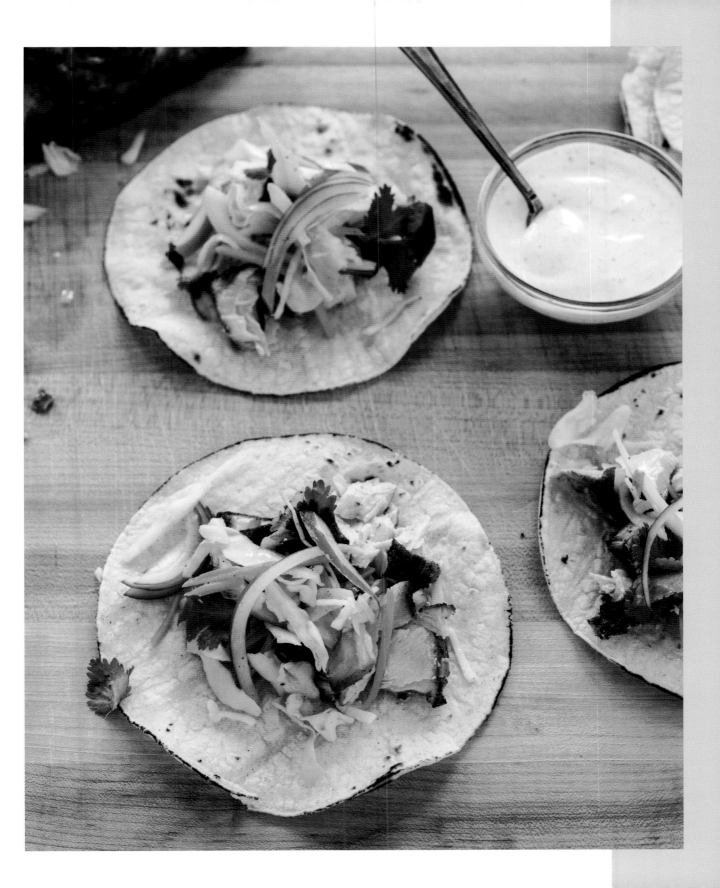

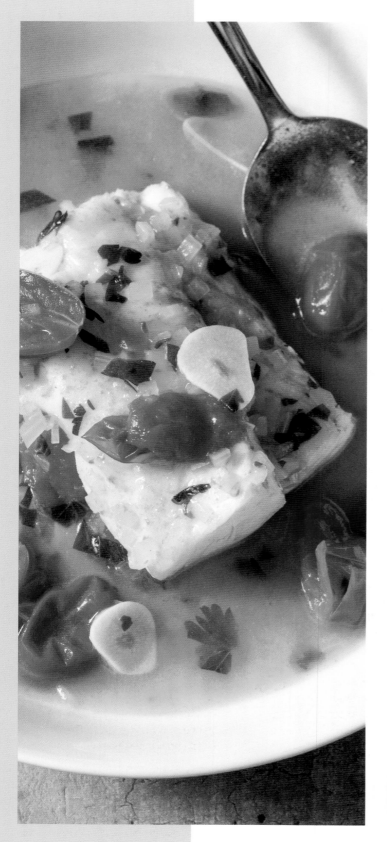

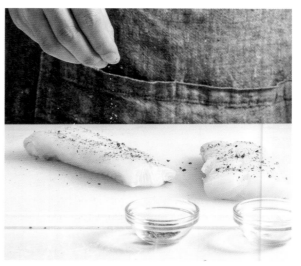

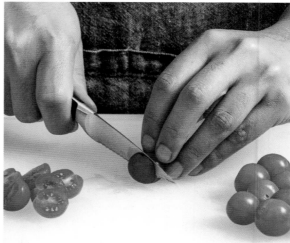

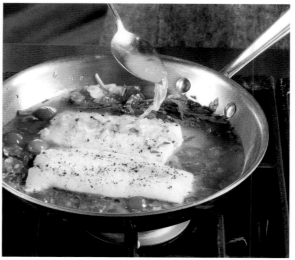

Pesce all'Acqua Pazza

SERVES 2

Why This Recipe Works This recipe is the essence of simplicity and really delivers on flavor. Pesce all'acqua pazza, or "fish in crazy water," refers to the centuries-old southern Italian tradition of cooking the day's catch in seawater. After building an aromatic base for poaching in the skillet, we spike the water-based broth with white wine for brightness and acidity and halved cherry tomatoes for sweetness and pops of color. For the fish, skin-on haddock fillets hold up nicely during simmering and suffuse the broth with rich flavor and body thanks to the abundant collagen in the skin. To ensure perfectly cooked fillets, poach them over low heat until they are nearly done and then slide the pan off the burner to finish the cooking. After just a few minutes, the haddock absorbs the heady flavor of the broth, and the broth is enriched by the fish. You can substitute skin-on fillets of other firm, white-fleshed fish such as sea bass, branzino, and red snapper for the haddock. Serve with crusty bread. You will need a 10-inch skillet with a tight-fitting lid for this recipe.

1 Sprinkle haddock all over with ¼ teaspoon salt and pepper and set aside.

2 Heat oil, garlic, and pepper flakes in 10-inch skillet over medium heat, stirring constantly, until garlic begins to sizzle gently, about 1½ minutes. Add onion, bay leaf, and remaining ¼ teaspoon salt and cook, stirring constantly, until onion just starts to soften, about 2 minutes. Add tomatoes and cook, stirring constantly, until tomatoes begin to soften, about 2 minutes. Stir in water, wine, parsley stems, and half of chopped parsley and bring to boil. Nestle haddock skin side down in liquid, moving aside solids as much as possible (it's fine if fillets fold over slightly at ends; liquid will not quite cover fillets). Spoon some liquid and solids over haddock. Reduce heat to low, cover, and simmer gently until fish registers 110 degrees at thickest point, 4 to 7 minutes. Let stand off heat, covered, until fish registers 130 degrees and is opaque and just cooked through, 3 to 7 minutes.

3 Divide haddock between 2 shallow soup bowls. Discard bay leaf and parsley stems; stir remaining chopped parsley into broth. Season broth with salt and pepper to taste. Spoon portion of broth and solids over each serving of haddock and serve immediately.

12 ounces skin-on haddock fillets, ¾ to 1 inch thick

½ teaspoon kosher salt, divided

⅛ teaspoon pepper

1 tablespoon extra-virgin olive oil

2 small garlic cloves, sliced thin

⅛ teaspoon red pepper flakes

½ small onion, chopped fine

1 small bay leaf

4 ounces cherry or grape tomatoes, halved

¾ cup water

2 tablespoons dry white wine

6 fresh parsley stems, plus 1½ tablespoons chopped fresh parsley, divided

PREP AHEAD
You can chop the onion and halve the cherry tomatoes up to 1 day ahead and refrigerate separately.

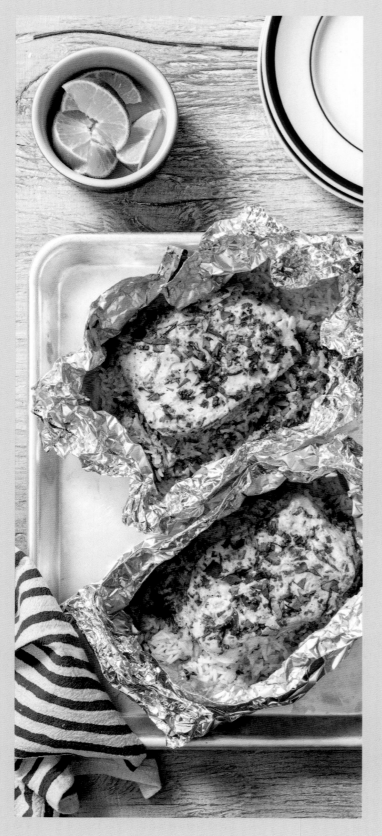

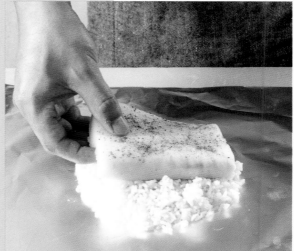

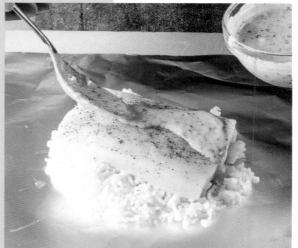

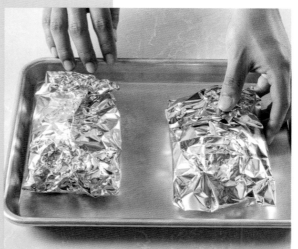

Easy Fish and Rice Packets with Coconut-Curry Sauce

SERVES 2 — SUPER EASY

Why This Recipe Works This is exactly the sort of fancy but weeknight-friendly recipe I know my patients want to make. There is very little prep required, and the clever combination of ingredients, plus cooking en papillote, delivers a main, a side, and a creamy sauce all at once—making it a good choice when cooking is the last thing you feel like doing. In the 15 minutes it takes to preheat your oven, you can easily assemble the packets. The coconut milk–based sauce, which includes Thai green curry paste, cilantro, and lime zest, does more than infuse the fish with flavor; it also provides a burst of color and transforms the rice into a rich, creamy accompaniment to the halibut. A sprinkle of cilantro and a squeeze of lime just before serving highlights the flavor of the sauce and brightens the dish. The packets are placed on a small, lightweight baking sheet, which is easy to maneuver into your oven. Note that you can also make this recipe in a toaster oven. The recipe can be easily doubled; you will need to use two small rimmed baking sheets or one larger baking sheet.

½   cup canned coconut milk

¼   cup minced fresh cilantro, divided

4   teaspoons Thai green curry paste

1   teaspoon grated lime zest, plus lime wedges

2   (6- to 8-ounce) skinless halibut fillets, ¾ to 1 inch thick

¼   teaspoon table salt

⅛   teaspoon pepper

2   cups cooked rice

1   Preheat oven to 400 degrees. Whisk coconut milk, 3 tablespoons cilantro, curry paste, and lime zest together in bowl.

2   Pat halibut dry with paper towels and sprinkle with salt and pepper. Cut two 14 by 12-inch rectangles of aluminum foil and lay them flat on counter. Mound 1 cup cooked rice in center of each piece of foil, then place fillets on top. Spoon coconut mixture over top of fillets, then tightly crimp foil into packets.

3   Set packets on small rimmed baking sheet, place on middle rack, and bake until halibut flakes apart when gently prodded with paring knife and registers 130 degrees, 18 to 20 minutes. (To check temperature, poke thermometer through foil of one packet and into halibut.)

— **TAKE AN 18-MINUTE BREAK** —

4   Carefully open packets, allowing steam to escape away from you. Sprinkle fillets with remaining 1 tablespoon cilantro and serve with lime wedges.

PREP AHEAD
You can assemble the fish packets up to 6 hours ahead and refrigerate.

MAKE IT EVEN EASIER
Use a rice cooker to make the rice, or use store-bought microwaveable rice.

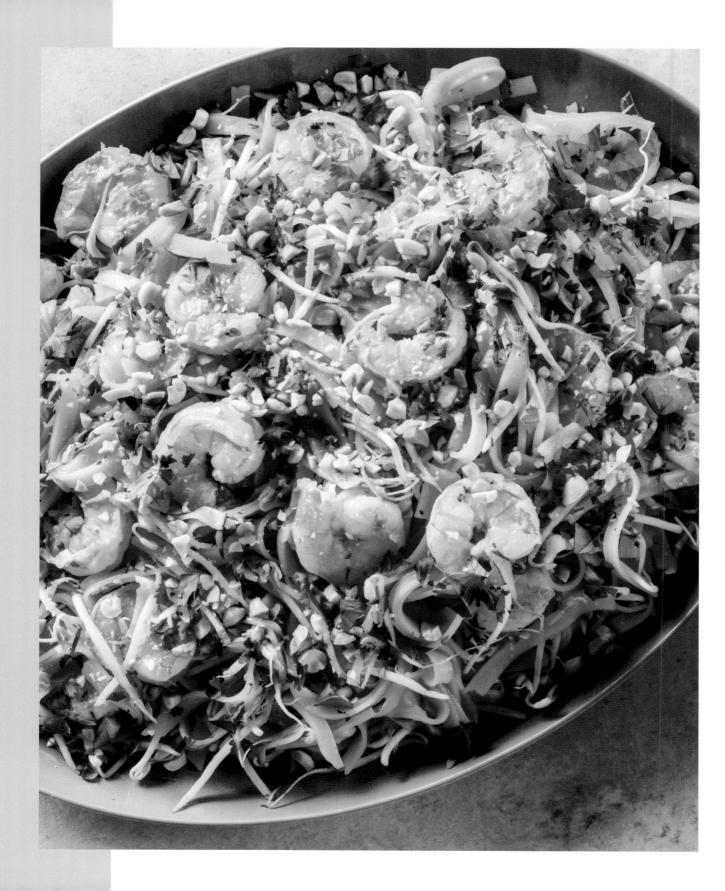

One-Pan Shrimp Pad Thai

SERVES 4 — SUPER EASY

Why This Recipe Works With a sweet-and-sour sauce; tender rice noodles; and plump, sweet shrimp, this easy take on Thailand's best-known noodles captures the essence of the beloved dish. This version streamlines the dish substantially without shortchanging flavor. There's no tamarind required in the sauce, which uses a simple combination of fish sauce, lime juice, and brown sugar. And shrimp alone was enough to give the pad thai heft—no need for dried shrimp in addition, or eggs. The noodles boast great texture as well, with crisp-fresh mung beans and chopped peanuts providing crunch in contrast with the juicy shrimp and just-chewy-enough rice noodles. To get the texture of the rice noodles just right, you must first soak them in hot water so they start to soften and then stir-fry them in the pan. Do not substitute other types of noodles for the rice noodles here.

1 Soak noodles in hot water until softened, about 15 minutes.

— TAKE A 15-MINUTE BREAK —

2 Combine lime juice, sugar, and fish sauce in bowl and set aside. Pat shrimp dry with paper towels. Heat oil in 12-inch nonstick skillet over medium heat until just beginning to smoke. Add shrimp and garlic and cook, stirring occasionally, until shrimp are pink, about 4 minutes. Transfer to plate.

3 Return now-empty skillet to medium heat. Drain noodles and add to skillet. Cook until any residual moisture has evaporated, about 2 minutes. Add lime juice mixture and cook until thickened slightly, about 4 minutes. Add shrimp and sprouts to skillet and cook until shrimp are cooked through, about 3 minutes. Transfer to bowl, sprinkle with cilantro and peanuts, and serve with lime wedges.

8 ounces (⅜-inch-wide) rice noodles

⅓ cup lime juice (3 limes) plus wedges for serving

⅓ cup packed brown sugar

¼ cup fish sauce

1 pound peeled and deveined extra-large shrimp (21 to 25 per pound)

2 tablespoons vegetable oil

4 garlic cloves, minced

8 ounces (4 cups) mung bean sprouts

¼ cup chopped fresh cilantro

¼ cup dry-roasted peanuts, chopped

Asparagus and Goat Cheese Tart

SERVES 4

6 ounces thin asparagus, trimmed and cut on bias ¼ inch thick (1 cup)

2 scallions, sliced thin

3 tablespoons extra-virgin olive oil, divided

2 tablespoons chopped pitted kalamata olives

1 garlic clove, minced

¼ teaspoon grated lemon zest

¼ teaspoon table salt

¼ teaspoon pepper

3 ounces goat cheese, softened, plus 1 ounce crumbled

1 (9½ by 9-inch) sheet puff pastry, thawed

PREP AHEAD
You can cut up the asparagus, slice the scallions, and chop the olives up to 1 day ahead and refrigerate separately.

Why This Recipe Works This recipe convinced me that making tarts using store-bought puff pastry is the way to go, because it cuts out most of the prep involved in making dough from scratch, and the tart fits easily on a small, lightweight rimmed baking sheet. This tart takes just minutes to assemble and makes for an impressive brunch dish or a simple light supper. Cut the asparagus into small pieces to skip any precooking and then toss the pieces with olive oil, garlic, lemon zest, scallions, and olives to provide fresh flavors with a briny finish. To anchor these toppings, soft goat cheese provides a creamy base, with olive oil blended in for easy spreading. Finally, crumbling more cheese on top adds richness. To thaw frozen puff pastry, let it sit either in the refrigerator for 24 hours or on the counter for 30 to 60 minutes. Look for asparagus spears no thicker than ½ inch. Note that you can also make this recipe in a toaster oven. The recipe was developed using a light-colored rimmed baking sheet; if using a dark pan, start checking for doneness 5 minutes earlier than advised in step 3.

1 Preheat oven to 425 degrees. Line small rimmed baking sheet with parchment paper. Combine asparagus, scallions, 1 tablespoon oil, olives, garlic, lemon zest, salt, and pepper in bowl. In separate bowl, mix softened goat cheese and 1 tablespoon oil until smooth.

— TAKE A 15-MINUTE BREAK—

2 Unfold pastry onto lightly floured counter and roll out to 11½ by 9-inch rectangle. Lightly brush outer ½ inch of pastry with water to create border, then fold border toward center, pressing gently to seal. Transfer pastry to prepared sheet.

3 Spread goat cheese mixture in even layer over center of pastry, avoiding folded border. Scatter asparagus mixture over goat cheese, then top with crumbled goat cheese. Bake, on middle rack, until pastry is puffed and bottom and sides are golden and asparagus is crisp-tender, about 22 minutes.

— TAKE A 22-MINUTE BREAK—

4 Transfer tart to wire rack and let cool for 10 minutes. Drizzle with remaining 1 tablespoon oil. Cut into 4 equal pieces and serve.

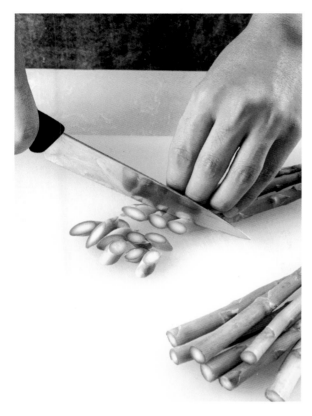

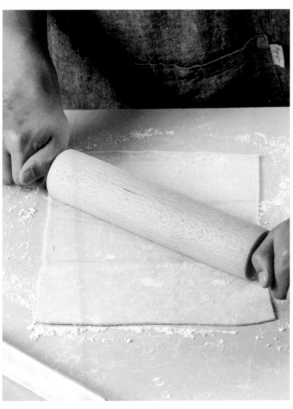

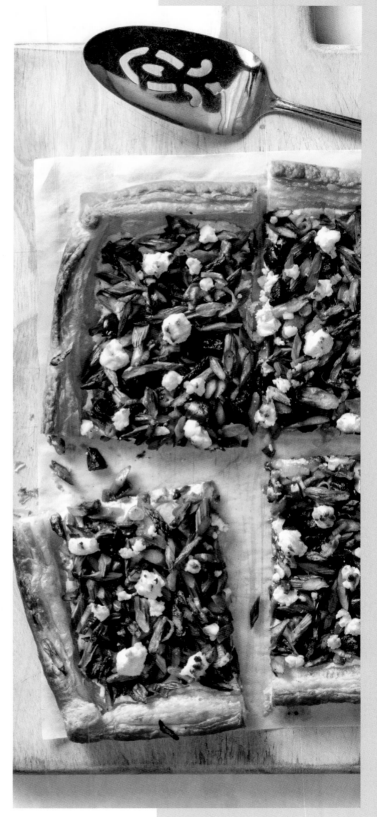

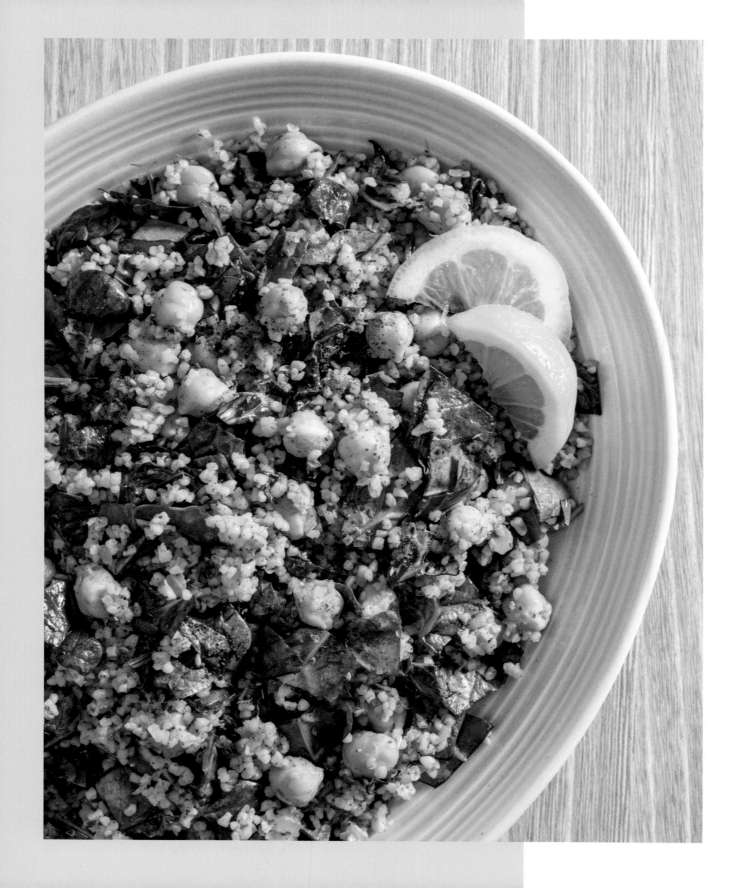

Instant Pot Bulgur with Spinach, Chickpeas, and Za'atar

SERVES 4 — SUPER EASY

Why This Recipe Works Hearty bulgur, nutty chickpeas, and fresh spinach come together in this light main or side dish, with a boost from the fragrant herbs, toasted sesame, and tangy sumac of the eastern Mediterranean spice blend za'atar. Fluffing the bulgur straight after cooking and then letting it sit (with a towel under the lid) is crucial to achieving perfectly cooked grains. The residual heat from the bulgur gently wilts the baby spinach without turning it gummy. When shopping, don't confuse bulgur with cracked wheat, which has a much longer cooking time and will not work in this recipe. Note that it will take the Instant Pot about 10 minutes to come up to pressure and start the cook cycle.

1 Using highest sauté function, heat 2 tablespoons oil in electric pressure cooker until shimmering. Add onion and salt and cook until onion is softened, about 5 minutes. Stir in garlic and 1 tablespoon za'atar and cook until fragrant, about 30 seconds. Stir in bulgur, chickpeas, and water.

2 Lock lid in place and close pressure release valve. Select high pressure cook function and cook for 1 minute.

— **TAKE AN 11-MINUTE BREAK** —

3 Turn off electric pressure cooker and quick-release pressure. Carefully remove lid, allowing steam to escape away from you. Gently fluff bulgur with fork. Lay clean dish towel over pot, replace lid, and let sit for 5 minutes. Add spinach, lemon juice, remaining 1 tablespoon za'atar, and remaining 1 tablespoon oil and toss gently to combine until spinach is wilted. Season with salt and pepper to taste. Serve with lemon wedges.

Ingredients

- 3 tablespoons extra-virgin olive oil, divided
- 1 onion, chopped fine
- ½ teaspoon table salt
- 3 garlic cloves, minced
- 2 tablespoons za'atar, divided
- 1 cup medium-grind bulgur, rinsed
- 1 (15-ounce) can chickpeas, rinsed
- 1½ cups water
- 5 ounces (5 cups) baby spinach
- 1 tablespoon lemon juice, plus lemon wedges for serving

PREP AHEAD

You can chop the onion up to 1 day ahead and refrigerate.

Stuffed Eggplant with Lentils, Pomegranate, and Ricotta

SERVES 2

3 tablespoons boiling water

3 tablespoons couscous

1 (1-pound) eggplant, halved lengthwise

2 tablespoons extra-virgin olive oil, divided

½ teaspoon cumin, divided

½ teaspoon table salt, divided

2 teaspoons pomegranate molasses, plus extra for serving

2 teaspoons lemon juice

1 (15-ounce) can lentils, rinsed

¼ cup fresh parsley leaves

2 tablespoons chopped toasted pistachios, plus extra for serving

¼ cup ricotta cheese

Why This Recipe Works This showstopping vegetarian main puts the spotlight on tender roasted eggplant halves that are stuffed with an easy-to-make lentil and couscous filling that is redolent of spices and herbs and boasts textural contrast. A 1-pound eggplant is the perfect size to serve two people. To help it release moisture and cook more quickly, it is important to first score its flesh and then roast it until tender but still sturdy enough not to collapse when filled. While the eggplant roasts, make a simple but flavorful filling of canned lentils (which require no additional time or prep) and quick-cooking couscous flavored with lemon, cumin, fresh parsley, and sweet-tart pomegranate molasses. Green pistachios add crunch and contrasting color, and dollops of ricotta contribute creamy richness. For an accurate measurement of boiling water, bring a kettle of water to a boil and then measure out the desired amount. Note that you can also make this recipe in a toaster oven. Serve sprinkled with pomegranate seeds and fresh parsley leaves, if desired.

1   Place parchment paper–lined small rimmed baking sheet on middle rack, and heat oven to 400 degrees. Combine boiling water and couscous in small bowl. Cover and let sit for 10 minutes.

— TAKE A 10-MINUTE BREAK —

2   Fluff couscous with fork and season with salt and pepper to taste; set aside.

3   Score flesh of each eggplant half in 1-inch diamond pattern, about 1 inch deep. Brush scored sides of eggplant with 1 tablespoon oil and sprinkle with ¼ teaspoon cumin and ¼ teaspoon salt. Arrange eggplant cut sides down on hot sheet and roast until flesh is tender, about 45 minutes.

— TAKE A 45-MINUTE BREAK —

4   Transfer eggplant cut sides down to paper towel–lined baking sheet and let drain.

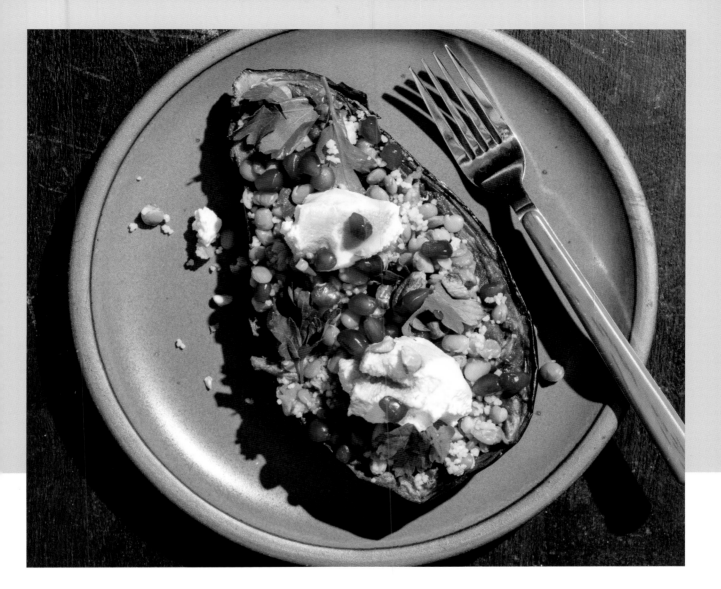

5 Whisk pomegranate molasses, lemon juice, remaining 1 tablespoon oil, remaining ¼ teaspoon cumin, and remaining ¼ teaspoon salt together in large bowl. Add couscous, lentils, parsley, and pistachios and toss to combine. Season with salt and pepper to taste.

6 Transfer eggplant cut sides up to serving plates. Using 2 forks, gently push eggplant flesh to sides to make room for filling. Gently mound lentil mixture into eggplant halves and pack lightly with back of spoon. Dollop ricotta evenly over lentils. Sprinkle with extra pistachios and drizzle with extra pomegranate molasses before serving.

PREP AHEAD

You can assemble the lentil filling up to 1 day ahead and refrigerate; make sure to stir to recombine before filling the eggplant. You can toast and chop the pistachios up to 1 day ahead.

MAKE IT EVEN EASIER

Buy pistachios already toasted or toast them in the microwave (see page 37).

Easy Air-Fryer Mains

These easy but dressed-up main dishes make the most of the air fryer. All of them serve two, but if your air fryer has a capacity of 6 quarts or more, you can double a recipe and still cook it in a single batch. However, it is critical to leave enough room for air circulation around the ingredients to ensure even cooking. If you have a smaller air fryer (less than 6 quarts) and are doubling a recipe, you will need to cook in batches.

Air-Fryer Roasted Bone-In Chicken Breasts
Serves 2

- 2 (12-ounce) bone-in split chicken breasts, trimmed
- 1 teaspoon extra-virgin olive oil
- ½ teaspoon table salt
- ¼ teaspoon pepper

Pat chicken dry with paper towels, rub with oil, and sprinkle with salt and pepper. Arrange breasts skin side down in air-fryer basket, spaced evenly apart, alternating ends. Place basket in air fryer and set temperature to 350 degrees. Cook until chicken registers 160 degrees, 20 to 25 minutes, flipping and rotating breasts halfway through cooking. Transfer chicken to serving platter, tent with aluminum foil, and let rest for 5 minutes. Serve.

TAKE IT UP A NOTCH
Serve with Lemon-Basil Salsa Verde

Whisk ¼ cup minced fresh parsley, ¼ cup chopped fresh basil, 3 tablespoons extra-virgin olive oil, 1 tablespoon rinsed and minced capers, 1 tablespoon water, 2 minced garlic cloves, 1 rinsed and minced anchovy fillet, ½ teaspoon grated lemon zest and 2 teaspoons juice, and ⅛ teaspoon salt together in bowl. Salsa can be refrigerated for up to 2 days ahead. Makes about ¾ cup.

Air-Fryer Sweet and Smoky Pork Tenderloin with Roasted Butternut Squash
Serves 2

Note that butternut squash that you buy cubed is usually not in uniform pieces. Cut the pieces so they are all the same size, ideally ¾-inch pieces.

- 1¼ pounds cubed butternut squash (5 cups)
- 1 tablespoon unsalted butter, melted, divided
- ⅛ teaspoon plus ½ teaspoon table salt, divided
- ⅛ teaspoon plus ½ teaspoon pepper, divided
- 3½ teaspoons molasses, divided
- 1 teaspoon smoked paprika
- 1 garlic clove, minced
- 1 (1-pound) pork tenderloin, trimmed and halved crosswise
- 1 teaspoon grated lime zest plus 1 teaspoon juice
- 2 tablespoons pepitas, toasted
- 1 tablespoon minced fresh chives

1   Toss squash with 1½ teaspoons melted butter, ⅛ teaspoon salt, and ⅛ teaspoon pepper in large bowl; transfer to air-fryer basket. Place basket in air fryer and set temperature to 350 degrees. Cook squash for 8 minutes, tossing halfway through cooking.

2   Meanwhile, microwave 3 teaspoons molasses, paprika, garlic, remaining ½ teaspoon salt, and remaining ½ teaspoon pepper in now-empty bowl until fragrant, about 30 seconds, stirring halfway through microwaving. Pat pork dry with paper towels, add to molasses mixture, and toss to coat.

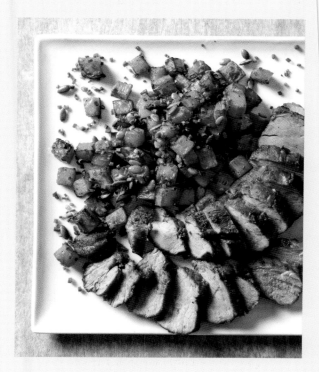

Air-Fryer Crispy Breaded Boneless Pork Chops
Serves 2

- ¾ cup panko bread crumbs
- 2 tablespoons unsalted butter, melted
- 1 large egg
- 2 tablespoons Dijon mustard
- 1 tablespoon all-purpose flour
- 1½ teaspoons dry mustard
- ½ teaspoon garlic powder
- ¼ teaspoon table salt
- ¼ teaspoon cayenne pepper
- 2 (8-ounce) boneless pork chops, 1½ inches thick, trimmed
  Lemon wedges

1 Toss panko with melted butter in bowl until evenly coated. Microwave, stirring frequently, until light golden brown, about 2 minutes; transfer to shallow dish. Whisk egg, Dijon mustard, flour, dry mustard, garlic powder, salt, and cayenne together in second shallow dish.

2 Pat chops dry with paper towels. Using sharp knife, cut 2 slits, about 2 inches apart, through fat on edges of each chop. Cut 1⁄16-inch-deep slits, spaced ½ inch apart, in crosshatch pattern on both sides of chops. Working with 1 chop at a time, dip in egg mixture, letting excess drip off, then coat with panko mixture, pressing gently to adhere.

3 Lightly spray base of air-fryer basket with vegetable oil spray. Arrange chops in prepared basket, spaced evenly apart. Place basket in air fryer and set temperature to 400 degrees. Cook until pork registers 140 degrees, about 15 minutes, flipping and rotating chops halfway through cooking. Serve with lemon wedges.

3 Stir squash, then arrange tenderloin pieces on top. (Tuck thinner tail end of tenderloin under itself as needed to create uniform pieces.) Return basket to air fryer and cook until pork registers 140 degrees, about 18 minutes, flipping and rotating tenderloin pieces halfway through cooking. Transfer pork to large plate, tent with aluminum foil, and let rest while finishing squash.

4 Whisk lime zest and juice, remaining 1½ teaspoons melted butter, and remaining ½ teaspoon molasses together in medium bowl. Add squash, pepitas, and chives and toss to coat. Season with salt and pepper to taste. Slice pork ½ inch thick and serve with squash.

PREP AHEAD
You can trim and cut the pork up to 1 day ahead and refrigerate. You can toast the pepitas up to 1 day ahead; you can also toast the pepitas in the microwave (see page 37).

PREP AHEAD
You can trim and score the pork chops up to 1 day ahead and refrigerate.

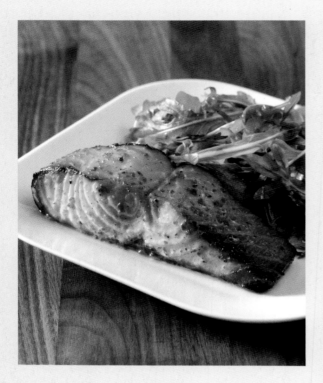

Place basket in air fryer and set temperature to 400 degrees. Cook salmon until center is still translucent when checked with tip of paring knife and registers 125 degrees (for medium-rare), 10 to 14 minutes, using sling to rotate fillets halfway through cooking.

4   Using sling, carefully remove salmon from air fryer. Slide fish spatula along underside of fillets and transfer to individual serving plates, leaving skin behind. Serve.

VARIATIONS

Hoisin-Glazed Salmon

Omit orange zest. Substitute 2 tablespoons hoisin sauce for marmalade, 1 tablespoon rice vinegar for orange juice, and ⅛ teaspoon ground ginger for mustard.

Honey Chipotle–Glazed Salmon

Omit orange zest and juice. Substitute 2 tablespoons honey for marmalade and 2 teaspoons minced canned chipotle chile in adobo sauce for mustard.

MAKING A FOIL SLING FOR AIR FRYER

Fold 1 long sheet of aluminum foil so it is 4 inches wide. Lay the sheet of foil widthwise across the basket, pressing the foil up and into the sides of the basket. Fold the excess foil as needed so that the edges of the foil are flush with the top of the basket.

Air-Fryer Orange Mustard–Glazed Salmon

Serves 2

- 1 tablespoon orange marmalade
- ¼ teaspoon grated orange zest plus 1 tablespoon juice
- 2 teaspoons whole-grain mustard
- 2 (6-to 8-ounce) skin-on salmon fillets, 1½ inches thick
- ¼ teaspoon table salt
- ⅛ teaspoon pepper

1   Make foil sling for air-fryer basket. Lightly spray foil and basket with vegetable oil spray.

2   Combine marmalade, orange zest and juice, and mustard in bowl. Pat salmon dry with paper towels and sprinkle with salt and pepper. Brush tops and sides of fillets evenly with glaze. Arrange fillets skin side down on sling in prepared basket, spaced evenly apart.

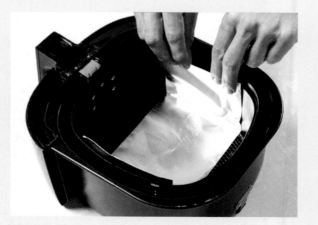

Air-Fryer Crunchy Cod Fillets

Serves 2

- ⅓ cup panko bread crumbs
- 1 teaspoon vegetable oil
- 1 small shallot, minced
- 1 small garlic clove, minced
- ½ teaspoon minced fresh thyme or ⅛ teaspoon dried
- ½ teaspoon table salt, divided
- ¼ teaspoon plus ⅛ teaspoon pepper, divided
- 1 tablespoon minced fresh parsley
- 1 large egg yolk
- 1 tablespoon mayonnaise
- ¼ teaspoon grated lemon zest, plus lemon wedges for serving
- 2 (8-ounce) skinless cod fillets, 1¼ inches thick

1 Make foil sling for air-fryer basket. Lightly spray foil and basket with vegetable oil spray.

2 Toss panko with oil in bowl until evenly coated. Stir in shallot, garlic, thyme, ¼ teaspoon salt, and ⅛ teaspoon pepper. Microwave, stirring frequently, until panko is light golden brown, about 2 minutes. Transfer to shallow dish and let cool slightly; stir in parsley. Whisk egg yolk, mayonnaise, lemon zest, and ⅛ teaspoon pepper together in bowl.

3 Pat cod dry with paper towels and sprinkle with remaining ¼ teaspoon salt and remaining ⅛ teaspoon pepper. Arrange fillets skinned side down on plate and brush tops evenly with mayonnaise mixture. (Tuck thinner tail ends of fillets under themselves as needed to create uniform pieces.) Working with 1 fillet at a time, dredge coated side in panko mixture, pressing gently to adhere. Arrange fillets crumb side up on sling in prepared basket, spaced evenly apart. Place basket in air fryer and set temperature to 300 degrees. Cook until cod registers 130 degrees, 12 to 16 minutes, using sling to rotate fillets halfway through cooking. Using sling, carefully remove cod from air fryer. Serve with lemon wedges.

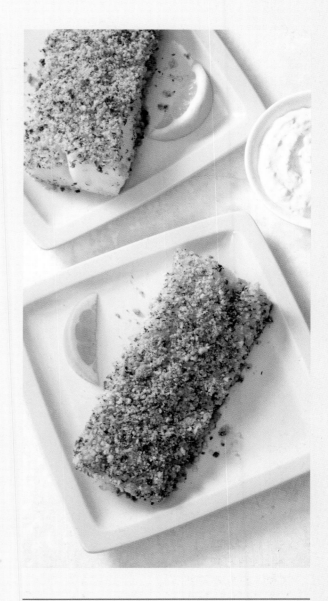

PREP AHEAD
You can mince the shallot up to 1 day in advance and refrigerate until using.

TAKE IT UP A NOTCH
Serve with Chipotle Mayonnaise (page 186).

Easy Sides

to Round Out Your Meal

* Try these recipes first if today is not one of your better days and you need a soul-refilling side dish with a high return on your energy investment.

Everyday Rice Pilaf

SERVES 4 TO 6 — SUPER EASY

Why This Recipe Works When you want a rice side dish with a little more flavor than plain rice, this pilaf should be your go-to recipe. It's very easy, and there is nearly a half-hour of walkaway time during which you can rest or turn your attention to the main course. Rinsing the rice before cooking removes excess starch and helps prevent clumping and then toasting the rice with chopped onion and extra-virgin olive oil for a few minutes in the pan at the outset deepens its flavor. Instead of following the typical ratio that's printed on the package (1 cup rice to 2 cups water), using a little less liquid delivers better results. Placing a dish towel under the lid while the rice finishes cooking off the heat absorbs excess moisture and locks in fluffiness. A nonstick saucepan works best, although a traditional saucepan will also work.

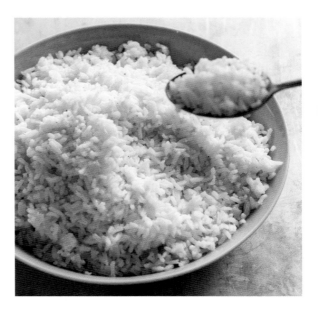

  2 **tablespoons extra-virgin olive oil**
  1 **onion, chopped fine**
  ¼ **teaspoon table salt**
1½ **cups long-grain white rice, rinsed**
2¼ **cups water**

1 Heat oil in large saucepan over medium heat until shimmering. Add onion and salt and cook until softened, about 5 minutes. Stir in rice and cook, stirring often, until edges of grains begin to turn translucent, about 3 minutes.

2 Stir in water and bring to simmer. Reduce heat to low, cover, and continue to simmer until rice is tender and water is absorbed, about 17 minutes.

— TAKE A 17-MINUTE BREAK —

3 Remove saucepan from heat and lay clean folded dish towel underneath lid. Let sit for 10 minutes.

— TAKE A 10-MINUTE BREAK —

4 Fluff rice with fork, season with salt and pepper to taste, and serve.

VARIATIONS

Rice Pilaf with Apricots and Almonds
Add ¼ teaspoon crumbled saffron threads (optional) with onion in step 1. Sprinkle ¼ cup chopped dried apricots over cooked rice before letting rice sit in step 3. Just before serving, stir in ¼ cup toasted slivered almonds.

Spiced Rice Pilaf with Ginger, Dates, and Parsley
Add 1½ teaspoons minced fresh ginger, 1 minced garlic clove, ⅛ teaspoon ground cinnamon, and ⅛ teaspoon ground cardamom to saucepan after cooking onion in step 1. Cook until fragrant, about 30 seconds. Before serving, stir in ¼ cup chopped dried dates and 1½ tablespoons minced fresh parsley

---

PREP AHEAD
You can chop the onion up to 1 day ahead and refrigerate.

Simple White Rice

SERVES 4 TO 6 — SUPER EASY

Why This Recipe Works Everyone should have a recipe that delivers perfect white rice, the essential base for myriad stir-fries or curries. For long-grain rice with distinct grains, rinse the rice of excess starch first. A nonstick saucepan works best, although a traditional saucepan will also work.

 2 cups long-grain white rice
 1 tablespoon unsalted butter
 3 cups water
 1 teaspoon table salt

1   Rinse rice in colander or fine-mesh strainer under cold running water until water runs clear. Place colander over bowl and set aside.

2   Melt butter in large saucepan over medium heat. Add rice and cook, stirring constantly, until grains become chalky and opaque, about 2 minutes. Add water and salt, increase heat to high, and bring to boil, swirling saucepan to blend ingredients. Reduce heat to low, cover, and simmer until all liquid is absorbed, about 19 minutes.

— TAKE A 19-MINUTE BREAK —

3   Off heat, remove lid and place dish towel folded in half over saucepan; replace lid. Let stand for about 12 minutes.

— TAKE A 12-MINUTE BREAK —

4   Fluff rice with fork and serve.

VARIATION
Simple White Rice for Two
Reduce rice to ¾ cup, butter to 1 teaspoon, water to 1¼ cups, and salt to ¼ teaspoon. Cook rice in small saucepan, using cooking times listed in recipe.

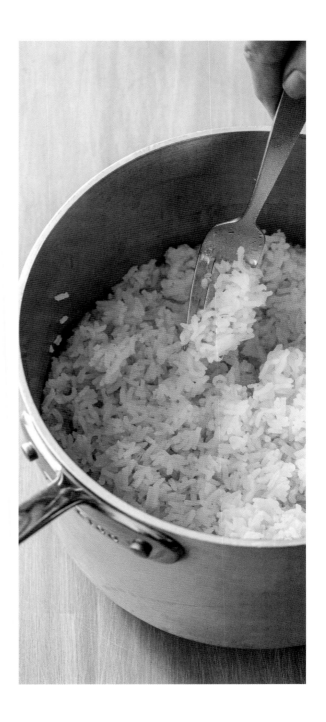

Sesame Sushi Rice

SERVES 4 TO 6 — SUPER EASY

Why This Recipe Works Even if you aren't adventurous enough to make your own sushi, you definitely need this recipe for sushi rice. Sushi rice, when seasoned, is so pleasantly sticky and tangy that it makes an ideal partner for many recipes, from stir-fries to fish, especially salmon. To achieve the right amount of stickiness and chew without gumminess, simmer the water and rice together (along with seasoned rice vinegar) before removing it from the heat, still covered, to finish cooking gently and evenly. Stirring in scallions, a hefty dose of toasted sesame oil, and sesame seeds at the end brings this rice to the next level. A nonstick saucepan works best, although a traditional saucepan will also work.

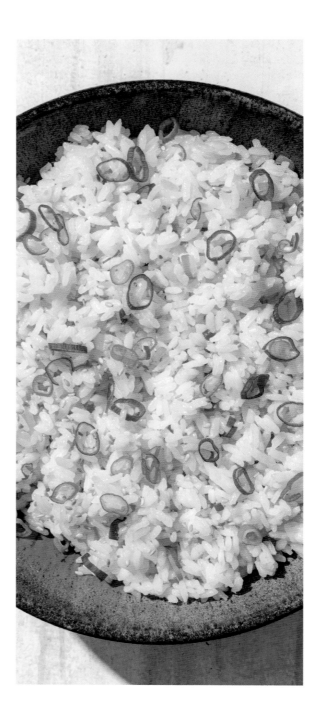

2½ cups water
2 cups sushi or short-grain white rice
2 teaspoons seasoned rice vinegar
1 teaspoon table salt
2 scallions, sliced thin
2 tablespoons toasted sesame oil
1 tablespoon sesame seeds, toasted

1 Bring water, rice, vinegar, and salt to boil in medium saucepan over high heat. Cover, reduce heat to low, and cook until liquid is absorbed, about 15 minutes.

— TAKE A 15-MINUTE BREAK —

2 Remove rice from heat and let sit, covered, until tender, about 15 minutes.

— TAKE A 15-MINUTE BREAK —

3 Fluff rice with fork; stir in scallions, oil, and sesame seeds and serve.

Hands-Off Baked Brown Rice

SERVES 2 — SUPER EASY

Why This Recipe Works Brown rice can definitely be a bit "finicky," but this foolproof method allows you to bake the rice in a loaf pan and gives you 50 minutes of free time while that is happening. Baking the rice allows more precise temperature control than cooking on the stovetop, and the even heat eliminates the risk of scorching. A loaf pan handily contains two servings of rice and creates the ideal amount of surface area for evaporation. Bringing the water to a boil before adding it to the pan also speeds up the cooking time. For an accurate measurement of boiling water, bring a full kettle of water to a boil and then measure out the desired amount. Note that you can also make this recipe in a toaster oven. Our preferred loaf pan measures 8½ by 4½ inches; if you use a 9 by 5-inch loaf pan, start checking for doneness 5 minutes early.

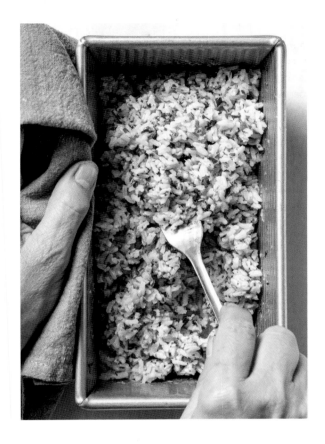

1¼ cups boiling water or vegetable broth
¾ cup long-grain, medium-grain, or short-grain brown rice, rinsed
2 teaspoons extra-virgin olive oil
¼ teaspoon table salt

1 Preheat oven to 375 degrees. Combine boiling water, rice, oil, and salt in 8½ by 4½-inch loaf pan. Cover pan tightly with double layer of aluminum foil. Bake, on middle rack, until rice is tender and no water remains, about 50 minutes.

— TAKE A 50-MINUTE BREAK —

2 Remove pan from oven and fluff rice with fork, scraping up any rice that has stuck to bottom. Cover pan with clean dish towel, then re-cover loosely with foil. Let rice sit for 10 minutes.

— TAKE A 10-MINUTE BREAK —

3 Season with salt and pepper to taste. Serve.

VARIATION

Hands-Off Baked Brown Rice with Parmesan, Lemon, and Herbs

Add ½ cup grated Parmesan cheese, 2 tablespoons minced fresh parsley, 2 tablespoons chopped fresh basil, and ¼ teaspoon grated lemon zest plus ¼ teaspoon juice to pan when fluffing rice in step 2.

TAKE IT UP A NOTCH

Use a flavored olive oil like chile, fennel, or rosemary oil.

Garlicky Fried Rice with Bok Choy

SERVES 4 TO 6

Why This Recipe Works This is a recipe for those who have discovered the beauty of a good rice cooker (see page 47) that makes it easy to have perfectly cooked rice on hand any time. This is such a delicious main or side dish that it is absolutely worth planning ahead so you have some cooked rice in the fridge for a quick meal. I love that this dish combines a green vegetable (baby bok choy) with rice in an ultra-aromatic base loaded with garlic (which does the heavy lifting), fish sauce, and lime juice and zest. Cooking the rice undisturbed at the end is key to getting those magical crispy bits, so don't go stir-crazy. You will need a 12-inch nonstick skillet with a tight-fitting lid for this recipe.

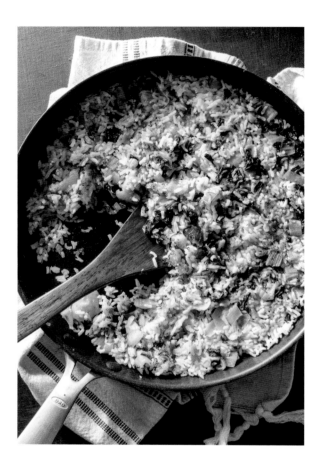

> 3 tablespoons vegetable oil, divided
> 1½ pounds baby bok choy, halved lengthwise and sliced crosswise ½ inch thick
> ½ teaspoon table salt
> 10 garlic cloves, minced
> 4 cups cooked rice
> 2 tablespoons fish sauce
> 1 teaspoon grated lime zest plus 1½ tablespoons juice
> ¼ teaspoon pepper

1   Heat 1 tablespoon oil in 12-inch nonstick skillet over medium-high heat until just smoking. Add bok choy and salt and cook until beginning to soften and char in spots, 2 to 4 minutes. Stir in garlic and cook until fragrant, about 30 seconds. Stir in rice, remaining 2 tablespoons oil, fish sauce, lime zest and juice, and pepper.

2   Firmly press rice mixture into compact, even layer. Cover and cook, without stirring, until rice begins to crisp, about 2 minutes. Uncover, reduce heat to medium, and continue to cook until bottom of rice is golden brown, about 5 minutes. Season with salt and pepper to taste, and serve.

PREP AHEAD
You can slice the bok choy up to 1 day ahead and refrigerate. You can make the fried rice up to 1 day ahead and refrigerate. To reheat, microwave in covered bowl until heated through, 2 to 4 minutes.

MAKE IT EVEN EASIER
Make the rice in your rice cooker or buy rice off the steam table at your local market.

Cauliflower Rice

SERVES 4 TO 6

Why This Recipe Works I always encourage my patients to eat more vegetables, and this easy-to-make cauliflower rice is a great way to do that. The key to making it is to blitz the florets in a food processor until transformed into perfect rice-size granules. To make cauliflower rice foolproof, work in batches to make sure all the florets break down evenly. Shallot and a small amount of vegetable broth boost the flavor. To ensure that the cauliflower is tender but still maintains a rice-like chew, it is best to steam it first in a covered pot and then finish cooking it uncovered to evaporate any remaining moisture for beautifully fluffy cauliflower rice.

2	pounds cauliflower florets, cut into 1-inch pieces (6 cups)
1	tablespoon extra-virgin olive oil
1	shallot, minced
½	cup vegetable or chicken broth
¾	teaspoon table salt
2	tablespoons minced fresh parsley

1 Working in 2 batches, pulse cauliflower florets in food processor until finely ground into ¼- to ⅛-inch pieces, 6 to 8 pulses, scraping down sides of bowl as needed; transfer to bowl.

2 Heat oil in large saucepan over medium-low heat until shimmering. Add shallot and cook until softened, about 3 minutes. Stir in cauliflower, broth, and salt. Cover and cook, stirring occasionally, until cauliflower is tender, about 13 minutes.

3 Uncover and continue to cook, stirring occasionally, until cauliflower rice is almost completely dry, about 3 minutes. Off heat, stir in parsley and season with salt and pepper to taste. Serve.

VARIATIONS
Mexican Cauliflower Rice
For a spicier rice, include a portion of the chile seeds.

Substitute ½ minced jalapeño and 1 small minced garlic clove for shallot. Substitute cilantro for parsley. Add ½ teaspoon ground cumin and ½ teaspoon ground coriander to saucepan with jalapeño and add ½ teaspoon lime juice to cauliflower with cilantro.

Cauliflower Rice with Almonds and Mint
Substitute mint for parsley. Add ⅛ teaspoon ground cardamom, ⅛ teaspoon ground cinnamon, and ⅛ teaspoon ground turmeric to saucepan with shallot. Add 2 tablespoons toasted sliced almonds to cauliflower with mint.

Cauliflower Rice for Two
Reduce cauliflower florets to 1 pound, oil to 1 teaspoon, minced shallot to 1 tablespoon, broth to ¼ cup, salt to ¼ teaspoon, and parsley to 1 tablespoon. Cook in small saucepan, using cooking times listed in recipe.

PREP AHEAD
You can mince the shallot up to 1 day ahead and refrigerate. Cauliflower rice can be refrigerated for up to 3 days. To reheat, microwave in covered bowl until heated through, 1 to 3 minutes, fluffing with fork halfway through microwaving.

MAKE IT EVEN EASIER
Buy cauliflower florets.

Classic Couscous

SERVES 4 TO 6 — SUPER EASY

Why This Recipe Works The beauty of couscous is that it practically cooks itself. So why bother with those dusty boxes of ready-to-cook couscous with dubious flavoring packages? It is far better to stock your pantry with a big cannister of high-quality fresh couscous. Then all you need is the right ratio of couscous to water or broth and a simple method, and you'll have perfect couscous in 12 minutes flat. Toasting the couscous grains in butter first deepens their flavor and helps them cook up fluffy and separate. Replacing half the cooking liquid with broth bumps up the flavor even further. Do not substitute pearl couscous here; it requires a much different cooking method.

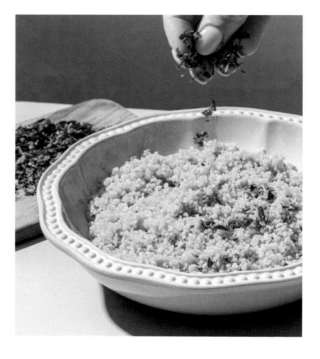

  2 **tablespoons unsalted butter**
  2 **cups couscous**
  1 **cup water**
  1 **cup vegetable or chicken broth**
  ½ **teaspoon table salt**

Melt butter in medium saucepan over medium-high heat. Add couscous and cook, stirring frequently, until grains are just beginning to brown, about 5 minutes. Add water, broth, and salt and stir briefly to combine. Cover, remove pan from heat, and let stand until grains are tender, about 7 minutes. Uncover, fluff grains with fork, and season with salt and pepper to taste. Serve.

VARIATIONS

Couscous with Curry and Mint

Stir 1½ teaspoons curry powder and 2 minced garlic cloves into toasted couscous and cook until fragrant, about 15 seconds, before adding liquids and salt. Gently fold 2 tablespoons minced fresh mint into couscous before serving.

Herbed Couscous for Two

Omit water. Reduce butter to 1 tablespoon, couscous to ⅓ cup, and broth to ½ cup. Once couscous is toasted, transfer to medium bowl. Sauté 1 minced garlic clove and 1 minced shallot in 1 tablespoon extra-virgin olive oil in saucepan until golden, about 3 minutes. Add broth and bring to boil. Pour over couscous in bowl. Stir ¼ cup minced fresh parsley into couscous when fluffing.

PREP AHEAD

You can make the couscous up to 2 days ahead and refrigerate; bring to room temperature before serving.

Farro Risotto with Fennel and Radicchio

SERVES 4 TO 6

Why This Recipe Works If you haven't tried farro, you will be surprised by its nutty, wheaty flavor and pleasant chew. It's very healthy and filling, and endlessly variable, making it a great option for salads and side dishes. Here, the farro is cooked risotto style (instead of boiling and draining)—which is actually how most Italians cook farro (the dish is called farrotto). Farro cooks faster than rice but requires frequent stirring to ensure even cooking. That said, the cooking time is just a little over 20 minutes. Onion, garlic, thyme, and fennel flavor the risotto, and you can certainly take a break after softening these aromatics in the saucepan. While it's traditional to finish risotto with butter and Parmesan, these mask the nutty flavors of farro; fresh parsley and balsamic vinegar are the perfect complement to the grain. Stirring in radicchio at the end preserves its assertive flavor which stands up so well to the hearty farro. Be sure to stir the farro often in step 2. Do not substitute pearled, quick-cooking, or presteamed farro (check the ingredient list on the package) for the whole farro.

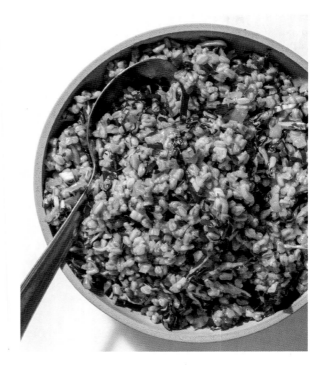

- 1 tablespoon extra-virgin olive oil
- 1 onion, chopped fine
- 1 fennel bulb, halved, cored, and chopped fine
- ¼ teaspoon table salt
- 3 garlic cloves, minced
- 1 teaspoon minced fresh thyme
- 1½ cups whole farro
- 2 cups vegetable or chicken broth
- 1½ cups water
- ½ small head radicchio, sliced thin
- 2 tablespoons minced fresh parsley
- 2 teaspoons balsamic vinegar

1 Combine oil, onion, fennel, and salt in large saucepan. Cover and cook over medium-low heat, stirring occasionally, until vegetables are softened, about 9 minutes. Stir in garlic and thyme and cook until fragrant, about 30 seconds. Turn off heat.

— TAKE A 15-MINUTE BREAK —

2 Add farro to saucepan and cook over medium-low heat until lightly toasted, about 2 minutes. Stir in broth and water and bring to simmer. Reduce heat to low and continue to simmer, stirring often, until farro is tender, about 22 minutes.

3 Stir in radicchio, parsley, and vinegar. Season with salt and pepper to taste, and serve.

PREP AHEAD
You can chop the onion and fennel and slice the radicchio up to 1 day ahead and refrigerate separately.

Barley with Celery and Miso

SERVES 4

Why This Recipe Works If you are looking for an easy side dish that is a bit unusual, this barley recipe is one to try. While the barley cooks unattended, you can whisk together an umami-packed dressing with rice vinegar, miso, soy sauce, sesame oil, and vegetable oil. Fresh ginger and garlic complete the flavor profile, and brown sugar adds balancing sweetness, while red pepper flakes add heat. Once the barley is cooked, let it cool briefly on a rimmed baking sheet, which allows it to dry thoroughly, then toss it with the dressing as well as aromatics and herbs to create a flavorful, hearty side. The cooking time for pearled barley will vary from product to product, so start checking the barley for doneness after about 20 minutes.

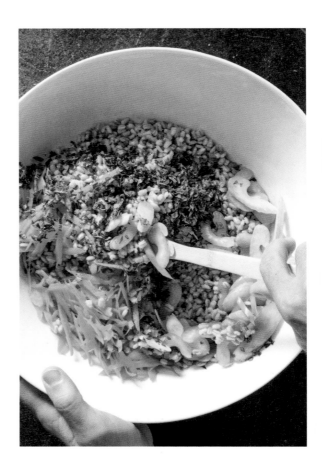

¾ cup pearled barley
   Table salt for cooking barley
1½ tablespoons seasoned rice vinegar
1½ teaspoons white miso paste
1½ teaspoons soy sauce
1½ teaspoons toasted sesame oil
1½ teaspoons vegetable oil
 1 teaspoon grated fresh ginger
 1 garlic clove, minced
½ teaspoon packed brown sugar
¼ teaspoon red pepper flakes
 1 celery rib, sliced thin on bias
 1 carrot, peeled and grated
¼ cup minced fresh cilantro

1 Line small rimmed baking sheet with parchment paper and set aside. Bring 2 quarts water to boil in large saucepan. Add barley and 1½ teaspoons salt and cook, adjusting heat to maintain gentle boil, until barley is tender with slight chew, about 22 minutes.

2 Whisk vinegar, miso, soy sauce, sesame oil, vegetable oil, ginger, garlic, sugar, and pepper flakes together in large bowl.

3 Drain barley. Transfer to prepared sheet and spread into even layer. Let stand until no longer steaming, about 6 minutes. Add barley to bowl with dressing and toss to coat. Add celery, carrot, and cilantro and stir to combine. Season with salt and pepper to taste. Serve.

PREP AHEAD
You can slice the celery and grate the ginger and carrot up to 1 day ahead and refrigerate separately.

Creamy Orzo with Boursin

SERVES 2 — SUPER EASY

Why This Recipe Works This extra-creamy pasta side for two is just the thing to cozy up to after a long day, and it is so easy to make. It also pairs well with the simplest of main courses like pan-seared salmon, roast chicken, and seared pork chops, making a satisfying weeknight dinner easy to pull off. The secret? A few tablespoons of Boursin cheese, which adds both herby flavor and creaminess in a flash. Cooking the orzo on the stovetop with a little garlic, oil, and broth yields a dish that's all the more comforting thanks to its ease. Using a relatively small amount of broth means that there is no need to wait long to achieve the creamy, saucy consistency we prefer; stirring the orzo encourages it to release its starch into the cooking liquid, and as a result it thickens up almost as if by magic. This recipe can be doubled, but you will need to use a large saucepan.

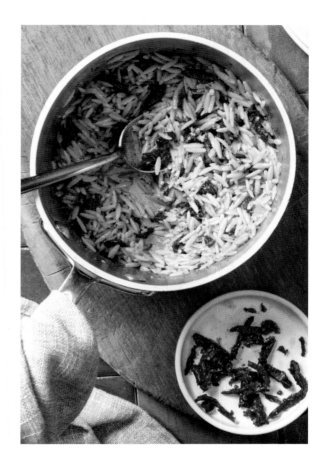

> 1 tablespoon extra-virgin olive oil
> ½ cup orzo
> 1 garlic clove, minced
> 1¾ cups vegetable or chicken broth, plus extra as needed
> 3 tablespoons Boursin

1 Cook oil, orzo, and garlic in small saucepan over medium heat until fragrant, about 1 minute. Stir in broth, bring to simmer, and cook, stirring often, until orzo is tender, about 19 minutes.

2 Off heat, vigorously stir in Boursin until creamy. Adjust consistency with extra hot broth as needed and season with salt and pepper to taste. Serve.

VARIATIONS

Orzo with Pesto and Sun-Dried Tomatoes

Substitute 1 tablespoon pesto for Boursin. Stir in ¼ cup thinly sliced oil-packed sun-dried tomatoes before serving.

Orzo with Shallot, Capers, and Dill

Omit garlic and Boursin. Cook 1 small minced shallot in oil until softened, about 2 minutes, before adding orzo. Stir 1 tablespoon rinsed capers and 1 tablespoon chopped fresh dill into orzo before serving.

Easy Cuban Black Beans

SERVES 2 — SUPER EASY

Why This Recipe Works I love shortcuts in the kitchen, as long as they don't sacrifice quality. When it comes to beans, the canned variety is frequently the best way to go: They are quick and easy but also offer the added bonus of utilizing their body-building bean liquid, also known in plant-based circles as aquafaba. This recipe draws its inspiration from Cuba, where spiced black beans are a staple. A quick sofrito of shallot, garlic, and bell pepper combined with cumin and oregano adds plenty of earthy flavor to simple canned black beans. Mashing some of the beans gives them a creamy texture, but leaving a portion whole keeps the dish from becoming soup. Serve with lime wedges; sour cream; and sliced avocado, if desired.

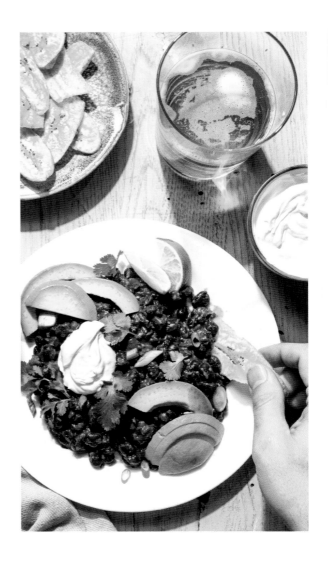

1	tablespoon vegetable oil
1	large shallot, minced
½	green bell pepper, chopped fine
2	garlic cloves, minced
¼	teaspoon dried oregano
¼	teaspoon ground cumin
⅛	teaspoon pepper
1	(15-ounce) can black beans, drained with liquid reserved, divided

1 Heat oil in medium saucepan over medium heat until shimmering. Add shallot and bell pepper and cook until softened and beginning to brown, about 5 minutes. Stir in garlic, oregano, cumin, and pepper and cook until fragrant, about 30 seconds. Turn off heat.

— TAKE A 10-MINUTE BREAK —

2 Add ½ cup beans and all reserved bean liquid to saucepan and mash with potato masher until mostly smooth. Stir in remaining beans. Cook over medium heat until warmed through, about 2 minutes. Season with salt and pepper to taste. Serve.

PREP AHEAD

You can mince the shallot and chop the pepper up to 1 day ahead and refrigerate separately. Cooked black beans can be refrigerated for up to 2 days.

Garlicky Braised Chickpeas

SERVES 2 — SUPER EASY

Why This Recipe Works This nutritious and super-easy side dish is an homage to the power and versatility of canned chickpeas. This dish, which tastes like it takes hours, can actually be on your table in less than 15 minutes. Consisting of little more than chickpeas and sticky-sweet toasted garlic, it has the toasty, lemony flavor of hummus with the hearty savor of whole beans. The bean liquid already present in a can of chickpeas helps thicken the rich sauce that clings to and glazes the chickpeas as it reduces. You will need an 8- or 10-inch skillet with a tight-fitting lid for this recipe.

- 2 tablespoons extra-virgin olive oil
- 2 garlic cloves, sliced thin
- 1 large shallot, minced
- 1 (15-ounce) can chickpeas
- 1 tablespoon minced fresh parsley, cilantro, or chives
- 1 teaspoon lemon juice, plus lemon wedges for serving

1   Cook oil and garlic in 8- or 10-inch skillet over medium-low heat, stirring occasionally, until garlic turns pale gold, about 2 minutes. Stir in shallot and cook until softened, about 2 minutes. Stir in chickpeas and their liquid; cover; and cook until chickpeas have warmed through, about 2 minutes.

2   Uncover; increase heat to medium; and simmer until liquid has reduced slightly, about 3 minutes. Off heat, stir in parsley and lemon juice and season with salt and pepper to taste. Serve with lemon wedges.

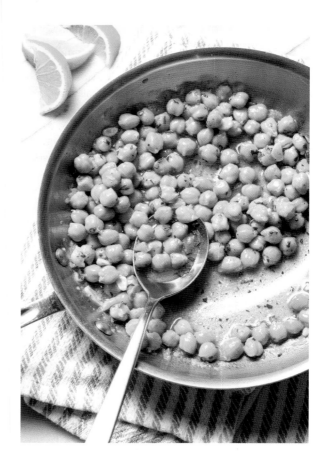

PREP AHEAD
You can mince the shallot up to 1 day ahead and refrigerate. Braised chickpeas can be refrigerated for up to 2 days.

TAKE IT UP A NOTCH
Drizzle with flavored olive oil, serve with yogurt, and/or sprinkle with herbs. Add cooked pasta and/or wilted greens such as spinach, kale, or Swiss chard, or serve over a swoosh of lemony yogurt with a side of pita.

Bean Gratin with Rosemary Parmesan

SERVES 4

Why This Recipe Works This is yet another hearty side dish that will encourage you to keep your pantry stocked with canned beans. It delivers a warm casserole of white beans infused with rosemary and enriched with Parmesan with very little cooking time. In traditional versions of this appealing Tuscan dish, dried beans are gently cooked for hours over low heat, allowing the beans to break down and bind together. To make this more practical as a side dish for four (and much faster), the key is to use convenient, time-saving canned beans. Mashing some of the beans before adding them to the dish gives the finished product the creamy, saucy texture of long-simmered beans. Broiling the beans in broth allows them to absorb the rich, savory flavor. You will need an 8-inch square broiler-safe baking dish or pan for this recipe. Note that you can also make this recipe in a toaster oven. This recipe can be easily doubled using a 13 by 9-inch broiler-safe baking pan. Depending on your broiler strength, you may need to increase or decrease cooking time to get the desired effect.

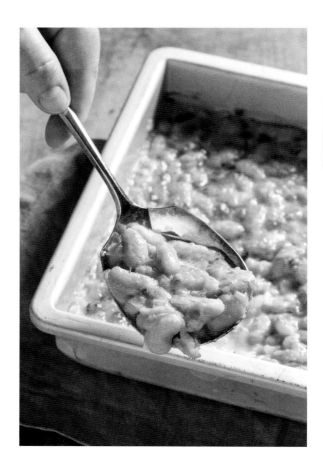

1 onion, chopped fine
2 tablespoons extra-virgin olive oil
3 garlic cloves, minced
1 teaspoon minced fresh rosemary or
   ¼ teaspoon dried
2 (15-ounce) cans white or cannellini beans,
   rinsed, divided
½ cup vegetable or chicken broth
2 ounces grated Parmesan cheese (1 cup)

1 Microwave onion, oil, garlic, and rosemary in medium bowl, stirring occasionally, until onion is softened, about 5 minutes.

2 Place rack 8 inches from broiler and preheat broiler. Add ⅔ cup beans to bowl with onion mixture and mash with potato masher until smooth. Stir in broth and remaining whole beans until combined.

3 Transfer mixture to 8-inch square broiler-safe baking dish or pan and sprinkle evenly with Parmesan. Broil until mixture is bubbling around edges and cheese is golden brown, about 6 minutes. Transfer dish to wire rack and let cool slightly before serving.

PREP AHEAD
You can chop the onion up to 1 day ahead and refrigerate.

Pan-Steamed Asparagus with Garlic

SERVES 6 — SUPER EASY

Why This Recipe Works Asparagus is one of my go-to sides because it always seems to elevate even the simplest meal. Here the asparagus steams in a small amount of water in a skillet along with butter, salt, and garlic. Once the water evaporates, the asparagus is perfectly crisp-tender and glossed with garlicky butter. This recipe works best with asparagus spears that are about ½ inch thick. If using thinner spears, reduce the uncovered cooking time to 1½ to 2 minutes. You will need a 12-inch skillet with a tight fitting lid for this recipe. This recipe can easily be halved; use a 10-inch skillet.

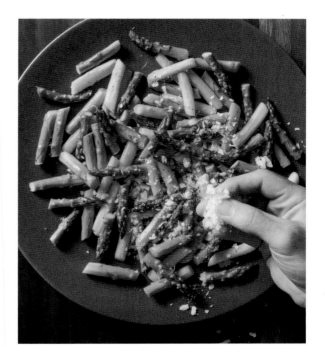

- 2 pounds asparagus
- 1 tablespoon unsalted butter
- 2 tablespoons water
- 1 garlic clove, minced
- ½ teaspoon table salt

1 Trim bottom inch of asparagus spears; discard trimmings. Peel bottom halves of spears until white flesh is exposed. Cut spears on bias into 2-inch lengths. Melt butter in 12-inch nonstick skillet over medium-high heat. Add water, garlic, and salt and stir to combine. Add asparagus, shaking skillet to evenly distribute. Cover and cook, without stirring, for 2 minutes.

2 Uncover and continue to cook, stirring occasionally, until skillet is almost dry and asparagus is crisp-tender, about 3 minutes. Transfer to bowl and serve.

VARIATIONS

Pan-Steamed Asparagus with Mint and Almonds

Combine ¼ cup chopped fresh mint, 2 teaspoons sherry vinegar, and ¼ teaspoon smoked paprika in small bowl. Stir mint mixture into asparagus and sprinkle with ¼ cup sliced almonds, toasted, cooled, and lightly crushed, just before serving.

Pan-Steamed Asparagus with Lemon and Parmesan

Combine 1 teaspoon grated lemon zest plus 1 tablespoon juice and ¼ teaspoon pepper in small bowl. Stir lemon zest mixture into asparagus and sprinkle with ¼ cup shredded Parmesan before serving.

Pan-Steamed Asparagus with Shallots and Herbs

Substitute ¼ cup minced shallots for garlic. Stir ¼ cup chopped fresh chives and 2 teaspoons chopped fresh dill into asparagus before serving.

PREP AHEAD
You can trim the asparagus up to 1 day ahead and refrigerate, wrapped in a damp dish towel.

Roasted Baby Carrots with Sage and Walnuts

SERVES 4 — SUPER EASY

Why This Recipe Works Bagged baby carrots are
a real time saver for home cooks, but if you are counting on them to be the star of a dish versus playing a
supporting role, as in a stew or a braise, you need a plan.
This recipe makes the most of them in two ways:
Tossing them with microwaved butter and honey adds
richness and sweetness, and spreading them on a
very hot (preheated) small rimmed baking sheet jump-
starts the cooking, allowing them to reach caramelized
perfection in 20 minutes. You do have to shake the
baking sheet once or twice during this cooking time
to ensure even cooking, but you certainly don't need
to stand by the oven that whole time. Note that you
can also make this recipe in a toaster oven.

1½ tablespoons unsalted butter
 1 tablespoon honey
 1 (16-ounce) bag baby carrots
 ¼ cup walnuts, toasted and chopped
1½ teaspoons finely chopped fresh sage

1   Preheat oven to 475 degrees. Heat small rimmed
baking sheet in oven, on middle rack, for 10 minutes.
Microwave butter and honey in medium bowl until
butter melts, about 1 minute.

2   Toss carrots with butter mixture in bowl. Spread
carrots on heated baking sheet. Return baking sheet to
oven and roast, shaking pan occasionally, until carrots
are browned and tender, about 20 minutes. Return
carrots to empty bowl and toss with walnuts and sage.
Season with salt and pepper. Serve.

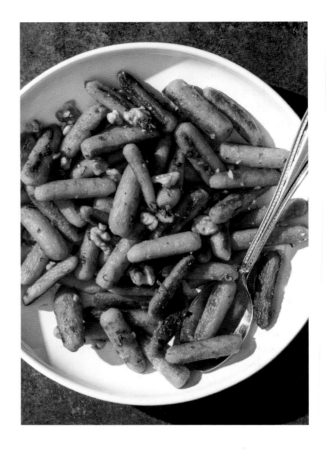

PREP AHEAD
You can toast and chop the walnuts up to 1 day ahead;
You can also toast the walnuts in the microwave (see
page 37).

Skillet-Charred Broccoli

SERVES 4

Why This Recipe Works Believe it or not, charred broccoli is my 6-year-old daughter's favorite side dish. What I like about it is that the process of charring gives broccoli a deeply roasted, lightly smoky flavor and crispy edges. Using a heavy hand with extra-virgin olive oil— a full 6 tablespoons—is the key to creating super-crispy florets. Barely stirring the broccoli for the first portion of the cooking allows it to develop dark, frizzled edges. You do have to stir it more frequently toward the end of cooking so that all the pieces are equally browned and tender. Smoked paprika plays up the natural smokiness of the charred broccoli, and some fragrant basil adds freshness for a side dish that is anything but ordinary— and well worth the little time spent minding the stove. The skillet may look very full when you add the broccoli in step 1, but the pieces of broccoli will shrink as they cook. In step 2, the broccoli pieces will begin to look very dark; this is OK.

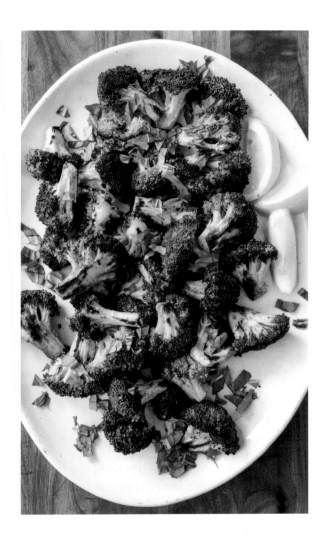

6	tablespoons extra-virgin olive oil
1½	pounds broccoli florets, cut into 2-inch pieces
1	teaspoon smoked paprika
¾	teaspoon table salt
½	teaspoon ground coriander
¼	teaspoon pepper
2	tablespoons chopped fresh basil
	Lemon wedges

1 Heat oil in 12-inch nonstick skillet over medium heat until shimmering. Add broccoli, paprika, salt, coriander, and pepper and stir to combine. Cook until broccoli is dark brown and crispy in spots, about 15 minutes, stirring every 5 minutes.

2 Continue to cook until broccoli is tender and well charred, about 7 minutes, stirring once every 2 to 3 minutes as needed. Transfer broccoli to platter. Season with salt and pepper to taste. Sprinkle with basil and serve with lemon wedges.

PREP AHEAD
You can cut up the broccoli up to 1 day ahead and refrigerate.

MAKE IT EVEN EASIER
Buy broccoli florets.

Garlicky Broccolini

SERVES 4 — SUPER EASY

Why This Recipe Works Broccolini, a nice alternative to broccoli, requires very little prep and cooks quickly. Here, it is steam-cooked in a small amount of water to emerge emerald green and perfectly cooked in just 5 minutes. A simple combination of minced garlic and red pepper flakes sautéed in a little oil right in the skillet after the broccolini is cooked, plus a sprinkling of Parmesan cheese before serving, elevates this simple side. Halving the bottom 2 inches of the thicker broccolini stalks lengthwise ensures that the stalks cook evenly. You will need a 12-inch nonstick skillet with a tight-fitting lid for this recipe.

- 2 tablespoons extra-virgin olive oil
- 2 garlic cloves, minced
- ⅛ teaspoon red pepper flakes
- ⅓ cup water
- ½ teaspoon table salt
- 1 pound broccolini, trimmed, bottom 2 inches of stems thicker than ½ inch halved lengthwise
- 2 tablespoons grated Parmesan cheese

1   Combine oil, garlic, and pepper flakes in bowl. Bring water and salt to boil in 12-inch nonstick skillet. Add broccolini; cover; reduce heat to medium-low; and cook until bright green and tender, about 5 minutes.

2   Uncover and cook until liquid evaporates, about 30 seconds. Clear center of skillet, add garlic mixture, and cook, mashing mixture into skillet, until fragrant, about 30 seconds. Stir garlic mixture into broccolini. Transfer to platter, sprinkle with Parmesan, and serve.

PREP AHEAD
You can prep the broccolini up to 1 day ahead and refrigerate.

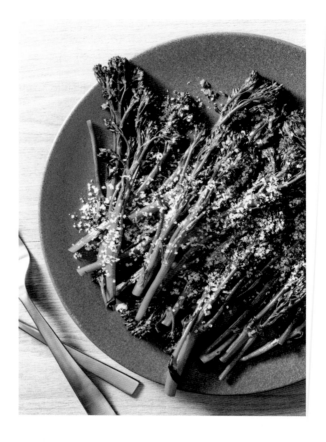

VARIATIONS

Broccolini with Shallots
Combine 2 tablespoons extra-virgin olive oil, 2 teaspoons minced shallot, 1 teaspoon grated lemon zest, 1 teaspoon minced fresh thyme, and ¼ teaspoon pepper in bowl. Replace garlic mixture with shallot mixture.

Broccolini with Capers and Lemon
Combine 2 tablespoons extra-virgin olive oil, 1 tablespoon rinsed and minced capers, 1 teaspoon grated lemon zest, and ¼ teaspoon pepper in bowl. Replace garlic mixture with caper mixture.

Instant Pot Braised Whole Cauliflower

SERVES 6

Why This Recipe Works Whole braised cauliflower is a showstopper. Here, you first make an intensely savory cooking liquid of garlic, optional anchovies, ras el hanout, and tomatoes in the Instant Pot. Deep cuts in the cauliflower stem allow the liquid and heat to reach the center, which renders the whole head perfectly tender. Note that it will take 10 minutes for the Instant Pot to come up to pressure and start the cook cycle.

- 2 tablespoons extra-virgin olive oil
- 6 garlic cloves, minced
- 3 anchovy fillets, rinsed and minced (optional)
- 2 teaspoons ras el hanout
- ⅛ teaspoon red pepper flakes
- 1 (28-ounce) can whole peeled tomatoes, drained with juice reserved, chopped coarse
- 1 large head cauliflower (3 pounds)
- ½ cup pitted brine-cured green olives, chopped coarse
- ¼ cup golden raisins
- ¼ cup fresh cilantro leaves
- ¼ cup pine nuts, toasted

1 Using highest sauté function, cook oil; garlic; anchovies (if using); ras el hanout; and pepper flakes in electric pressure cooker until fragrant, about 3 minutes. Turn off electric pressure cooker, then stir in tomatoes and reserved juice.

2 Trim outer leaves of cauliflower and cut stem flush with bottom florets. Using paring knife, cut 4-inch-deep cross in stem. Nestle cauliflower stem side down into pot and spoon some of sauce over top. Lock lid in place and close pressure release valve. Select high pressure cook function and cook for 3 minutes.

— TAKE A 13-MINUTE BREAK —

3 Turn off electric pressure cooker and quick-release pressure. Carefully remove lid, allowing steam to escape away from you. Using tongs and slotted spoon, transfer

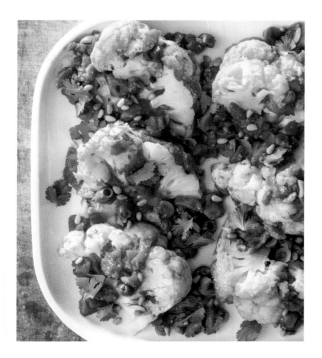

cauliflower to serving dish and tent with aluminum foil. Stir olives and raisins into sauce and cook, using highest sauté function, until sauce has thickened slightly, about 5 minutes. Season with salt and pepper to taste. Cut cauliflower into wedges and spoon some of sauce over top. Sprinkle with cilantro and pine nuts. Serve, passing remaining sauce separately.

PREP AHEAD

You can drain and chop the tomatoes (reserve the liquid), chop the olives, and toast the pine nuts up to 1 day ahead. (Refrigerate the tomatoes and their liquid and the olives separately.) You can also toast the pine nuts in the microwave (see page 37).

MAKE IT EVEN EASIER

Use 1½ teaspoons anchovy paste instead of anchovies.

Elote

SERVES 2

Why This Recipe Works This Mexican-style street corn, charred and slathered with a mixture of mayonnaise, queso fresco, lime juice, garlic, and more is a staple at every street fair in New York City, where I live. To bring this messy street food into a home kitchen, broiling corn on the cob in the oven instead of heading out to the grill keeps things easy. Brushing the corn with oil helps create good charring. Note that you can also make this recipe in a toaster oven, and the recipe can be easily doubled. Depending on your broiler strength, you may need to increase or decrease the cooking time. Feta cheese can be substituted for the queso fresco.

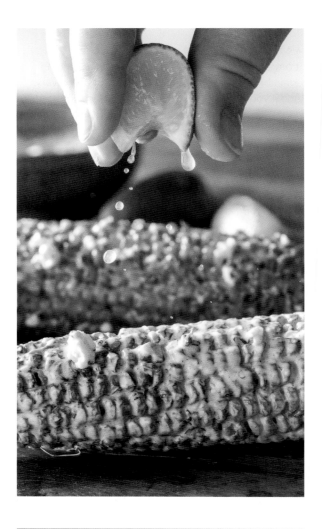

2 ears corn, husks and silk removed, stalks left intact
1 teaspoon extra-virgin olive oil
3 tablespoons mayonnaise
1 tablespoon crumbled queso fresco
1 tablespoon minced fresh cilantro
1 teaspoon lime juice, plus lime wedges for serving
1 small garlic clove, minced
¼ teaspoon chili powder
Pinch table salt

1 Position rack 6 inches from broiler element and preheat broiler. Brush corn all over with oil and transfer to aluminum foil–lined small rimmed baking sheet. Broil corn until well browned on 1 side, about 10 minutes. Flip corn and broil until browned on opposite side, about 10 minutes longer.

2 Meanwhile, whisk mayonnaise, queso fresco, cilantro, lime juice, garlic, chili powder, and salt in bowl until incorporated. Remove corn from oven and brush evenly on all sides with mayonnaise mixture. Season with salt and pepper to taste. Serve corn with lime wedges and any extra mayonnaise mixture.

PREP AHEAD
You can make the mayonnaise mixture up to 1 day ahead and refrigerate.

MAKE IT EVEN EASIER
Buy already shucked corn.

Sautéed Snow Peas with Lemon and Parsley

SERVES 4 — SUPER EASY

Why This Recipe Works Sweet, grassy snow peas are the star component in this superspeedy side. Make it once and I'm certain you will turn to it again and again because it is simplicity itself, and easy to vary. And if you organize your ingredients before you start to cook, everything comes together very quickly. Adding a sprinkle of sugar, salt, and pepper and cooking the peas without stirring for a short time helps to achieve a flavorful sear; you then continue to cook them, stirring constantly, until they are just crisp-tender. To boost flavor, clear the center of the pan and quickly sauté a mixture of minced shallot, oil, and lemon zest before stirring everything together. A squeeze of lemon juice and a sprinkling of parsley just before serving keeps the snow peas fresh and bright.

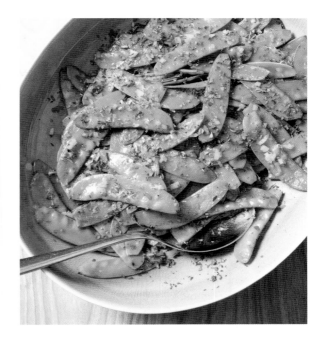

1	tablespoon vegetable oil, divided
1	small shallot, minced
1	teaspoon finely grated lemon zest plus 1 teaspoon juice, divided
¼	teaspoon table salt
⅛	teaspoon pepper
⅛	teaspoon sugar
12	ounces snow peas, strings removed
1	tablespoon minced fresh parsley

1 Combine 1 teaspoon oil, shallot, and lemon zest in bowl. In separate bowl, combine salt, pepper, and sugar.

2 Heat remaining 2 teaspoons oil in 12-inch nonstick skillet over high heat until just smoking. Add snow peas; sprinkle with salt mixture; and cook, without stirring, for 30 seconds. Stir briefly, then cook, without stirring, for 30 seconds. Continue to cook, stirring constantly, until peas are crisp-tender, about 2 minutes.

3 Push peas to sides of skillet. Add shallot mixture to center and cook, mashing mixture into skillet, until fragrant, about 30 seconds. Stir shallot mixture into peas. Stir in lemon juice and parsley and season with salt and pepper to taste. Serve.

VARIATIONS

Sautéed Snow Peas with Garlic, Cumin, and Cilantro

Add 2 minced garlic cloves and ½ teaspoon toasted and cracked cumin seeds to shallot mixture in step 1. Substitute ½ teaspoon lime zest for lemon zest, lime juice for lemon juice, and cilantro for parsley.

Sautéed Snow Peas with Lemongrass and Basil

Substitute 2 teaspoons minced fresh lemongrass for lemon zest, lime juice for lemon juice, and basil for parsley.

PREP AHEAD
You can mince the shallot and prep the snow peas up to 1 day ahead and refrigerate separately.

Skillet-Charred Green Beans

SERVES 2 — SUPER EASY

Why This Recipe Works Green beans are often sold loose, so it's easy to buy the precise amount you need, making them a great option when cooking for two—but how can you turn an average green bean side into something special? Answer: Burn them (partially, that is). When blistered and browned, beans have a light chew and concentrated flavor. Many skillet-charred green bean recipes require precooking the green beans before charring them in the skillet; this hybrid skillet method allows you to first steam and then char them without changing the cooking vessel. First, cook the beans covered with a small amount of water, steaming them until crisp-tender. After uncovering the beans, the oil chars their outsides, giving them a deep, almost smoky flavor. Once the beans finish cooking, you just toss them in lemon zest and juice for a bright hit of citrus flavor. You will need a 10- or 12-inch nonstick skillet with a tight-fitting lid for this recipe.

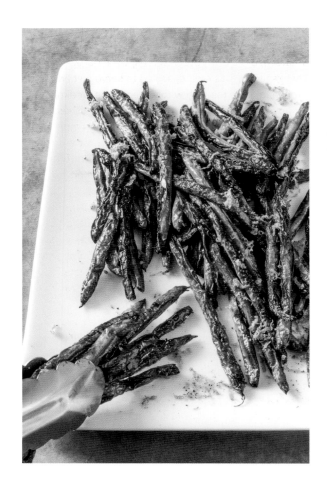

12	ounces trimmed green beans
2	tablespoons water
1	tablespoon extra-virgin olive oil
⅛	teaspoon table salt
⅛	teaspoon pepper
½	teaspoon grated lemon zest plus 1 teaspoon juice

1   Combine green beans, water, oil, salt, and pepper in 10- or 12-inch nonstick skillet. Cover and cook over medium-high heat, shaking skillet occasionally, until water has evaporated, about 7 minutes.

2   Uncover and continue to cook until green beans are blistered and browned, about 2 minutes. Off heat, stir in lemon zest and juice and season with salt and pepper to taste. Serve.

MAKE IT EVEN EASIER
Buy trimmed green beans.

TAKE IT UP A NOTCH
Sprinkle with chopped or slivered almonds. Drizzle with chili oil, harissa, or Herb-Yogurt Sauce (page 63).

Garlic-Parmesan Mashed Potatoes

SERVES 2

Why This Recipe Works For most of us, mashed potatoes, never mind garlic and Parmesan mashed potatoes, are a dish reserved for special occasions like Thanksgiving. This recipe, scaled to serve just two and simplified, puts the dish within reach on a weeknight for anyone with back issues because there is less of everything to deal with, and the method is simple. The first step is to simmer and drain sliced potatoes in a saucepan (not a large pot) and remove them. Then to get truly complex garlic flavor without roasting garlic, it is added in three ways: a garlic paste sautéed in butter for clean, mellow flavor; a small amount of rehydrated garlic powder for complex, lightly roasted flavor; and a very small amount of raw garlic paste for assertiveness. In order to maximize the garlic powder's flavor, it is important to first bloom it in water to reactivate the enzyme that produces the compound allicin, which is responsible for garlic's characteristic flavor.

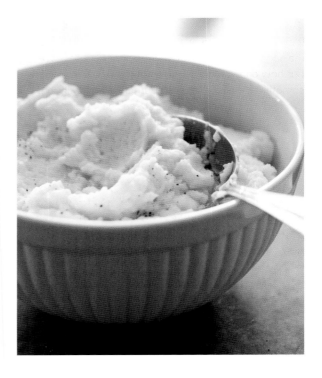

1	pound Yukon Gold potatoes, peeled and sliced ½ inch thick
¼	teaspoon garlic powder
2	tablespoons unsalted butter, cut into 2 pieces
½	teaspoon garlic, minced to paste, divided
1	ounce grated Parmesan cheese (½ cup)
½	teaspoon table salt
¼	teaspoon pepper
⅓	cup warm whole milk

1   Place potatoes in medium saucepan, add water to cover by 1 inch, and bring to simmer over medium-high heat. Adjust heat to maintain gentle simmer and cook until paring knife can be easily slipped in and out of potatoes, about 20 minutes.

— TAKE A 20-MINUTE BREAK —

2   Drain potatoes. Combine garlic powder and ¼ teaspoon water in small bowl. Melt butter in now-empty saucepan over medium-low heat.

Stir in ⅜ teaspoon garlic paste and garlic powder mixture; cook, stirring constantly, until fragrant and golden, about 1 minute. Transfer butter mixture to medium bowl and thoroughly stir in Parmesan, salt, pepper, and remaining ⅛ teaspoon garlic paste.

3   Place again-empty saucepan over low heat. Using potato masher, mash potatoes until almost smooth. Using rubber spatula, stir in butter mixture until incorporated. Stir in warm milk until incorporated. Season with salt and pepper to taste; serve immediately.

PREP AHEAD

You can peel and slice the potatoes up to 1 day ahead and refrigerate, covered with water in a bowl.

Baked Potatoes

SERVES 1–4 — SUPER EASY

Why This Recipe Works I never felt the need for a recipe for a baked potato, but then again I never really thought mine were perfect. Enter this clever method you can use for baking one to four russet potatoes. It is slightly more work than simply tossing potatoes in the oven and hoping for the best, but it isn't hard and makes a world of difference. Coating the potatoes in salty water just before baking gives the skin a light flavor and appetizing crunch, and then elevating them on a wire rack ensures even cooking all the way through from the increased airflow. Baking the potatoes in a very hot oven prevents a leathery film from forming underneath the peel. Once the potatoes reach 205 degrees (the temperature at which they reach their ideal doneness), remove them from the oven, brush the skins with oil, and bake for an additional 10 minutes. This method ensures potatoes with a crispy skin and perfectly fluffy interiors. Note that you can bake the potatoes in a toaster oven. Serve with a flavored butter or your favorite toppings. Do not increase salt or water in step 1 when scaling up.

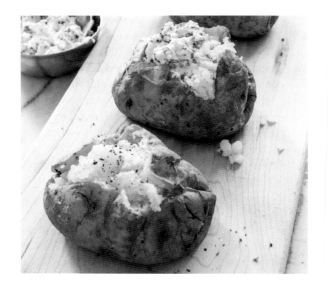

2   tablespoons table salt for brining
1–4 (7- to 9-ounce) russet potatoes, unpeeled,
     lightly pricked with fork in 6 places
1   teaspoon vegetable oil

1   Preheat oven to 450 degrees. Dissolve salt in ½ cup water in large bowl. Place potatoes in bowl and toss so exterior of potatoes is evenly moistened. Transfer potatoes to wire rack set in small rimmed baking sheet and bake, on middle rack, until center of potatoes registers 205 degrees, about 1 hour.

— TAKE A 1-HOUR BREAK —

2   Remove potatoes from oven and brush tops and sides with oil. Return potatoes to oven and continue to bake for 10 minutes.

— TAKE A 10-MINUTE BREAK —

3   Remove potatoes from oven and, using paring knife, make 2 slits, forming X, in each potato. Using clean dish towel, hold ends and squeeze slightly to push flesh up and out. Season with salt and pepper to taste. Serve immediately.

TAKE IT UP A NOTCH
Serve with Blue Cheese–Pepper Butter
Mash 2 tablespoons softened unsalted butter, 1 tablespoon crumbled blue cheese, and ¼ teaspoon pepper together in bowl. You can make the butter up to 1 week ahead and refrigerate, sealed in plastic wrap. Makes enough for 2 potatoes.

Serve with Lemon-Thyme Butter
Mash 2 tablespoons softened unsalted butter, 1 teaspoon minced fresh thyme, ¼ teaspoon grated lemon zest, and ¼ teaspoon juice together in bowl. You can make the butter up to 1 week ahead and refrigerate, sealed in plastic wrap, until using. Makes enough for 2 potatoes.

Braised Red Potatoes with Lemon and Chives

SERVES 4

Why This Recipe Works I love to make a big sheet pan of golden, crispy roasted potatoes, especially when I have company, but I know bending down to get a big sheet pan into and out of the oven for a side dish would be a nonstarter for most of my patients. But what if you could get red potatoes with the creamy interiors created by steaming and the crispy browned exteriors produced by roasting—without doing either? That's the result promised by recipes for braised red potatoes, but they rarely deliver. This recipe, however, makes good on that promise. Halved small red potatoes, along with butter and salted water (plus thyme for flavoring), are simmered in a 10-inch skillet until their interiors are perfectly creamy and the water is fully evaporated. Letting the potatoes continue to cook in the now-dry skillet until their cut sides brown in the butter develops the rich flavor and crisp edges of roasted potatoes. These crispy, creamy potatoes are so good they need only a minimum of seasoning: Simply toss with some minced garlic (softened in the simmering water along with the potatoes), lemon juice, chives, and pepper. Use small red potatoes measuring about 1½ inches in diameter.

1	pound small red potatoes, unpeeled, halved
1½	cups water
2	tablespoons unsalted butter
2	garlic cloves, peeled
2	sprigs fresh thyme
½	teaspoon table salt
1	teaspoon lemon juice
⅛	teaspoon pepper
4	teaspoons minced fresh chives

1 Arrange potatoes in single layer, cut side down, in 10-inch nonstick skillet. Add water, butter, garlic, thyme sprigs, and salt and bring to simmer over medium-high heat. Reduce heat to medium, cover, and simmer until potatoes are just tender, about 15 minutes. Turn off heat and uncover skillet.

— TAKE A 15-MINUTE BREAK —

2 Transfer garlic to cutting board; discard thyme sprigs. Place skillet over medium-high heat and vigorously simmer potatoes, swirling skillet occasionally, until water evaporates and butter starts to sizzle, about 15 minutes. Mince garlic to paste, transfer to bowl, and stir in lemon juice and pepper.

3 Continue to cook potatoes, swirling skillet frequently, until butter browns and cut sides of potatoes turn spotty brown, about 5 minutes. Off heat, add garlic mixture and chives and toss to thoroughly coat. Serve immediately.

VARIATIONS

Braised Red Potatoes with Miso and Scallions
Reduce salt to ¼ teaspoon. Substitute 2 teaspoons red miso for lemon juice and 2 thinly sliced scallions for chives.

Braised Red Potatoes with Dijon and Tarragon
Substitute 1½ teaspoons Dijon mustard for lemon juice and 2 teaspoons minced fresh tarragon for chives.

PREP AHEAD
You can halve the potatoes up to 1 day ahead and refrigerate, covered with water in a bowl.

Easy Air-Fryer Sides

There are many reasons to cook vegetables in your air fryer, and not just fried renditions of them. The air fryer's convection heat ably cooks vegetables of all kinds—without hogging valuable oven or stovetop space. The other appeal of using the air-fryer to make vegetable sides is that it frees you up to focus on your main course or make a beautiful salad.

Air-Fryer Roasted Asparagus
Serves 4

- 1 pound asparagus, trimmed and halved crosswise
- 1 teaspoon extra-virgin olive oil
- ⅛ teaspoon table salt
- ⅛ teaspoon pepper
- Lemon wedges

Toss asparagus with oil, salt, and pepper in bowl; transfer to air-fryer basket. Place basket in air fryer and set temperature to 400 degrees. Cook asparagus until tender and bright green, 6 to 8 minutes, tossing halfway through cooking. Season with salt and pepper to taste. Serve with lemon wedges.

PREP AHEAD
You can trim and halve the asparagus up to 1 day ahead and refrigerate, wrapped in a damp dish towel.

TAKE IT UP A NOTCH
Serve with Mint-Orange Gremolata
Combine 2 tablespoons minced fresh mint, 2 tablespoons minced fresh parsley, 2 teaspoons grated orange zest, 1 minced garlic clove, and pinch cayenne pepper in bowl. Makes about ⅓ cup.

Serve with Tarragon-Lemon Gremolata
Combine 2 tablespoons minced fresh tarragon, 2 tablespoons minced fresh parsley, 2 teaspoons grated lemon zest, and 1 minced garlic clove in bowl. Makes about ⅓ cup.

Air-Fryer Brussels Sprouts
Serves 4

If you are buying loose Brussels sprouts, select those that are about 1½ inches long. Quarter Brussels sprouts longer than 2½ inches. If desired, add 3 thinly sliced shallots to the Brussels sprouts when adding to the air fryer.

- 1 pound Brussels sprouts, trimmed and halved
- 1 tablespoon extra-virgin olive oil
- ¼ teaspoon table salt
- ⅛ teaspoon pepper
- Lemon wedges

Toss Brussels sprouts with oil, salt, and pepper in bowl; transfer to air-fryer basket. Place basket in air fryer and set temperature to 350 degrees. Cook Brussels sprouts until tender; well browned; and crispy, about 22 minutes, tossing halfway through cooking. Season with salt and pepper to taste. Serve with lemon wedges.

PREP AHEAD
You can trim and halve the Brussels sprouts up to 1 day ahead and refrigerate.

MAKE IT EVEN EASIER
Buy trimmed and halved Brussels sprouts.

TAKE IT UP A NOTCH
Serve with Lemon-Chive Dipping Sauce
Whisk ¼ cup mayonnaise, 1 tablespoon minced fresh chives, ½ teaspoon grated lemon zest plus 2 teaspoons juice, ½ teaspoon Worcestershire sauce, ½ teaspoon Dijon mustard, and ¼ teaspoon garlic powder together in bowl. Dipping sauce can be refrigerated for up to 2 days. Makes about ⅓ cup.

Air-Fryer Roasted Eggplant with Capers, Oregano, and Garlic

Serves 4

If baby eggplant is unavailable, two 1-pound eggplants can be substituted; halve it lengthwise before slicing it crosswise. If your air fryer is smaller than 6 quarts, you may need to cook in batches.

- 4 baby eggplants (8 to 10 ounces each), sliced into 1-inch-thick rounds
  Olive oil spray
- ½ teaspoon table salt
- ¼ teaspoon pepper
- 2 tablespoons extra-virgin olive oil
- 2 teaspoons capers, rinsed and minced
- 2 teaspoons minced fresh oregano
- 1 large garlic clove, minced
- 1 teaspoon grated lemon zest plus 4 teaspoons juice

1   Lightly spray both sides of eggplant with oil spray and sprinkle with salt and pepper. Arrange eggplant in even layer in air-fryer basket (pieces may overlap). Place basket in air fryer and set temperature to 350 degrees. Cook until eggplant is deep golden brown, about 18 minutes, flipping eggplant halfway through cooking.

2   Whisk oil, capers, oregano, garlic, and lemon zest and juice together in large bowl. Add eggplant and toss gently to combine. Serve warm or at room temperature.

PREP AHEAD

Roasted eggplant can be refrigerated for up to 3 days. Let come to room temperature before serving.

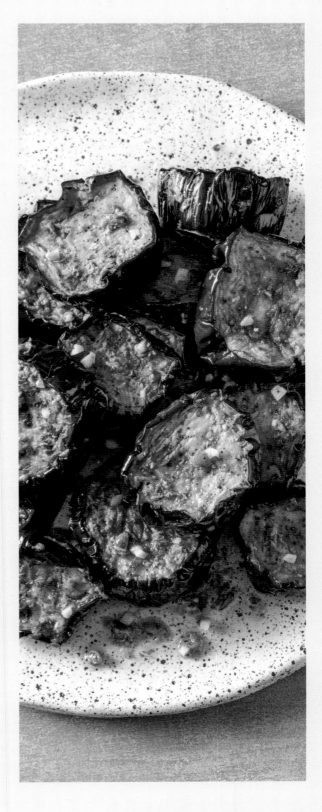

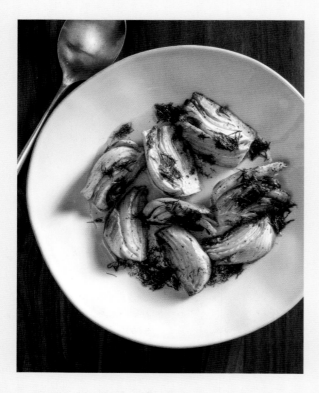

Air-Fryer Roasted Fennel with Orange-Honey Dressing

Serves 4

Look for fennel bulbs that measure 3½ to 4 inches in diameter and weigh around 1 pound with the stalks; trim so that the bulb remains intact.

2 fennel bulbs, base lightly trimmed, 2 tablespoons fronds chopped coarse, stalks discarded
¼ cup extra-virgin olive oil, divided
1 tablespoon water
½ teaspoon table salt
½ teaspoon pepper
4 teaspoons honey
1 tablespoon white wine vinegar
¼ teaspoon grated orange zest plus 1 tablespoon juice

1 Cut fennel bulbs lengthwise through core into 8 wedges (do not remove core). Whisk 2 tablespoons oil, water, salt, and pepper in large bowl until salt has dissolved. Add fennel wedges and toss gently to coat.

2 Arrange fennel wedges cut side down in air-fryer basket (wedges may overlap). Place basket in air fryer and set temperature to 350 degrees. Cook until fennel is tender and well browned, about 16 minutes, flipping wedges halfway through cooking.

3 Whisk fennel fronds, honey, vinegar, orange zest and juice, and remaining 2 tablespoons oil together in bowl. Season with salt and pepper to taste. Transfer fennel to serving platter and drizzle with dressing. Serve.

PREP AHEAD

You can trim and chop the fennel bulbs up to 1 day ahead and refrigerate.

Air-Fryer French Fries

Serves 4

Frequently tossing the potatoes ensures the most even cooking and browning. Tossing the fries in a bowl, rather than in the basket, yields the best results and the fewest broken fries. Do not clean out the tossing bowl while you are cooking; the residual oil helps the crisping process.

1½ pounds russet potatoes, peeled
2 tablespoons vegetable oil, divided
½ teaspoon table salt

1 Cut potatoes lengthwise into ½-inch-thick planks. Stack 3 or 4 planks and cut into ½-inch-thick sticks; repeat with remaining planks.

2 Submerge potatoes in large bowl of water and rinse to remove excess starch. Drain potatoes and repeat process as needed until water remains clear. Cover potatoes with hot tap water and let sit for 10 minutes. Drain potatoes, transfer to paper towel–lined rimmed baking sheet, and thoroughly pat dry.

3 Toss potatoes with 1 tablespoon oil in clean, dry bowl, then transfer to air-fryer basket. Place basket in air fryer, set temperature to 350 degrees, and cook for 8 minutes. Transfer potatoes to now-empty bowl and toss gently to redistribute. Return potatoes to air fryer

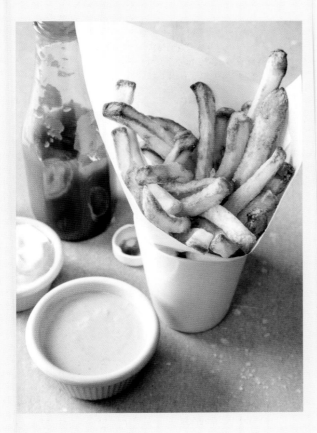

Air-Fryer Roasted Green Beans with Sun-Dried Tomatoes and Sunflower Seeds
Serves 4

- 1 pound trimmed green beans, halved
- 2 teaspoons extra-virgin olive oil, divided
- ⅛ teaspoon table salt
- ⅛ teaspoon pepper
- ½ cup torn fresh basil
- ⅓ cup oil-packed sun-dried tomatoes, rinsed, patted dry, and chopped
- 1 tablespoon lemon juice
- 2 ounces goat cheese, crumbled (½ cup)
- ¼ cup roasted sunflower seeds

1 Toss green beans with 1 teaspoon oil, salt, and pepper in bowl; transfer to air-fryer basket. Place basket in air fryer and set temperature to 400 degrees. Cook green beans until crisp-tender, about 14 minutes, tossing halfway through cooking.

2 Toss green beans with remaining 1 teaspoon oil, basil, sun-dried tomatoes, and lemon juice in large bowl. Season with salt and pepper to taste. Transfer to serving dish and sprinkle with goat cheese and sunflower seeds. Serve.

PREP AHEAD
You can trim and halve the green beans up to 1 day ahead and refrigerate.

MAKE IT EVEN EASIER
Buy trimmed green beans and jarred, chopped sun-dried tomatoes.

and cook until softened and potatoes have turned from white to blond (potatoes may be spotty brown at tips), about 8 minutes.

4 Transfer potatoes to now-empty bowl and toss with salt and remaining 1 tablespoon oil. Return potatoes to air fryer, increase temperature to 400 degrees, and cook until golden brown and crispy, about 18 minutes, tossing gently in bowl to redistribute every 5 minutes. Transfer fries to large plate and season with salt and pepper to taste. Serve immediately.

TAKE IT UP A NOTCH
Serve with Sriracha Dipping Sauce
Whisk ¼ cup mayonnaise, 1 tablespoon sriracha, 1 tablespoon lime juice, 1½ teaspoons grated fresh ginger, and ⅛ teaspoon soy sauce together in bowl. Dipping sauce can be refrigerated for up to 2 days. Makes about ⅓ cup.

Easy Slow-Cooker Sides

When you are serving four or more, and especially when you are cooking for friends and family and want to be part of the conversation, it pays to relegate a side dish to your trusty slow cooker, where the work can be done earlier in the day. This frees you up to enjoy your company when they arrive and eliminates last minute stress or the need to be chained to the stove monitoring roasted potatoes or stirring polenta. Here is an assortment of company-worthy sides that work perfectly in a slow cooker.

Slow-Cooker Red Potatoes with Rosemary and Garlic

Serves 4 to 6

Look for small red potatoes measuring 1 to 2 inches in diameter. This recipe can be easily doubled in a 7-quart slow cooker; you will need to increase the cooking time range by 1 hour.

- 2   pounds small red potatoes, unpeeled
- 2   tablespoons extra-virgin olive oil, divided
- 3   garlic cloves, minced
- ½   teaspoon table salt
- ¼   teaspoon pepper
- 1   teaspoon minced fresh rosemary

1   Combine potatoes, 1 tablespoon oil, garlic, salt, and pepper in slow cooker. Cover and cook until potatoes are tender, 5 to 6 hours on low or 3 to 4 hours on high.

— TAKE A BREAK —

2   Stir in rosemary and remaining 1 tablespoon oil. Season with salt and pepper to taste. Serve.

PREP AHEAD
Potatoes can be held on warm or low setting for up to 2 hours.

Slow-Cooker Creamy Polenta

Serves 6

Coarse-ground degerminated cornmeal such as yellow grits (with uniform grains the size of couscous) works best in this recipe. Avoid instant or quick-cooking products, as well as whole-grain, stone-ground, and regular cornmeal.

- 3   cups water, plus extra as needed
- 1   cup whole milk
- 1   cup coarse-ground cornmeal
- 2   garlic cloves, minced
- 1   teaspoon table salt
- 1   sprig fresh rosemary (optional)
- 2   ounces grated Parmesan cheese (1 cup)
- 2   tablespoons unsalted butter

1   Lightly coat slow cooker with vegetable oil spray. Whisk water, milk, cornmeal, garlic, and salt together in prepared slow cooker. Cover and cook until polenta is tender, 3 to 4 hours on low or 2 to 3 hours on high.

— TAKE A BREAK —

2   Nestle rosemary sprig, if using, into polenta; cover; and let steep for 10 minutes; discard rosemary sprig. Whisk Parmesan and butter into polenta until combined. Season with salt and pepper to taste. Serve.

PREP AHEAD
Polenta can be held on warm or low setting for up to 2 hours; adjust consistency with extra hot water as needed before serving.

Slow-Cooker Parmesan Risotto

Serves 6

You will need an oval slow cooker for this recipe.

- 1 onion, chopped fine
- 4 tablespoons unsalted butter, divided
- 3 garlic cloves, minced
- 1 teaspoon minced fresh thyme or ¼ teaspoon dried
- ½ teaspoon table salt
- 5 cups vegetable or chicken broth, divided, plus extra as needed
- ½ cup dry white wine
- 2 cups arborio rice
- 2 ounces grated Parmesan cheese (1 cup)
- 2 tablespoons minced fresh chives
- 1 teaspoon lemon juice

1 Lightly coat slow cooker with vegetable oil spray. Microwave onion, 2 tablespoons butter, garlic, thyme, and salt in bowl, stirring occasionally, until onion is softened, about 5 minutes; transfer to prepared slow cooker.

2 Microwave 2 cups broth and wine in 4-cup liquid measuring cup until steaming, about 5 minutes. Stir broth mixture and rice into slow cooker. Gently press 16 by 12-inch sheet of parchment paper onto surface of broth mixture, folding down edges as needed. Cover and cook until rice is almost fully tender and all liquid is absorbed, 2 to 3 hours on high.

— TAKE A 2- TO 3-HOUR BREAK —

3 Microwave remaining 3 cups broth in now-empty measuring cup until steaming, about 5 minutes. Discard parchment. Slowly stream broth into rice, stirring gently, until liquid is absorbed and risotto is creamy, about 1 minute. Gently stir in remaining 2 tablespoons butter, Parmesan, chives, and lemon juice until combined. Adjust consistency with extra hot broth as needed. Season with salt and pepper to taste. Serve.

PREP AHEAD

You can chop the onion up to 1 day ahead and refrigerate.

Slow-Cooker Brown Rice with Peas, Feta, and Mint

Serves 6

For an accurate measurement of boiling water, bring a full kettle of water to a boil and then measure out the desired amount. You will need an oval slow cooker for this recipe.

- 3 cups boiling water
- 2 cups long-grain brown rice, rinsed
- 1 tablespoon unsalted butter
- ½ teaspoon table salt
- 1 cup frozen peas, thawed
- 2 ounces feta cheese, crumbled (½ cup)
- ¼ cup chopped fresh mint
- 2 teaspoons lemon juice

1 Lightly spray inside of slow cooker with vegetable oil spray. Combine boiling water, rice, butter, and salt in slow cooker. Gently press 16 by 12-inch sheet of parchment paper onto surface of water, folding down edges as needed. Cover and cook until rice is tender and all water is absorbed, 1 to 2 hours on high.

— TAKE A 1- TO 2-HOUR BREAK —

2 Discard parchment. Fluff rice with fork, then gently fold in peas, feta, mint, and lemon juice. Season with salt and pepper to taste. Serve.

PREP AHEAD

You can crumble the feta cheese up to 1 day ahead and refrigerate.

Sauces

*That Jump-Start
Dinner*

* Try these recipes first if today is not one of your better days and you need a soul-refilling recipe with high return on your energy investment.

Pesto Sauces

MAKES ABOUT 1½ CUPS
ENOUGH FOR 2 POUNDS PASTA

Able to dress up just about anything, pesto is one of the most versatile sauces you can make. And a food processor allows you to make it in minutes once your ingredients are prepped. I remember the first time I made pesto: I couldn't believe something so good could come from so few components. Pestos can be prepared with a variety of ingredients—traditional basil, other herbs and greens like parsley, arugula, and kale, and even potent ingredients like sun-dried tomatoes and olives. The pesto recipes here make a large quantity, so you can stock your freezer with them, making a weeknight pasta dinner super easy. They are also great to have on hand to dollop on pizza or grilled chicken or fish, swirl into soup, spread on a sandwich, or to make bruschetta—just to name a few ideas. In addition to a flavorful base, there are a few basic requirements: Use a high-quality extra-virgin olive oil (its flavor will really shine through) and add some type of nuts or seeds (to give the pesto richness and body). When you're tossing the pesto with cooked pasta, it is important to add some pasta cooking water to achieve the proper sauce consistency. See page 288 for a method for cooking pasta for two using a large saucepan. See page 37 for a method for toasting nuts in the microwave. To make prep work easier, use your kitchen shears to remove basil and parsley leaves.

PREP AHEAD

You can refrigerate these pestos for up to 3 days or freeze for up to 2 months. To prevent browning, press plastic wrap flush to surface or top with thin layer of olive oil. Bring to room temperature before using.

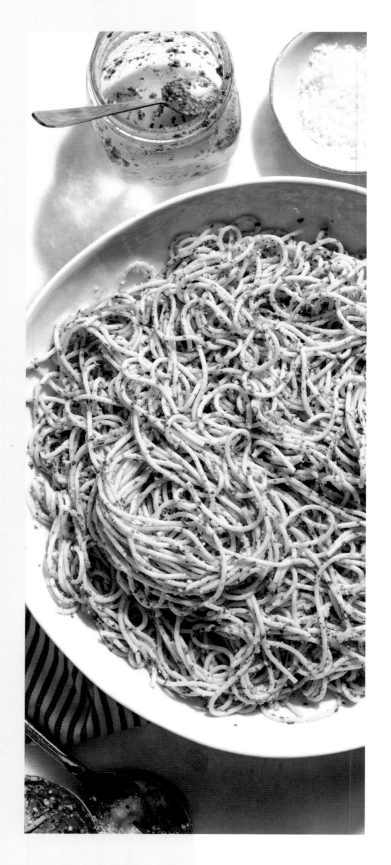

Classic Basil Pesto

This classic pesto tastes great slathered on a wrap or panini or used as a base for bruschetta.

- 4 cups fresh basil leaves
- ¼ cup fresh parsley leaves
- ½ cup pine nuts, toasted
- 6 garlic cloves, peeled
- 1 cup plus 2 tablespoons extra-virgin olive oil
- 1 ounce grated Parmesan cheese (½ cup)

Process basil, parsley, pine nuts, and garlic in food processor until finely chopped, about 1 minute, scraping down sides of bowl as needed. With processor running, slowly add oil until incorporated. Transfer pesto to bowl, stir in Parmesan, and season with salt and pepper to taste.

VARIATIONS

Toasted Walnut and Parsley Pesto

Omit basil and increase parsley to ¾ cup. Substitute 2 cups toasted walnuts for pine nuts.

Arugula and Ricotta Pesto

Part-skim ricotta can be substituted here, but do not use nonfat ricotta or the pesto will be dry and gummy.

Substitute 2 cups baby arugula for basil and increase parsley to 2 cups. Reduce Parmesan to ¼ cup and stir ⅔ cup whole-milk ricotta cheese into pesto with Parmesan.

Kale and Sunflower Seed Pesto

This assertive pesto makes a great topping for pizza or bruschetta and is delicious tossed with roasted potatoes or carrots, served with gnocchi, or spooned over grilled swordfish or steak.

- 4 ounces baby kale (2 cups)
- 1 cup fresh basil leaves
- ½ cup raw sunflower seeds, toasted
- 2 garlic cloves, peeled
- 1 teaspoon red pepper flakes (optional)
- ½ cup plus 2 tablespoons extra-virgin olive oil
- 1½ ounces grated Parmesan cheese (¾ cup)

Process kale; basil; sunflower seeds; garlic; and pepper flakes, if using, in food processor until finely chopped, about 1 minute, scraping down sides of bowl as needed.

With processor running, slowly add oil until incorporated. Transfer pesto to bowl, stir in Parmesan, and season with salt and pepper to taste.

Green Olive and Orange Pesto

This pesto is great swirled into hummus or spooned over fish. Use high-quality green olives here.

- 1½ cups fresh parsley leaves
- ½ cup slivered almonds, toasted
- ½ cup pitted brine-cured green olives
- 2 garlic cloves, peeled
- ½ teaspoon grated orange zest plus 2 tablespoons juice
- ½ cup plus 2 tablespoons extra-virgin olive oil
- 1½ ounces grated Parmesan cheese (¾ cup)

Process parsley, almonds, olives, garlic, and orange zest and juice in food processor until finely chopped, about 1 minute, scraping down sides of bowl as needed. With processor running, slowly add oil until incorporated. Transfer pesto to bowl, stir in Parmesan, and season with salt and pepper to taste.

Sun-Dried Tomato Pesto

This pesto is great as a filling for rolled chicken breasts and pork tenderloin or spooned over simply prepared broccoli rabe. It also brings a grilled cheese sandwich to the next level: Simply slather some on the bread before adding the cheese and cooking the sandwich.

- 1 cup oil-packed sun-dried tomatoes, patted dry and chopped
- ¼ cup walnuts, toasted
- 3 garlic cloves, peeled
- ½ cup plus 2 tablespoons extra-virgin olive oil
- 1 ounce grated Parmesan cheese (½ cup)

Process tomatoes, walnuts, and garlic in food processor until finely chopped, about 1 minute, scraping down sides of bowl as needed. With processor running, slowly add oil until incorporated. Transfer pesto to bowl, stir in Parmesan, and season with salt and pepper to taste.

Pasta Sauces

Here are a variety of pasta sauces that are quite versatile and easy to prep and cook. A couple of them make large batches, so you can stock your freezer with portions, ensuring that dinner—be it a simple bowl of pasta or a recipe like lasagna that uses a sauce—is in easy reach. I rely on these at home more than I care to admit; they are perfect for those tough days when you need something delicious to sustain you.

Below you will find a method for perfectly cooking pasta for two in a large saucepan. And see page 291 for a method for cooking a pound of pasta directly in sauce thinned with water in a skillet (several from this chapter will work). Make sure to reserve some of the starchy pasta water if you are boiling your pasta as it will help thicken the sauce.

HOW TO COOK PASTA FOR TWO

This method allows you to cook a smaller amount of pasta in far less water in a large saucepan instead of a larger pot. Any pasta shape will work with this method. If using long-strand pasta, loosely wrap it in a dish towel and then press the bundle against the corner of a counter to break the noodles in half.

½ pound pasta
   Table salt for cooking pasta

Bring 2 quarts water to boil in large saucepan. Add 1½ teaspoons salt and pasta and cook, stirring occasionally, until al dente. Drain and serve with sauce.

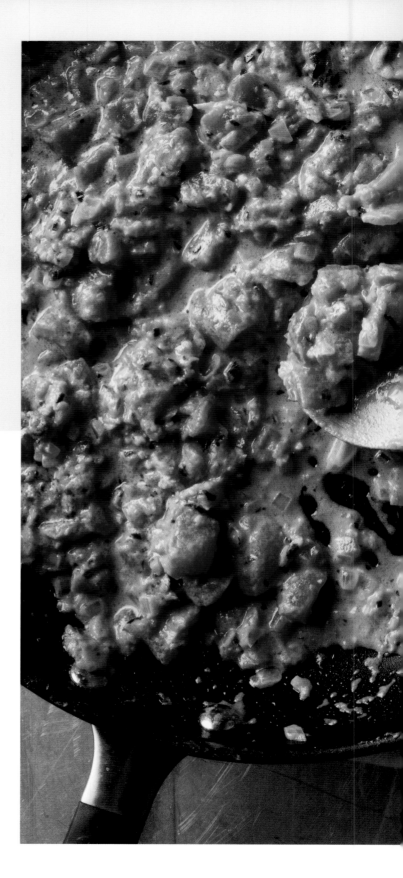

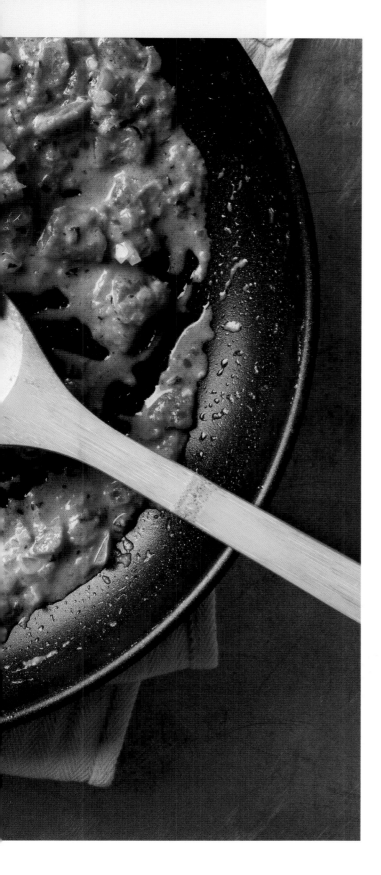

Pomodoro Sauce

Makes about 4 cups — ***enough for 1 pound pasta***

Tomatoes meet cream in this classic sauce that is also characterized by an assertive tomato flavor and chunky texture. The sauce is quintessentially Italian in its simplicity—it's quick to make but packs a flavor punch that belies its basic ingredient list. A hefty amount of aromatics gives the sauce great backbone, and the heavy cream offers instant velvety richness. Canned diced tomatoes have great tomato flavor and are a perfect way to get the right chunky texture since they hold their shape nicely during the cooking time.

- 2 tablespoons extra-virgin olive oil
- 1 onion, chopped fine
- 2 teaspoons dried oregano
- 4 garlic cloves, minced
- ½ teaspoon red pepper flakes
- 1 (28-ounce) can diced tomatoes
- ⅔ cup heavy cream
- ½ teaspoon table salt

Heat oil in medium saucepan over medium heat until shimmering. Add onion and cook until softened and lightly browned, about 6 minutes. Stir in oregano, garlic, and pepper flakes and cook until fragrant, about 30 seconds. Stir in tomatoes and their juice, cream, and salt. Bring to simmer and cook, stirring occasionally, until reduced to about 4 cups, about 15 minutes. Season with salt and pepper to taste.

VARIATION

Pomodoro Sauce with Fennel and Capers

Omit salt. Increase garlic to 6 cloves. Substitute 1 thinly sliced fennel bulb for onion, 1 teaspoon minced fresh thyme for pepper flakes, and white wine for cream. Add 1 tablespoon rinsed capers to saucepan with tomatoes.

PREP AHEAD

You can chop the onion up to 1 day ahead and refrigerate. You can refrigerate the sauce for up to 1 week or freeze for up to 2 months.

Slow-Cooker Classic Marinara

Makes about 10 cups — enough for 3 pounds pasta

Stocking your freezer with homemade marinara sauce is a great way to ensure that dinner is within reach on busy nights—or whenever you don't feel like spending much time in the kitchen. Plus, the marinara has many uses beyond saucing pasta. Use it on a pizza, or to make lasagna, chicken or eggplant Parmesan, or any other dish calling for a simple tomato sauce. And the slow cooker is a great way to make a big batch, so you always have marinara on hand. The key is to choose the right tomato products since there is no evaporation possible during the long cooking time as there would be if made on the stovetop. A combination of three different tomato products (tomato paste, crushed tomatoes, and tomato puree) does the trick. The concentrated products (paste and puree) provide strong, complex flavor without adding unwanted water. To ensure the right depth of flavor overall without any stovetop work, microwave the aromatics with oil and the tomato paste before adding them to the slow cooker. A little sugar added at the end of the cooking time balances the acidity of this brightly flavored sauce.

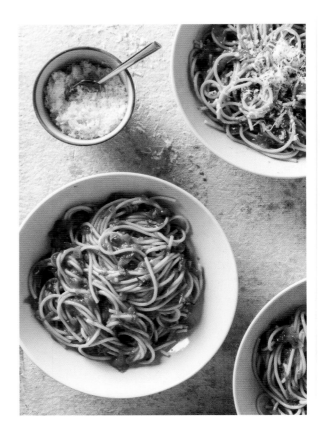

- 2   onions, chopped fine
- 6   garlic cloves, minced
- 2   tablespoons tomato paste
- 2   tablespoons extra-virgin olive oil
- 2   teaspoons dried oregano
- 1   teaspoon table salt
- 2   (28-ounce) cans crushed tomatoes
- 1   (28-ounce) can tomato puree
- ½   cup dry red wine
- 2   teaspoons sugar, plus extra for seasoning
    Chopped fresh basil

1   Microwave onions, garlic, tomato paste, oil, oregano, and salt in bowl, stirring occasionally, until onions are softened, about 5 minutes; transfer to slow cooker. Stir in tomatoes, tomato puree, and wine. Cover and cook until sauce is deeply flavored, 8 to 10 hours on low or 5 to 7 hours on high.

—   **TAKE A BREAK**   —

2   Stir sugar into sauce. Season with salt, pepper, and extra sugar to taste. Before serving, stir in 2 tablespoons basil for every 5 cups sauce.

PREP AHEAD

You can chop the onions up to 1 day ahead and refrigerate. You can refrigerate the sauce for up to 1 week or freeze for up to 2 months; stir in basil after reheating.

TAKE IT UP A NOTCH
Mussels Marinara

Combine 2 cups sauce and 2 pounds mussels in 12-inch skillet, cover, and cook over medium heat for 10 to 12 minutes, until mussels have opened and are cooked through. Discard any mussels that have not opened. Serve with crusty bread. Serves 2 to 3.

Puttanesca Sauce

Makes about 3 cups   —   enough for 1 pound pasta

This vibrant pasta sauce has its roots in Naples and, as legend has it, originated with the "ladies of the night." It is certainly a robust sauce given its combination of anchovy fillets, red pepper flakes, olives, and capers. I love it for its bright flavors but also because it can be easily assembled and requires only 10 minutes simmering time, making it the perfect pantry pasta sauce for the healthy back kitchen. Feel free to use 2 teaspoons anchovy paste instead of the fillets.

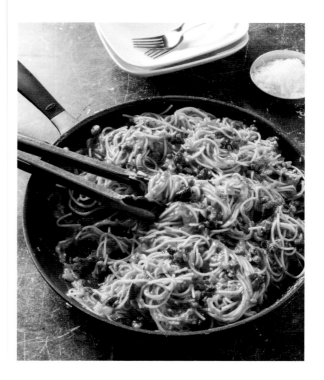

- 2 tablespoons unsalted butter
- ¼ cup finely chopped onion
- 4 anchovy fillets, rinsed and minced
- ½ teaspoon red pepper flakes
- ½ teaspoon table salt
- ¼ teaspoon dried oregano
- 2 garlic cloves, minced
- 1 (28-ounce) can crushed tomatoes
- ¼ teaspoon sugar
- ¼ cup pitted kalamata olives, chopped
- 3 tablespoons capers, rinsed and minced
- 1 tablespoon extra-virgin olive oil

1 Melt butter in medium saucepan over medium-low heat. Add onion, anchovies, pepper flakes, salt, and oregano and cook, stirring occasionally, until onion is softened and lightly browned, about 4 minutes. Stir in garlic and cook until fragrant, about 30 seconds.

2 Stir in tomatoes and sugar, bring to simmer, and cook until thickened slightly, about 10 minutes. Off heat, stir in olives, capers, and oil. Season with salt and pepper to taste.

PREP AHEAD

You can chop the onion, anchovies, olives, and capers up to 1 day ahead and refrigerate separately. You can refrigerate the sauce for up to 1 week or freeze for up to 2 months.

HOW TO MAKE SKILLET PASTA MARINARA, PUTTANESCA, OR ARRABBIATA

This handy method allows you to cook pasta in the sauce instead of filling and draining a large pot. Any pasta shape will work with the method. If using long-strand pasta, loosely wrap half of it in a dish towel and then press the bundle against a corner of a counter to break the noodles in half; repeat with the remaining noodles.

Combine 3 cups sauce, 2 cups water, and 1 pound pasta in 12-inch skillet and bring to simmer over medium-high heat. Reduce heat to medium; cover; and cook, stirring often, until pasta is al dente. Top with chopped parsley and serve with grated Parmesan. Serves 4 to 6.

Arrabbiata Sauce

Makes about 3 cups — enough for 1 pound pasta

This easy-to-make sauce replicates the long-simmered flavor of traditional tomato sauce, but with a spicy kick. It starts with onions—finely diced for more surface area—that are caramelized in butter for added richness. Dried herbs and garlic complete the base flavors. Canned crushed tomatoes, which require no chopping or pureeing, are the bulk of the sauce, and a pinch of sugar rounds out their tang.

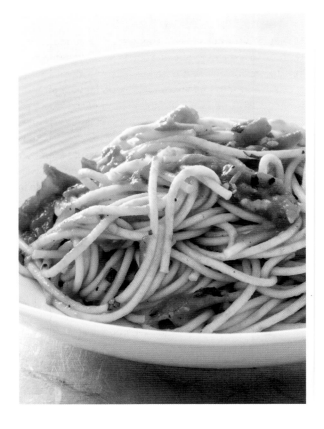

2	tablespoons unsalted butter
¼	cup finely chopped onion
¼–¾	teaspoon red pepper flakes
½	teaspoon table salt
¼	teaspoon dried oregano
4	garlic cloves, minced
1	(28-ounce) can crushed tomatoes
¼	teaspoon sugar
2	tablespoons chopped fresh parsley
1	tablespoon extra-virgin olive oil

1   Melt butter in medium saucepan over medium-low heat. Add onion, pepper flakes, salt, and oregano and cook, stirring occasionally, until onion is softened and lightly browned, about 4 minutes. Stir in garlic and cook until fragrant, about 30 seconds.

2   Stir in tomatoes and sugar, bring to simmer, and cook until thickened slightly, about 10 minutes.

—   TAKE A 10-MINUTE BREAK   —

3   Off heat, stir in parsley and oil and season with salt and pepper to taste.

PREP AHEAD

You can chop the onion up to 1 day ahead and refrigerate. You can refrigerate the sauce for up to 1 week or freeze for up to 2 months.

TAKE IT UP A NOTCH

Shrimp Arrabbiata

Bring 1 cup Arrabbiata Sauce to simmer in 10-inch skillet over medium heat. Add ½ pound peeled and deveined extra-large shrimp and cook for 3 to 5 minutes, until shrimp are opaque. Serve over pasta or polenta. Serves 2. See method for cooking pasta for two in a saucepan on page 288.

Slow-Cooker Bolognese

Makes about 7 cups — enough for 2 pounds pasta

Bolognese is the king of pasta sauces and the ultimate comfort food. I rarely have a leisurely afternoon to make it, as it takes a fair amount of minding the stove to first incorporate the milk and then the wine into the meat, not to mention the long simmering time. This easy, big-batch slow-cooker recipe has all the flavor and rich meatiness of traditional versions but needs less attention. So it's perfect for the healthy back kitchen, and you will feel rich indeed when you have batches of Bolognese in your freezer. To solve the problem of how to incorporate the dairy that tenderizes the meat and gives Bolognese its hallmark richness, an unconventional solution is key: a panade, which is typically a mixture of bread and milk, but here, cream provides extra richness. Mix the meat and panade and add it raw to the slow cooker. At the end of hours of hands-off cooking, you'll have a rich Bolognese with concentrated flavor and a tender texture that rivals a long-simmering stovetop version. If you cannot find meatloaf mix, substitute ¾ pound 85 percent lean ground beef and ¾ pound ground pork.

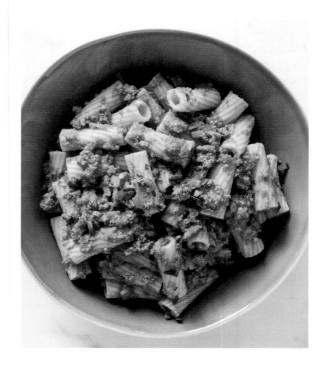

1½	tablespoons unsalted butter
½	onion, chopped fine
½	carrot, peeled and chopped fine
2	tablespoons minced celery
2	tablespoons tomato paste
2	garlic cloves, minced
⅛	teaspoon dried thyme
¼	cup dry white wine
1½	slices hearty white sandwich bread, torn into 1-inch pieces
½	cup heavy cream
¼	teaspoon table salt
¼	teaspoon pepper
1½	pounds meatloaf mix
1	(28-ounce) can crushed tomatoes

1   Melt butter in 10-inch skillet over medium heat. Add onion, carrot, and celery and cook until softened and lightly browned, about 9 minutes. Stir in tomato paste, garlic, and thyme and cook until fragrant, about 1 minute. Stir in wine, scraping up any browned bits; transfer to slow cooker.

2   Mash bread, cream, salt, and pepper into paste in large bowl using fork. Add meatloaf mix and knead with hands until well combined. Stir meatloaf mixture and tomatoes into slow cooker until combined. Cover and cook until meat is tender, 9 to 10 hours on low or 6 to 7 hours on high.

— **TAKE A BREAK** —

3   Using large spoon, skim fat from surface of sauce. Break up any remaining large pieces of meat with spoon. Season with salt and pepper to taste. Serve.

PREP AHEAD
You can chop the onion, carrot, and celery up to 1 day ahead and refrigerate separately. You can refrigerate the sauce for up to 1 week or freeze for up to 2 months.

MAKE IT EVEN EASIER
Buy mirepoix and substitute it for the onion, carrot, and celery; you will need ¾ cup.

Simmering Sauces 101

Supermarkets now carry a variety of jarred simmering sauces, but homemade versions taste worlds better and are easy to make. Unlike stir-fry sauces, which are added at the very end of fast-cooking stir-fries, these sauces are used as cooking mediums, so they can infuse food with flavor more thoroughly. I cannot think of an easier way to put a fresh and highly flavorful dinner on the table with very little work. Plus, it is fun to mix and match chicken, fish, shrimp, or tofu with a variety of homemade simmering sauces. You can also add vegetables and fresh herbs. Each of these sauces makes 4 cups of sauce, so you will be able to stash some in the freezer to use later since 1 to 2 cups of sauce (depending on the protein used) is enough to serve four. You can also halve the sauce amounts if serving just two. You can make these simmering sauces in a medium saucepan, but you will need either a 10- or 12-inch skillet when combining sauce and protein depending on whether you are cooking for two or four.

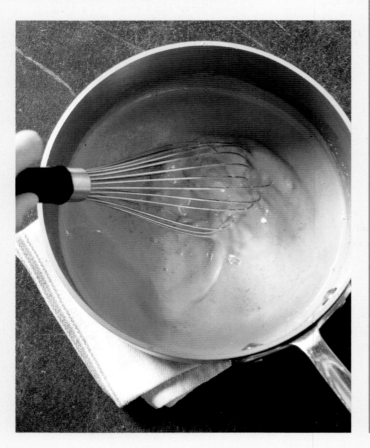

START WITH THE RIGHT CUT AND BROWN IF NECESSARY

For quick simmers, lean boneless, skinless chicken breasts, fish fillets, shrimp, and tofu require little preparation besides a sprinkle of salt and pepper. Bone-in chicken breasts or thighs require trimming, browning, and a longer simmering time. Make sure to pat proteins dry before browning or simmering.

ADD SAUCE, SIMMER, AND COOK

If making your sauce from scratch (versus using sauce that has been frozen and thawed) follow the chart at right and make sure it has simmered for the required amount of time before adding protein. Bring frozen and thawed sauces to a simmer before adding protein. Position protein in an even layer in the skillet, and make sure to bring the sauce and protein to a simmer on the stovetop before continuing to ensure even heating. And unless you are cooking delicate fish, you should stir or flip the protein halfway through cooking.

ADD VEGETABLES IF DESIRED

If using quick-cooking proteins, you can add vegetables like thawed frozen peas, snow peas, small broccoli or cauliflower florets, or greens like spinach or thinly sliced baby bok choy in the last 5 minutes of cooking. For boneless chicken, you can add 1-inch pieces of potatoes, sliced carrots, green beans, sliced bell pepper strips, or sliced celery at the beginning; for bone-in chicken, add these vegetables in the last 15 minutes of the cooking time. Stir in fresh herbs like parsley and cilantro just before serving.

PREP AHEAD

All simmering sauces can be refrigerated for up to 1 day ahead or frozen for up to 2 months.

How To Use Simmering Sauces
ENOUGH FOR 4 SERVINGS

If serving just 2, cut the protein amounts in half, use half the sauce amount, and cook in a 10-inch skillet.

PROTEIN AND PREPARATION	SAUCE AMOUNT AND TYPES	COOKING INSTRUCTIONS AND PAIRINGS
4 boneless, skinless chicken breasts or 8 boneless, skinless thighs *Trimmed*	2 cups Cacciatore, Simple Curry, Ginger-Sesame (and variations), Extra-Spicy, Sweet and Tangy, or Mole-Style Simmering Sauce	Simmer chicken in sauce, covered, in 12-inch skillet over medium-low heat until chicken breasts register 160 degrees or chicken thighs register 195 degrees, 15 to 20 minutes. Serve over rice, couscous, pasta, or polenta depending on sauce used.
2 pounds bone-in chicken pieces *Trimmed, browned in a skillet, and skin removed*	2 cups Cacciatore, Simple Curry, Ginger-Sesame (and variations), Sweet and Tangy, or Mole-Style Simmering Sauce	Simmer chicken in sauce, covered, in 12-inch skillet over medium-low heat until chicken breasts register 160 degrees, 20 to 25 minutes, and/or chicken thighs/drumsticks register 195 degrees, 45 to 50 minutes. Serve over rice, couscous, pasta, or polenta depending on sauce used.
4 skinless fish fillets, 1 to 1½ inches thick	2 cups Simple Curry, Ginger-Sesame (and variations), Extra-Spicy, Sweet and Tangy, or Mole-Style Simmering Sauce	Simmer fish in sauce, covered, in 12-inch skillet over medium-low heat until fish flakes apart when gently prodded with paring knife, about 10 minutes. Serve over rice.
1 pound peeled and deveined extra-large shrimp (21 to 25 per pound)	1 cup Simple Curry, Ginger-Sesame (and variations), Extra-Spicy, or Sweet and Tangy Simmering Sauce	Simmer shrimp in sauce in 12-inch skillet over medium-low heat until shrimp are opaque throughout, 3 to 5 minutes. Serve over rice.
1 pound extra-firm tofu *Cut into ¾-inch-thick cubes and drained for 20 minutes on paper towels*	1 cup Simple Curry, Ginger-Sesame (and variations), Extra-Spicy, Sweet and Tangy, or Mole-Style Simmering Sauce	Simmer tofu in sauce, covered, in 12-inch skillet, over medium-low heat until heated through, about 15 minutes. Serve over rice.

Cacciatore Simmering Sauce

Makes about 4 cups

This rustic tomato sauce, also known as "hunter-style" (cacciatore means hunter in Italian), features earthy mushrooms, garlic, onion, and red wine as well as a hefty amount of oregano. It is traditionally paired with chicken, although you could certainly just toss it with pasta alone. Chicken cacciatore requires some simmering time, especially if using bone-in chicken, but the sauce itself couldn't be easier and requires only 15 minutes cooking time once you add the tomatoes.

2 tablespoons extra-virgin olive oil
1 onion, chopped fine
6 ounces cremini mushrooms, thinly sliced
2 tablespoons minced fresh oregano or 2 teaspoons dried
4 garlic cloves, minced
1 (28-ounce) can diced tomatoes
⅔ cup dry red wine
½ teaspoon table salt

1   Heat oil in medium saucepan over medium heat until shimmering. Add onion and mushrooms and cook until vegetables are dry and lightly browned, about 10 minutes. Stir in oregano and garlic and cook until fragrant, about 30 seconds. Stir in tomatoes and their juice, wine, and salt. Bring to simmer and cook, stirring occasionally, until reduced to about 4 cups, about 15 minutes.

2   Season with salt and pepper to taste.

PREP AHEAD

You can chop the onion and slice the mushrooms up to 1 day ahead and refrigerate separately. You can make the sauce up to 1 day ahead or freeze for up to 2 months.

MAKE IT EVEN EASIER
Buy sliced mushrooms.

Simple Curry Simmering Sauce

Makes about 4 cups

This curry sauce is heavily dependent on spices and other aromatics, so it pays to first bloom them to bring out their flavors. The sauce pairs well with nearly any protein (see chart on page 295) and also vegetables such as thawed frozen peas, small diced potatoes or sweet potatoes, cauliflower florets, sliced carrots, or thawed pearl onions. For a spicier sauce, use Madras curry powder.

¼ cup vegetable oil
1 onion, chopped fine
6 garlic cloves, minced
2 tablespoons grated fresh ginger
2 tablespoons curry powder
3½ cups vegetable or chicken broth
1 cup heavy cream
1 tablespoon cornstarch
2 teaspoons honey

1   Heat oil in medium saucepan over medium heat until shimmering. Add onion and cook until softened, about 5 minutes. Stir in garlic, ginger, and curry powder and cook until fragrant, about 1 minute. Stir in broth; bring to simmer; and cook, stirring occasionally, until reduced to about 3 cups, about 22 minutes.

2   Whisk cream, cornstarch, and honey in bowl until cornstarch and honey have dissolved and no lumps remain, then whisk mixture into sauce. Return to simmer and cook until slightly thickened, about 3 minutes. Season with salt and pepper to taste.

PREP AHEAD

You can chop the onion and grate the ginger up to 1 day ahead and refrigerate separately. You can make the sauce up to 1 day ahead or freeze for up to 2 months.

Ginger-Sesame Simmering Sauce

Makes about 4 cups

This crave-worthy simmering sauce will transform just about any protein you choose (see chart on page 295). It is very ginger forward in flavor given that it uses a hefty 2 tablespoons grated fresh ginger. Scallions are sautéed along with the ginger to build a solid base and then a combination of water, fragrant oyster sauce, and a little soy sauce creates the sauce itself. With just 6 minutes of simmering, all the flavors meld beautifully. For the right consistency, a mixture of cornstarch and water provides the requisite silkiness.

- 2 scallions, minced
- 6 garlic cloves, minced
- 2 tablespoons grated fresh ginger
- 2 teaspoons vegetable oil
- 3¾ cups water, divided
- ½ cup oyster sauce
- 1 tablespoon soy sauce
- 2½ tablespoons cornstarch
- 2 tablespoons sesame seeds, toasted
- 2 tablespoons toasted sesame oil

1 Cook scallions, garlic, ginger, and vegetable oil in medium saucepan over medium heat, stirring frequently, until fragrant but not browned, about 2 minutes. Stir in 3½ cups water, oyster sauce, and soy sauce. Bring to simmer and cook until flavors meld and sauce has reduced to about 4 cups, about 6 minutes.

2 Whisk remaining ¼ cup water and cornstarch in bowl until no lumps remain. Whisk mixture into sauce and simmer until slightly thickened, about 2 minutes. Off heat, whisk in sesame seeds and sesame oil.

VARIATIONS

Sichuan Peppercorn–Ginger Simmering Sauce

You can crack the peppercorns using a mortar and pestle.

Omit sesame seeds. Add 1½ tablespoons cracked Sichuan peppercorns to saucepan with scallions.

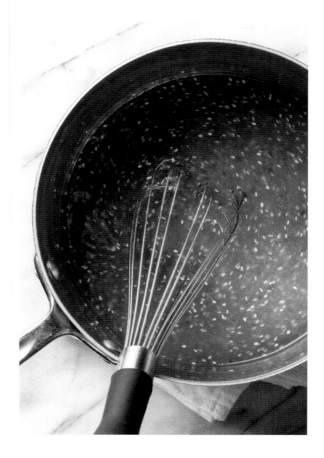

Orange-Chile Simmering Sauce

For a spicier sauce, use the larger amount of chiles.

Substitute 2 to 4 dried Thai bird chiles, toasted and coarsely chopped, for scallions. Reduce ginger to 2 teaspoons. Stir 1 tablespoon grated orange zest into sauce with sesame seeds.

PREP AHEAD

You can mince the scallions and grate the ginger up to 1 day ahead and refrigerate separately. You can toast the sesame seeds up to 1 day ahead. You can make the sauce up to 1 day ahead or freeze for up to 2 months.

MAKE IT EVEN EASIER

Buy toasted sesame seeds.

Extra-Spicy Simmering Sauce

Makes about 4 cups

Dried bird or arbol chiles give this sharp and sweet sauce a distinctive punch of heat that is tempered by a cup of Chinese black vinegar. Equal amounts of oyster and hoisin sauce round out the salty-sweet profile: Hoisin, made with fermented soybean paste, is thick and sweet with warm spices, while oyster sauce, made from oyster extract, is salty and just mildly sweet. Broth, instead of water, adds overall savory notes to this balanced and delicious sauce that perfectly coats proteins like tofu, shrimp, chicken, and fish (see chart on page 295).

- 6 dried Thai bird or arbol chiles, stemmed
- 2½ cups vegetable or chicken broth, divided
- 1 cup Chinese black vinegar or unseasoned rice vinegar
- ½ cup oyster sauce
- ½ cup hoisin sauce
- 2 tablespoons cornstarch
- ⅓ cup toasted sesame oil

1 Toast chiles in medium saucepan over medium-high heat, stirring frequently, until fragrant, about 4 minutes. Stir in 2¼ cups broth, vinegar, oyster sauce, and hoisin sauce and bring to simmer. Cook, stirring occasionally, until flavors meld and sauce has reduced to about 4 cups, about 10 minutes.

2 Whisk remaining ¼ cup broth and cornstarch in bowl until no lumps remain. Whisk mixture into sauce and simmer until slightly thickened, about 2 minutes. Off heat, whisk in sesame oil.

PREP AHEAD

You can make the sauce up to 1 day ahead or freeze for up to 2 months.

Sweet and Tangy Simmering Sauce

Makes about 4 cups

When a milder simmering sauce is called for, this sweet and tangy one with a base of pineapple juice is the one to make. Many stir-fries marry chunks of pineapple with a sweet soy-based sauce, a combination that is superappealing. This simmering sauce takes the same approach, where the sweetness of the juice, brown sugar, and ketchup is balanced with a hefty amount of soy sauce and rice vinegar. Two tablespoons of grated fresh ginger plus garlic ensures that it doesn't tilt into too-sweet territory. This sauce is especially good paired with chicken and tofu, but you can pair it with shrimp or fish as well (see chart on page 295).

- 3 cups pineapple juice, divided
- ⅓ cup soy sauce
- ⅓ cup ketchup
- ⅓ cup unseasoned rice vinegar
- ⅓ cup packed light brown sugar
- 2 tablespoons grated fresh ginger
- 4 garlic cloves, minced
- 2 teaspoons chili-garlic sauce
- 3 tablespoons cornstarch

1 Bring 2¾ cups pineapple juice, soy sauce, ketchup, vinegar, sugar, ginger, garlic, and chili-garlic sauce to simmer in medium saucepan over medium heat. Cook, stirring occasionally, until flavors meld and sauce has reduced to about 4 cups, about 10 minutes.

2 Whisk remaining ¼ cup pineapple juice and cornstarch in bowl until no lumps remain. Whisk mixture into sauce and simmer until slightly thickened, about 2 minutes.

PREP AHEAD

You can grate the ginger up to 1 day ahead and refrigerate. You can make the sauce up to 1 day ahead or freeze for up to 2 months.

Mole-Style Simmering Sauce

Makes about 4 cups

There are many styles of mole in Mexico, and this simmering sauce aims to capture the appeal and essence of one of the most famous. Mole poblano is known for its combination of chiles, chocolate, raisins, and nuts and seeds, but this version comes together without all of the work normally required. The first step is to toast dried, chopped chiles and set them aside. Next, soften onion and bloom spices (cinnamon and cloves) with garlic before adding chopped semi-sweet chocolate. Chicken broth pulls the sauce together, along with savory diced tomatoes. Raisins add a backbone of welcome sweetness here. Once everything simmers long enough to blend the rich flavors together, an immersion blender (right in the saucepan) renders the sauce silky smooth. The sauce pairs well with chicken, tofu, and fish (see chart on page 295). It is also great spooned over roasted or grilled meat, used as a smothering sauce for burritos, or as a base for taco fillings.

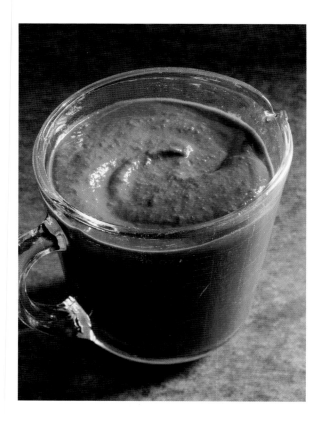

3   dried ancho chiles, stemmed, seeded, and chopped (¾ cup)

3   tablespoons vegetable oil

1   onion, chopped

2   garlic cloves, minced

½   teaspoon ground cinnamon

¼   teaspoon table salt

⅛   teaspoon ground cloves

1   ounce semisweet chocolate, chopped coarse

3   cups chicken broth

1   (14.5-ounce) can diced tomatoes, drained

¼   cup raisins

¼   cup dry-roasted peanuts

2   tablespoons sesame seeds, toasted

1   Toast ancho chiles in medium saucepan over medium-high heat, stirring frequently, until fragrant, 2 to 6 minutes; transfer to plate.

2   Heat oil in now-empty saucepan over medium heat until shimmering. Add onion and cook until softened, about 5 minutes. Stir in garlic, cinnamon, salt, and cloves and cook until fragrant, about 30 seconds. Add chocolate and stir until melted, about 30 seconds.

3   Stir in broth, tomatoes, raisins, peanuts, sesame seeds, and chiles and simmer until reduced to about 4 cups, about 30 minutes.

— **TAKE A 30-MINUTE BREAK** —

4   Off heat, using immersion blender, blend sauce until smooth, about 1 minute. Season with salt and pepper to taste.

PREP AHEAD

Chiles, onion, and chocolate can be chopped up to 1 day ahead and refrigerated separately. Sesame seeds can be toasted up to 1 day ahead. You can make the sauce up to 1 day ahead or freeze for up to 2 months.

MAKE IT EVEN EASIER

Use semisweet chocolate chips instead of the chocolate. Buy toasted sesame seeds.

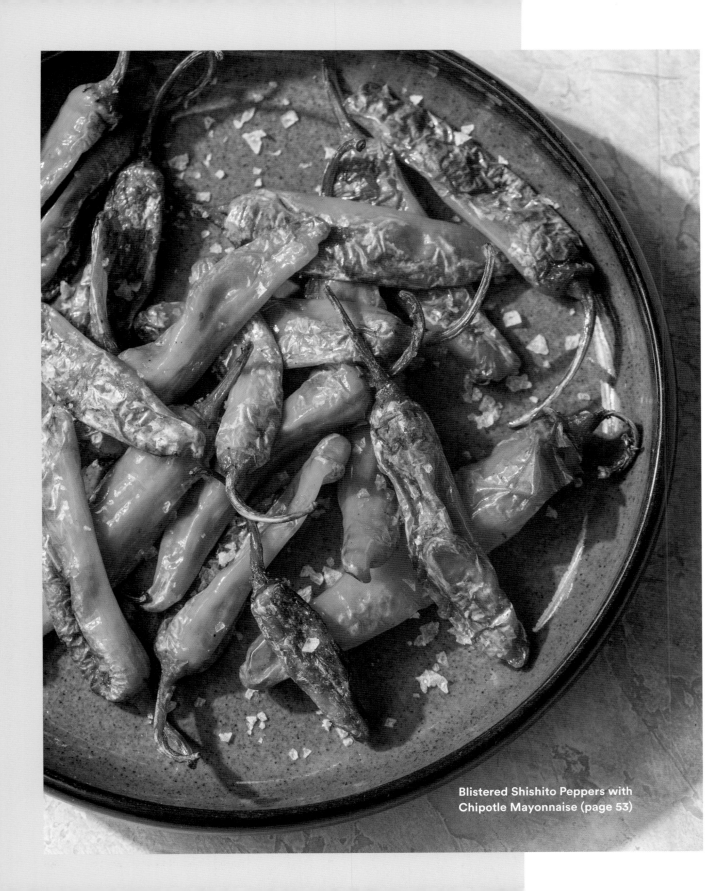

Blistered Shishito Peppers with
Chipotle Mayonnaise (page 53)

Nutritional Information for Our Recipes

To calculate the nutritional values of our recipes per serving, we used The Food Processor SQL by ESHA research. When using this program, we entered all the ingredients, using weights wherever possible. We also used our preferred brands in these analyses. Any ingredient listed as "optional" was excluded from the analyses. If there is a range in the serving size, we used the highest number of servings to calculate nutritional values. We did not include additional salt or pepper for food that's seasoned to taste.

	CALORIES	TOTAL FAT (G)	SAT FAT (G)	CHOL (MG)	SODIUM (MG)	TOTAL CARB (G)	DIETARY FIBER (G)	TOTAL SUGARS (G)	PROTEIN (G)
HOW TO COOK & EAT WELL DESPITE BACK PAIN									
Get Inspired by the Produce at the Farmers' Market									
Fresh Tomato Salsa (per ¼ cup)	15	0	0	0	0	3	1	2	1
Simple Tomato Salad with Capers and Parsley	90	7	1	0	260	5	2	3	1
Peach and Cucumber Salad with Mint	70	0	0	0	200	18	2	14	2
Raw Asparagus Salad with Pesto, Radishes, and Pecorino Romano	200	16	4	15	310	8	3	4	9
Zucchini Ribbon Salad with Shaved Parmesan	310	27	7	20	520	4	1	3	14
Peach Caprese Salad with Raspberry Vinaigrette	210	13	8	40	180	10	1	8	11
Baguette with Radishes, Butter, and Herbs	120	11	6	25	90	6	1	1	1
Golden Beets with Tahini-Lemon Vinaigrette and Pepitas	180	13	2	0	330	13	4	8	6
Green and Yellow Bean Salad with Sherry-Shallot Vinaigrette	140	11	1.5	0	200	8	3	4	2
Blistered Shishito Peppers with Chipotle Mayonnaise	260	27	3.5	10	200	3	1	2	1
Steamed Corn with Miso-Honey Butter	190	11	5	25	160	24	2	10	5
Skillet-Roasted Sugar Snap Peas with Soy Sauce and Sesame Seeds	100	4.5	0	0	135	9	3	4	4

	CALORIES	TOTAL FAT (G)	SAT FAT (G)	CHOL (MG)	SODIUM (MG)	TOTAL CARB (G)	DIETARY FIBER (G)	TOTAL SUGARS (G)	PROTEIN (G)
SALAD FOR DINNER									
Blue Cheese, Walnut, and Chicken Chopped Salad	580	42	8	105	290	8	4	2	43
Easy Slow-Cooker Poached Chicken (per 8 ounces)	280	6	1.5	165	420	1	0	0	52
Bibb Lettuce and Chicken Salad with Peanut Dressing	530	26	4	145	940	14	3	8	59
Perfect Poached Chicken (per 8 ounces)	270	6	1.5	165	100	0	0	0	51
Zucchini Noodle Chicken Salad with Ginger and Garam Masala	330	12	1.5	110	380	19	3	15	36
Herb-Yogurt Sauce (per ¼ cup)	40	2	1.5	10	30	4	0	3	2
Arugula Salad with Steak Tips and Gorgonzola	580	46	16	115	1000	8	2	4	35
Chef's Salad with Turkey, Salami, and Asiago	380	30	10	65	1140	9	4	4	21
Homemade Garlic Croutons (per ¼ cup)	45	1.5	0	0	140	6	0	1	1
Lemony Salmon and Roasted Beet Salad	600	44	9	185	660	10	2	6	40
Easy-Peel Hard-Cooked Eggs (per egg)	70	5	1.5	185	70	0	0	0	6
Smoked Salmon Niçoise Salad	470	20	7	295	330	25	4	5	45
Seared Scallop Salad with Snap Peas and Radishes	370	22	3	40	980	15	3	5	23
Warm Spiced Pearl Couscous Salad with Chorizo	1210	54	15	75	2240	139	11	38	43
Lentil Salad with Pomegranate and Walnuts	330	16	2	0	420	34	13	6	14
Lentil Salad with Spiced Carrots and Cilantro	300	11	1.5	0	480	37	14	7	14
Warm Broccoli, Chickpea, and Avocado Salad	550	40	5	0	1560	43	16	4	14
Barley Salad with Pomegranate, Pistachios, and Feta	550	20	5	20	520	85	15	20	14
Side Salad Inspiration									
Simplest Green Salad	130	14	2	0	0	1	0	0	1
Arugula Salad with Fennel and Shaved Parmesan	120	11	2	5	180	6	2	2	2
Mâche Salad with Cucumber and Mint	120	11	1.5	0	95	4	2	1	2
Radicchio, Endive, and Arugula Salad	70	7	1	0	55	3	1	1	1
Vinaigrettes That Jazz Up Everyday Side Salads									
Make-Ahead Vinaigrette (per tablespoon)	100	11	1.5	0	105	1	0	1	0
Make-Ahead Sherry-Shallot Vinaigrette (per tablespoon)	110	11	1.5	0	100	1	0	1	0
Make-Ahead Balsamic-Fennel Vinaigrette (per tablespoon)	110	11	1.5	0	100	2	0	2	0
Make-Ahead Cider-Caraway Vinaigrette (per tablespoon)	110	11	1.5	0	100	1	0	1	0

	CALORIES	TOTAL FAT (G)	SAT FAT (G)	CHOL (MG)	SODIUM (MG)	TOTAL CARB (G)	DIETARY FIBER (G)	TOTAL SUGARS (G)	PROTEIN (G)
SALAD FOR DINNER (CONT.)									
Raspberry Vinaigrette (per tablespoon)	90	8	1	0	80	5	0	5	0
Tahini-Lemon Dressing (per tablespoon)	80	9	1.5	0	150	1	0	0	1
Maple-Mustard Vinaigrette (per tablespoon)	60	5	1	0	240	4	0	3	0
Yogurt-Dill Dressing (per tablespoon)	30	2.5	1	0	115	0	0	0	1
STREAMLINED COMFORT CLASSICS									
Spatchcocked Roast Chicken with Rosemary and Garlic	630	46	12	195	790	0	0	0	49
Spatchcocked Roast Chicken with Sesame and Ginger	630	46	12	195	790	1	0	0	49
Instant Pot Chicken Tagine	260	9	1.5	105	600	18	4	8	26
Green Chicken Enchiladas	450	18	9	120	1380	34	2	10	39
Quick Pickled Shallots and Radishes (per 2 tablespoons)	10	0	0	0	95	3	0	1	0
Chicken, Spinach, and Artichoke Pot Pie	570	36	21	180	1060	30	7	6	34
Tuscan Steak with Garlicky Spinach	660	43	11	190	550	8	4	0	57
Modern Beef Pot Pie with Mushrooms and Sherry	770	43	14	150	990	34	2	7	58
Stovetop Classic Pot Roast with Potatoes and Carrots	710	44	17	200	1060	21	2	4	47
Slow-Cooker Shredded Beef Tacos	510	28	11	105	380	33	0	7	33
Tangy Coleslaw (per ¼ cup)	20	0	0	0	40	4	1	3	0
Glazed Meatloaf with Root Vegetables	680	38	13	220	1500	37	5	15	44
Slow-Cooker Brisket and Onions	590	36	14	200	310	6	1	2	56
Instant Pot Wine-Braised Short Ribs and Potatoes	280	11	3.5	40	700	28	3	6	17
Marmalade-Glazed Pork Loin	270	6	1.5	140	520	7	0	6	45
Pork Tenderloin Stroganoff	510	28	12	125	1300	31	1	5	33
Sizzling Garlic Shrimp	320	22	6	230	1100	5	1	1	24
Oven-Poached Side of Salmon	220	7	1.5	85	330	1	0	0	36
Fresh Tomato Relish (per 2 tablespoons)	25	1.5	0	0	240	2	1	1	1
Meaty Loaf Pan Lasagna	570	35	16	160	1550	29	2	7	34
Baked Spaghetti and Meatballs	820	31	9	80	1850	91	9	13	39
Skillet Ravioli with Meat Sauce	500	24	8	60	1500	41	4	14	33
Skillet Ziti with Sausage and Peppers	630	29	15	85	1700	55	4	6	41
Cheesy Tex-Mex Chili Mac	740	34	15	130	1050	64	3	10	47
Simple Stovetop Macaroni and Cheese	470	19	9	45	860	51	0	5	24
Grown-Up Stovetop Macaroni and Cheese	450	17	8	45	870	51	0	5	25

	CALORIES	TOTAL FAT (G)	SAT FAT (G)	CHOL (MG)	SODIUM (MG)	TOTAL CARB (G)	DIETARY FIBER (G)	TOTAL SUGARS (G)	PROTEIN (G)
STREAMLINED COMFORT CLASSICS (CONT.)									
Instant Pot Creamy Spring Vegetable Linguine	370	9	3.5	20	860	53	11	3	18
Unstuffed Shells with Butternut Squash and Leeks	800	37	21	100	820	88	7	8	28
Veggie Sheet Pan Pizza	690	35	12	45	1450	70	1	19	27
Three-Cheese Sheet Pan Pizza	700	39	15	50	1630	63	0	14	27
Meaty Sheet Pan Pizza	810	46	17	80	2000	64	0	15	37
HEARTY SOUPS & STEWS									
Sun-Dried Tomato and White Bean Soup	180	4.5	1	5	1030	26	7	2	12
Grilled Cheese Sandwich (per sandwich)	430	22	13	60	670	38	2	5	16
Creamy Chickpea and Roasted Garlic Soup	150	3	0	0	750	22	6	1	8
Crispy Garlic (per 2 tablespoons)	90	7	1	0	0	6	0	0	1
Easy Food-Processor Gazpacho	150	10	1.5	0	780	13	2	6	2
Cauliflower Soup	100	6	4	15	650	11	3	4	3
Crispy Capers (per 2 teaspoons)	40	4.5	0.5	0	135	0	0	0	0
Pasta e Piselli	400	14	4	15	1020	52	3	7	16
Tomato, Bulgur, and Red Pepper Soup	130	4	0.5	0	670	18	3	5	3
Easy Corn Chowder with Bacon	580	18	9	45	1190	96	10	12	18
Chicken Tortilla Soup	270	12	2	40	780	20	3	3	19
Almost-Instant Ginger Beef Ramen	300	13	4.5	35	1770	28	0	2	18
Beef and Barley Soup	540	15	4	80	2470	67	13	14	38
Easy Instant Pot Beef Stew with Mushrooms and Bacon	260	10	4	50	1120	20	2	7	24
Weeknight Beef Chili	460	29	8	75	1260	25	7	8	28
Slow-Cooker Pork Posole	230	8	2	50	1200	21	4	5	18
SKILLET MEALS									
Pan-Seared Chicken with Warm Bulgur Pilaf	640	24	7	190	740	45	8	3	62
Stir-Fried Chicken and Vegetables with Black Bean Garlic Sauce	360	13	1.5	125	790	15	1	8	44
Chicken Lo Mein with Bok Choy	370	15	2	110	1170	24	1	22	33
Caramelized Black Pepper Chicken	370	11	2	125	670	24	1	20	40
Chicken Curry with Tomatoes and Ginger	280	14	3	125	850	11	3	5	28

	CALORIES	TOTAL FAT (G)	SAT FAT (G)	CHOL (MG)	SODIUM (MG)	TOTAL CARB (G)	DIETARY FIBER (G)	TOTAL SUGARS (G)	PROTEIN (G)
SKILLET MEALS (CONT.)									
Chicken, Sun-Dried Tomato, and Goat Cheese Burgers	420	20	7	110	730	31	1	5	29
Sun-Dried Tomato and Caper Mayonnaise (per tablespoon)	200	21	3.5	10	820	1	0	0	0
Steak Tips with Spicy Cauliflower	510	34	9	135	720	8	3	4	46
Steak Tips with Ras el Hanout and Couscous	490	24	7	115	710	29	3	2	40
Pan-Seared Strip Steaks with Crispy Potatoes	760	46	10	120	830	33	3	2	57
Red Curry Pork Lettuce Wraps	630	30	10	115	680	51	1	2	36
Easy Salmon Burgers	380	28	6	80	430	2	1	0	29
Chipotle Mayonnaise (per tablespoon)	90	10	1.5	5	100	0	0	0	0
Salmon and Rice with Cucumber Salad	680	36	8	125	850	36	2	1	52
Braised Halibut with Leeks and Mustard	440	20	11	155	800	9	1	2	43
Red Curry Cod with Mushroom Rice	630	15	9	100	1180	70	2	4	50
Spicy Shrimp and Ramen with Peanuts	690	35	10	145	2990	65	3	7	31
Seared Scallops with Sage Butter Sauce and Squash	460	24	15	115	1500	34	5	5	30
Penne with Chicken, Mushrooms, and Gorgonzola	740	29	9	110	1070	68	3	4	41
Skillet Penne alla Vodka	460	13	6	25	500	69	3	11	13
Lemony Shrimp with Orzo, Feta, and Olives	490	14	5	240	2150	51	1	6	39
Fideos with Chickpeas	440	11	1.5	0	1070	69	6	11	14
Garlic Aioli (per 2 tablespoons)	200	23	3.5	35	150	0	0	0	1
Parmesan Polenta with Broccoli Rabe, Sun-Dried Tomatoes, and Pine Nuts	500	33	11	45	990	43	8	1	13
Stir-Fried Eggplant in Garlic-Basil Sauce	150	8	1	0	1420	18	3	11	3
Salad Bar Stir-Fry with Tofu	290	12	1.5	0	980	38	0	20	12
Xīhóngshì Chao Jīdàn	300	21	5	370	1110	12	0	7	14

SIMPLE MAINS THAT WON'T STRAIN YOUR BACK

	CALORIES	TOTAL FAT (G)	SAT FAT (G)	CHOL (MG)	SODIUM (MG)	TOTAL CARB (G)	DIETARY FIBER (G)	TOTAL SUGARS (G)	PROTEIN (G)
Slow-Cooker Citrus-Braised Chicken Tacos	420	10	2	160	1100	44	1	6	38
Avocado Crema (per tablespoon)	20	1.5	0	0	0	1	1	0	0
Slow-Cooker Sweet and Tangy Pulled Chicken Sandwiches	420	10	2	95	1000	42	2	18	40
Quick Pickle Chips (per ¼ cup)	30	0	0	0	420	7	0	5	0

	CALORIES	TOTAL FAT (G)	SAT FAT (G)	CHOL (MG)	SODIUM (MG)	TOTAL CARB (G)	DIETARY FIBER (G)	TOTAL SUGARS (G)	PROTEIN (G)
SIMPLE MAINS THAT WON'T STRAIN YOUR BACK (CONT.)									
Instant Pot Lemony Chicken Thighs with Fingerling Potatoes and Lemon	300	8	1.5	95	600	33	4	1	23
Chicken and Chorizo Paella	710	37	10	115	1600	52	5	6	44
Instant Pot Chicken Sausages with White Beans and Spinach	450	26	6	190	1210	23	6	4	27
Slow-Cooker Turkey Breast with Cherry-Orange Sauce	350	6	2	150	700	12	1	9	60
One-Pan Steak Fajitas	920	39	13	155	1890	79	4	11	62
Spice-Roasted Steaks	310	13	4	120	370	2	1	0	45
Steakhouse Spice Blend (per teaspoon)	5	0	0	0	0	1	1	0	0
Tex-Mex Spice Blend (per teaspoon)	5	0	0	0	0	1	1	0	0
Pork Burgers with Lime and Sriracha	530	29	9	105	470	30	0	5	36
Sriracha Mayonnaise (per tablespoon)	70	7	1	5	95	1	0	0	0
Salmon Tacos with Cilantro-Lime Slaw	340	12	3	60	1010	31	2	4	26
Pesce all'Acqua Pazza	240	8	1	90	980	8	2	3	29
Easy Fish and Rice Packets with Creamy Coconut-Curry Sauce	430	15	11	95	650	32	0	1	41
One-Pan Shrimp Pad Thai	510	14	2	180	1540	69	2	15	29
Asparagus and Goat Cheese Tart	440	34	15	20	480	33	3	3	12
Instant Pot Bulgur with Spinach, Chickpeas, and Za'atar	300	12	1.5	0	500	43	9	3	9
Stuffed Eggplant with Lentils, Pomegranate, and Ricotta	520	22	5	15	920	63	19	14	22
Easy Air-Fryer Mains									
Air-Fryer Roasted Bone-In Chicken Breasts	490	27	8	175	780	0	0	0	57
Lemon-Basil Salsa Verde (per ¼ cup)	130	14	2	0	210	1	0	0	1
Air-Fryer Sweet and Smoky Pork Tenderloin with Roasted Butternut Squash	490	15	6	165	880	39	6	14	53
Air-Fryer Crispy Breaded Boneless Pork Chops	580	22	11	275	840	27	0	1	58
Air-Fryer Orange Mustard–Glazed Salmon	520	32	7	125	540	8	0	7	46
Honey Chipotle–Glazed Salmon	520	32	7	125	670	8	0	4	47
Hoisin-Glazed Salmon	550	32	7	125	430	18	0	18	47
Air-Fryer Crunchy Cod Fillets	350	12	2	190	800	15	1	2	44

	CALORIES	TOTAL FAT (G)	SAT FAT (G)	CHOL (MG)	SODIUM (MG)	TOTAL CARB (G)	DIETARY FIBER (G)	TOTAL SUGARS (G)	PROTEIN (G)
EASY SIDES TO ROUND OUT YOUR MEAL									
Everyday Rice Pilaf	210	5	1	0	95	38	1	1	3
Rice Pilaf with Apricots and Almonds	260	7	1	0	100	45	2	6	5
Spiced Rice Pilaf with Ginger, Dates, and Parsley	230	5	1	0	100	43	2	5	4
Simple White Rice	240	2.5	1.5	5	390	49	1	0	4
Simple White Rice for Two	270	2.5	1.5	5	300	55	1	0	5
Sesame Sushi Rice	290	6	1	0	430	54	2	1	5
Hands-Off Baked Brown Rice	290	7	1	0	280	51	2	0	5
with Parmesan, Lemon, and Herbs	410	15	6	25	830	56	3	1	14
Garlicky Fried Rice with Bok Choy	230	7	1	0	510	36	2	2	5
Cauliflower Rice	60	3	0.5	0	390	9	3	3	3
Mexican Cauliflower Rice	60	3	0.5	0	390	8	3	3	3
Cauliflower Rice with Almonds and Mint	80	4	0.5	0	390	10	4	3	4
Cauliflower Rice for Two	80	3	0.5	0	420	12	5	5	5
Classic Couscous	250	4	2.5	10	320	45	3	0	7
Couscous with Curry and Mint	260	4.5	2.5	10	320	46	3	0	8
Herbed Couscous for Two	240	13	4.5	15	780	26	2	2	4
Farro Risotto with Fennel and Radicchio	210	4	0	0	350	40	6	6	7
Barley with Celery and Miso	190	4	0.5	0	1110	34	7	3	5
Creamy Orzo with Boursin	270	16	7	25	790	25	0	2	5
Orzo with Pesto and Sun-Dried Tomatoes	320	11	1.5	0	770	49	2	3	9
Orzo with Shallot, Capers, and Dill	190	7	1	0	760	26	1	2	4
Easy Cuban Black Beans	200	8	1	0	530	30	1	3	9
Garlicky Braised Chickpeas	270	17	2.5	0	400	23	7	1	8
White Bean Gratin with Rosemary and Parmesan	250	11	3	10	700	23	7	2	15
Pan-Steamed Asparagus with Garlic	45	2	1	5	190	6	3	3	4
with Mint and Almonds	60	4	1.5	5	210	4	2	2	3
with Lemon and Parmesan	60	3.5	2	10	290	4	2	2	3
with Shallots and Herbs	40	2	1	5	200	4	2	2	2
Roasted Baby Carrots with Sage and Walnuts	190	14	3.5	10	90	16	4	10	3
Skillet Charred Broccoli	240	22	3	0	490	9	4	3	5
Garlicky Broccolini	110	9	1.5	5	400	4	3	0	5
Broccolini with Shallots	110	9	1.5	5	400	4	3	1	5
Broccolini with Capers and Lemon	100	9	1.5	5	450	4	3	0	5

	CALORIES	TOTAL FAT (G)	SAT FAT (G)	CHOL (MG)	SODIUM (MG)	TOTAL CARB (G)	DIETARY FIBER (G)	TOTAL SUGARS (G)	PROTEIN (G)
EASY SIDES TO ROUND OUT YOUR MEAL (CONT.)									
Instant Pot Braised Whole Cauliflower	160	11	1	0	540	15	3	8	4
Elote (Mexican Street Corn)	270	22	3.5	10	260	19	2	5	5
Sautéed Snow Peas with Lemon and Parsley	70	3.5	0.5	0	140	8	0	4	3
with Garlic, Cumin, and Cilantro	80	4	0.5	0	140	9	0	4	3
with Lemongrass and Basil	70	3.5	0	0	150	7	0	4	2
Skillet Charred Green Beans	120	7	1	0	160	12	5	6	3
Garlic-Parmesan Mashed Potatoes	330	11	7	30	890	45	0	2	11
Baked Potatoes	210	1.5	0	0	310	46	3	2	5
Blue Cheese–Pepper Butter (per 1½ tablespoons)	120	13	8	35	50	0	0	0	1
Lemon-Thyme Butter (per tablespoon)	100	12	7	30	0	0	0	0	0
Braised Red Potatoes with Lemon and Chives	130	6	3.5	15	310	19	2	2	2
with Miso and Scallions	140	6	3.5	15	290	20	2	2	3
with Dijon and Tarragon	140	6	3.5	15	360	19	2	1	2
Easy Air-Fryer Sides									
Air-Fryer Roasted Asparagus	20	1	0	0	70	2	1	1	1
Mint-Orange Gremolata (per tablespoon)	5	0	0	0	0	1	0	0	0
Tarragon-Lemon Gremolata (per tablespoon)	5	0	0	0	0	1	0	0	0
Air-Fryer Brussels Sprouts	60	1.5	0	0	160	10	4	2	3
Lemon-Chive Dipping Sauce (per tablespoon)	100	11	1.5	5	110	1	0	0	0
Air-Fryer Roasted Eggplant with Capers, Oregano, and Garlic	120	7	1	0	340	14	6	7	2
Air-Fryer Roasted Fennel with Orange-Honey Dressing	180	14	2	0	360	15	4	11	2
Air-Fryer French Fries	190	7	1	0	310	31	2	1	4
Sriracha Dipping Sauce (per tablespoon)	100	11	1.5	5	220	1	0	1	0
Air-Fryer Roasted Green Beans with Sun-Dried Tomatoes and Sunflower Seeds	170	12	4	10	160	12	4	4	7
Easy Slow-Cooker Sides									
Slow-Cooker Red Potatoes with Rosemary and Garlic	150	5	0.5	0	230	25	3	2	3
Slow-Cooker Creamy Polenta	200	9	4.5	20	600	24	2	2	6
Slow-Cooker Parmesan Risotto	360	12	6	30	1000	53	2	1	10
Slow-Cooker Brown Rice with Peas, Feta, and Mint	280	6	3	15	310	50	3	2	7

	CALORIES	TOTAL FAT (G)	SAT FAT (G)	CHOL (MG)	SODIUM (MG)	TOTAL CARB (G)	DIETARY FIBER (G)	TOTAL SUGARS (G)	PROTEIN (G)
SAUCES THAT JUMP-START DINNER									
Pesto Sauces									
Classic Basil Pesto (per 2 tablespoons)	230	25	3.5	0	45	2	0	0	2
Toasted Walnut and Parsley Pesto (per 2 tablespoons)	320	35	4.5	0	45	4	1	1	4
Arugula and Ricotta Pesto (per 2 tablespoons)	250	27	4.5	10	40	3	1	0	3
Kale and Sunflower Seed Pesto (per 2 tablespoons)	150	16	2.5	5	65	2	1	0	2
Green Olive and Orange Pesto (per 2 tablespoons)	160	16	2.5	5	150	3	1	1	2
Sun-Dried Tomato Pesto (per 2 tablespoons)	170	17	2.5	0	90	5	1	0	2
Pasta Sauces									
Pomodoro Sauce (per cup)	250	21	10	45	640	13	3	6	3
Pomodoro Sauce with Fennel and Capers (per cup)	150	7	1	0	410	14	5	6	2
Slow-Cooker Classic Marinara (per cup)	100	3.5	0	0	590	17	4	9	3
Mussels Marinara	330	9	1.5	85	1260	22	2	6	38
Puttanesca Sauce (per cup)	240	19	6	25	1470	17	4	9	5
Arrabbiata Sauce (per cup)	60	4.5	2	5	250	6	1	3	1
Shrimp Arrabbiata	110	3.5	1	145	770	4	1	2	16
Slow-Cooker Bolognese (per cup)	400	29	13	95	380	13	2	6	20
Simmering Sauces									
Cacciatore Simmering Sauce (per cup)	160	7	1	0	640	14	3	6	3
Simple Curry Simmering Sauce (per cup)	390	36	16	70	680	16	2	6	3
Ginger-Sesame Simmering Sauce (per cup)	210	16	2.5	0	1380	15	2	0	5
Sichuan Peppercorn–Ginger Simmering Sauce (per cup)	140	9	1.5	0	1380	12	1	0	2
Orange-Chile Simmering Sauce (per cup)	210	16	2	0	1380	14	2	0	4
Extra-Spicy Simmering Sauce (per cup)	350	19	3	0	2170	42	0	26	2
Sweet and Tangy Simmering Sauce (per cup)	210	0	0	0	1770	51	1	37	2
Mole-Style Simmering Sauce (per cup)	360	25	4.5	0	740	32	7	15	8

Conversions & Equivalents

Some say cooking is a science and an art. We would say that geography has a hand in it, too. Flours and sugars manufactured in the United Kingdom and elsewhere will feel and taste different from those manufactured in the United States. So we cannot promise that the loaf of bread you bake in Canada or England will taste the same as a loaf baked in the States, but we can offer guidelines for converting weights and measures. We also recommend that you rely on your instincts when making our recipes. Refer to the visual cues provided. If the dough hasn't "come together in a ball" as described, you may need to add more flour—even if the recipe doesn't tell you to. You be the judge.

The recipes in this book were developed using standard U.S. measures following U.S. government guidelines. The charts below offer equivalents for U.S. and metric measures. All conversions are approximate and have been rounded up or down to the nearest whole number.

Example:

| 1 teaspoon | = | 4.9292 milliliters, rounded up to 5 milliliters |
| 1 ounce | = | 28.3495 grams, rounded down to 28 grams |

VOLUME CONVERSIONS:

U.S.	METRIC
1 teaspoon	5 milliliters
2 teaspoons	10 milliliters
1 tablespoon	15 milliliters
2 tablespoons	30 milliliters
¼ cup	59 milliliters
⅓ cup	79 milliliters
½ cup	118 milliliters
¾ cup	177 milliliters
1 cup	237 milliliters
1¼ cups	296 milliliters
1½ cups	355 milliliters
2 cups (1 pint)	473 milliliters
2½ cups	591 milliliters
3 cups	710 milliliters
4 cups (1 quart)	0.946 liter
1.06 quarts	1 liter
4 quarts (1 gallon)	3.8 liters

WEIGHT CONVERSIONS:

OUNCES	GRAMS
½	14
¾	21
1	28
1½	43
2	57
2½	71
3	85
3½	99
4	113
4½	128
5	142
6	170
7	198
8	227
9	255
10	283
12	340
16 (1 pound)	454

CONVERSIONS FOR COMMON BAKING INGREDIENTS:

Baking is an exacting science. Because measuring by weight is far more accurate than measuring by volume, and thus more likely to produce reliable results, in our recipes we provide ounce measures in addition to cup measures for many ingredients. Refer to the chart below to convert these measures into grams.

INGREDIENT	OUNCES	GRAMS
Flour		
1 cup all-purpose flour*	5	142
1 cup cake flour	4	113
1 cup whole-wheat flour	5½	156
Sugar		
1 cup granulated (white) sugar	7	198
1 cup packed brown sugar (light or dark)	7	198
1 cup confectioners' sugar	4	113
Cocoa Powder		
1 cup cocoa powder	3	85
Butter†		
4 tablespoons (½ stick or ¼ cup)	2	57
8 tablespoons (1 stick or ½ cup)	4	113
16 tablespoons (2 sticks or 1 cup)	8	227

* U.S. all-purpose flour, the most frequently used flour in this book, does not contain leaveners, as some European flours do. These leavened flours are called self-rising or self-raising. If you are using self-rising flour, take this into consideration before adding leaveners to a recipe.

† In the United States, butter is sold both salted and unsalted. We generally recommend unsalted butter. If you are using salted butter, take this into consideration before adding salt to a recipe.

OVEN TEMPERATURES:

FAHRENHEIT	CELSIUS	GAS MARK
225	105	¼
250	120	½
275	135	1
300	150	2
325	165	3
350	180	4
375	190	5
400	200	6
425	220	7
450	230	8
475	245	9

CONVERTING TEMPERATURES FROM AN INSTANT-READ THERMOMETER:

We include doneness temperatures in many of the recipes in this book. We recommend an instant-read thermometer for the job. Refer to the table above to convert Fahrenheit degrees to Celsius. Or, for temperatures not represented in the chart, use this simple formula:

Subtract 32 degrees from the Fahrenheit reading, then divide the result by 1.8 to find the Celsius reading.

Example:
"Roast chicken until thighs register 175 degrees."

To Convert:
175°F − 32 = 143°
143° ÷ 1.8 = 79.44°C, rounded down to 79°C

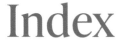

Index

Note: Page references in *italics* indicate photographs.

B

E

F

G

M

N

Neural foramen, 3
Nonstick skillets, 42
Noodles
    Almost-Instant Ginger Beef Ramen, 154, *155*
    Chicken Lo Mein with Bok Choy, 170, *171*
    One-Pan Shrimp Pad Thai, *240,* 241
    Pork Tenderloin Stroganoff, 112–13, *113*
    Red Curry Pork Lettuce Wraps, *184,* 185
    Spicy Shrimp and Ramen with Peanuts, 194–95, *195*
Nucleus pulposus, 3
Nuts
    toasting in microwave, 37
    see also specific nuts

O

Olive(s)
    Chicken and Chorizo Paella, 222–23, *223*
    Green, and Orange Pesto, 287
    Instant Pot Braised Whole Cauliflower, 271, *271*
    Instant Pot Chicken Tagine, *90,* 91
    Instant Pot Lemony Chicken Thighs with Fingerling
        Potatoes and Lemon, *220,* 221
    Orzo, and Feta, Lemony Shrimp with, 202, *203*
    Pan-Seared Chicken with Warm Bulgur Pilaf, 166–67, *167*
    Puttanesca Sauce, 291, *291*
    Smoked Salmon Niçoise Salad, 70–71, *71*
One-Pan Shrimp Pad Thai, *240,* 241
One-Pan Steak Fajitas, 228, *229*
Onions
    and Brisket, Slow-Cooker, 106–7, *107*
    chopping, 40
    Easy Instant Pot Beef Stew with Mushrooms and
        Bacon, *158,* 159
    One-Pan Steak Fajitas, 228, *229*
Orange
    -Cherry Sauce, Slow-Cooker Turkey Breast with,
        226, 227
    -Chile Simmering Sauce, 297
    and Green Olive Pesto, 287
    -Honey Dressing, Air-Fryer Roasted Fennel with,
        280, *280*
    -Mint Gremolata, 278

Orange *(cont.)*
    Mustard–Glazed Salmon, Air-Fryer, 250, *250*
    Slow-Cooker Citrus-Braised Chicken Tacos, 216–17, *217*
Oregano, Capers, and Garlic, Air-Fryer Roasted
    Eggplant with, 279, *279*
Oven-Poached Side of Salmon, 116–17, *117*
Ovens, placing pots and pans in, 53
Oyster sauce
    Extra-Spicy Simmering Sauce, 298
    Ginger-Sesame Simmering Sauce, 297, *297*
    Orange-Chile Simmering Sauce, 297
    Sichuan Peppercorn–Ginger Simmering Sauce, 297

P

Pad Thai, One-Pan Shrimp, *240,* 241
Paella, Chicken and Chorizo, 222–23, *223*
Pan-Seared Chicken with Warm Bulgur Pilaf, 166–67, *167*
Pan-Seared Strip Steaks with Crispy Potatoes, 182, *183*
Pan-Steamed Asparagus
    with Garlic, 267
    with Lemon and Parmesan, 267, *267*
    with Mint and Almonds, 267
    with Shallots and Herbs, 267
Pantry organization, 25
Paprika
    Tex-Mex Spice Blend, 231
Parmesan
    -Garlic Mashed Potatoes, 275, *275*
    and Lemon, Pan-Steamed Asparagus with, 267, *267*
    Lemon, and Herbs, Hands-Off Baked Brown Rice with,
        257, *257*
    Meaty Loaf Pan Lasagna, 118–19, *119*
    Polenta with Broccoli Rabe, Sun-Dried Tomatoes,
        and Pine Nuts, 206–7, *207*
    Risotto, Slow-Cooker, 283
    and Rosemary, White Bean Gratin with, 266, *266*
    Shaved, and Fennel, Arugula Salad with, 82
    Shaved, Zucchini Ribbon Salad with, *52,* 53
    Skillet Ziti with Sausage and Peppers, 124, *125*
    Unstuffed Shells with Butternut Squash and Leeks,
        132, 133
Parsley
    Arugula and Ricotta Pesto, 287
    Ginger, and Dates, Spiced Rice Pilaf with, 254
    Green Olive and Orange Pesto, 287